INFORMATION TECHNOLOGY IN MEDICAL DIAGNOSTICS III

Information Technology in Medical Diagnostics III

Metrological aspects of biomedical research

Editors

Waldemar Wójcik, Saygid Uvaysov and Andrzej Smolarz

Routledge
Taylor & Francis Group

Routledge is an imprint of the Taylor & Francis Group, an informa business

Typeset by MPS, Chennai, India

Published by: Routledge
Schipholweg 107C, 2316 XC Leiden, The Netherlands
e-mail: Pub.NL@taylorandfrancis.com
www.routledge.com – www.taylorandfrancis.com

ISBN: 978-0-367-76586-6 (Hbk)
ISBN: 978-1-003-16766-2 (eBook)
ISBN: 978-0-367-76589-7 (Pbk)
DOI: 10.1201/9781003167662

Table of contents

Preface

The science of a complex system of biomedical measurements is experiencing a period of rapid development. Progress in the right direction in solving metrological problems in medicine is possible if we systemically consider medical technology, using the formal approach. Its main principle is to determine the elements and rules of their interaction, which allows to introduce a mathematical system and represent any technology or object in the form of a structure on which it is possible to formulate necessary estimates and to declare synthesis processes, including metrological ones.

Development of effective measuring technologies and measuring tools of any complexity begins with the analysis of the information space of the object of observation. In the monograph, this part of the research is examined on the example of the analysis of the information space used for the study of knee joints of the organs of motion.

Within the framework of any medical technology, the following semantic link is valid: (state or result) = (therapeutic effect) · (state of the subject). Thus, the set of results of the technology is equivalent (with a confidence of 0.99) to the set of maps of the therapeutic effects of the set of states of the subject itself. Reliable diagnoses, measurements as well as therapeutic or surgical technologies must all be implemented with a small margin of error. The error is a numerical value. Thus, there is a need to form the notion of error for medical measurements, medical diagnostics or medical technology. The problem of biomedical measurements is associated with the solution of successive problems, which can be named in the following order: the problem of structuring, the problem of observability, the problem of measurability. Let us analyse how issues of structuring, observability and measurability are considered within the metrological aspects of biomedical measurements. The solution of metrological problems in medicine is possible if we consider medical technology systemically with the application of structural formal ideology. Its main principle is to determine the elements and rules of their interaction, which allows us to introduce an algebraic system and represent any technology, any object in the form of a structure on which it is possible to formulate the necessary estimates and declare processes of synthesis, including metrological ones.

This approach considers many examples. The first one is the metrological characteristics of the design of a pathospecific glaucoma diagnostic device. Glaucoma is an intraocular pressure pathology that causes irreversible neurodegenerative changes in retinal and optic nerve structures. It consists of "fast" and "slow" components. The significant spread of the disease and the degree of disability due to it are caused not only by the lack of therapy, but also by the inadequacy of diagnosis including the "painful" stage of the disease, the absence in the arsenal of a practical doctor of an accessible and sufficiently accurate automated method for assessing the state of compensation for hydro and hemodynamic parameters of the eye. This leads to untimely and inadequate administration of treatment and, as a consequence, to the progression of the disease. As before, the issues of distinguishing between the concepts of "health" and "norm" as applied to glaucoma remain insufficiently illuminated in the scientific literature. In medicine, an opinion is widespread about the state of "norm" as a single state, "the best of really possible homogeneous states". At the same time, studies in adult healthy people have shown that the "norm" in one age population can be heterogeneous and should be evaluated taking into account individual and typological properties and the peculiarities of the organisation of the systemic activity of the organism. This determines the purpose of the research, which consists in the development of a pathospecific measuring device for the diagnosis of glaucoma.

The principles of the structural information approach are also realised within the framework of metrological analysis in haematological studies. A class of bio-instrumental information and measurement systems is used in which the primary converter of the input is the biological object under study. It makes possible to specify the study of the properties of the bio object.

At present, laboratory diagnostics is an independent branch of medical science, which can claim objectivity if laboratory research is metrologically correct. The provision of clinical and laboratory research at the level of the clinical diagnostic laboratory is to develop and implement measures to prevent the negative impact of factors at the preanalytical, analytical and post-analytical stage. Development of an efficient and cost-effective management system for clinical and laboratory research is a modern solution to the issue of harmonisation of results and prompt correction of current clinical and laboratory diagnostic problems.

The study of the relationship between the size of uniaxial anisotropy formed in the electromagnetic field in haemoglobin solutions and its level in blood is also devoted to the issue of increasing the accuracy of laboratory tests. This is important in the study of blood chemical composition. The results obtained in this study indicate a close correlation between the hybrid parameters of optical radiation conductivity and tensors of haemoglobin material characteristics. This allows characterizing its composition employing magnetooptical reaction.

The development of adequate reference test signals for electroencephalographs is devoted to the issues of metrological certification of medical measuring instruments. It is realised based on structural schemes of algorithms for measuring the probabilistic characteristics of the stationary segment of the electroencephalogram in the simulation of the test signal. Numerous studies using EEG segmentation have found that EEGs consist of relatively stationary segments whose duration of the main mass varies between 0.2 and 12 seconds. Their classification according to spectral characteristics indicates the existence of a fairly compact set of typical segments, up to several dozen. As a result of the analysis of the research data, it can be concluded that to obtain an electroencephalographic signal model, non-parametric segmentation should be applied first, and then the statistical estimation of the obtained segments should be performed. The technology of non-parametric EEG segmentation has been developed based on the theory of analysis of moments of rapid changes or disturbances in time series with a clearly expressed chord-setting structure. The discrepancies thus determined are signs of boundaries between quasi-stationary fragments. The methodology of non-parametric analysis is based on two ideas. It has been proven that defining changes in any decomposition function of probabilistic characteristics can be reduced (with arbitrary accuracy) to determine changes in mathematical anticipation of some other sequence created from the original. The obtained structural diagrams of algorithms for calculating probabilistic characteristics will allow for metrological analysis and subsequent evaluation of errors at each stage of data processing.

Based on the developed concept, it is possible to conduct accelerated tests of electroencephalographic devices without the need to disconnect from the current operation and to automate all measurement processes, which significantly simplifies the service technician's work and minimizes the risk of human factor influence on the technical research process.

The metrological aspects of medical measurements are also considered in radiothermography in the complex diagnosis of inflammatory processes of the abdominal cavity. There is a need for accurate and timely diagnosis of inflammatory processes in the abdominal cavity by a non-invasive method in a form convenient for the physician without harmful effects on the body. At the same time, the polymorphism of clinical symptoms in combination with atypical manifestations of the disease imposes errors due to the method of conducting the study and subsequent hardware processing of the thermographic picture. In the work, a comparative metrological analysis of various methods of conducting thermographic studies was carried out. Such factors were considered as thermal imager resolution, thermal sensitivity, noise level (signal-to-noise ratio), affecting the quality of the received thermal image. A distinctive feature of non-invasive methods for studying the thermal radiation of bioobjects is their complete harmlessness and high information content. Radiotermometry (RTM-method) is a new method of medical diagnostics. The essence of the method is the non-invasive measurement of the deep temperatures of biological objects by recording the radio emission power of objects. The difference between the RTM method and the well-known physical methods of investigation (palpation, x-ray studies, ultrasound methods, tomography) lies in the fact that deviations are studied not in the anatomical structure of internal tissues but in deviation from normal metabolism processes that, in the case of inflammatory processes, affect the distribution temperatures in internal tissues.

Experimentally, the RTM method has been successfully tested in various fields of medicine: neurology and neurosurgery; cardiology; gastroenterology; traumatology and orthopaedics; combobustology; diagnosis of ENT diseases; endocrinology or gynaecology. The RTM-method has special perspectives in oncology – it is used for early diagnosis of breast cancer.

In each of the following cases, the infrared radiation method can be used. However, in the case of contact analysis of the reception of thermal radiation from biological objects, an unavoidable measurement error that arises from the reflection of radiation at the antenna-object boundary. The reflection coefficients can differ significantly from the differences in the dielectric properties of the radiating tissues. With absolute temperature measurements, it is necessary to take into account the effect of the mismatch between the contact antennas and the human body on the accuracy of measuring the radio-resistant temperatures of deep tissues or internal organs.

Temperature anomalies of internal tissues generate inflammatory and other processes, often preceded by structural changes, which is important for early diagnosis. In the early 1970s research was carried out for the first time on the visualisation of infrared radiation of the epigastric region and its dependence and distribution on the functional states of the stomach. This was followed by studies were that were crucial for substantiating the clinical application of remote thermal methods. Subsequently, thermography was widely used in non-invasive diagnostics in abdominal surgery, angiology, neurology, neoplasms of the breast, skin, muscular and bone tissue as well as the thyroid gland.

The first step in the determining of the medical system is its structuring. That means isolation of certain functional elements and a definition of all links between them. This is the basis for determining the functions of the whole system and assigning a system formal parameter. This formal parameter will be an exit of an output element: the output element assigns an output parameter. Then we choose the system function which can be formed by sequentially transferring of the input action, that is, the action of the environment from the entrance to the selected output. That was obviously for us that the entrance would be the place of contacting with the outside medium. Two chapters are then dedicated to the knee joint – the information space needed to describe its operation and objective parameterisation of the load on it. All this to prevent diseases associated with the violation of the distribution of loads on the knee joint, as well as in the case of correction of axial deformities of the lower limbs, surgical interventions were attempted in order to increase growth, with endoprosthetics, the manufacture of individual endoprostheses, in some cases the selection of orthopaedic footwear and insoles, or the load on the components of the knee joint.

The anatomical parametrisation of the passive exoskeleton of the upper limbs is devoted to the objective parameterisation of the biological information space as the basis for its effective work. The study presents the possibility of anatomical parametrisation of the EXZAR passive exoskeleton of the upper limb used for habilitation and rehabilitation of patients with upper flaccid vapours (mono) paresis. Interest in exoskeletons of extremities is dictated by practical necessity. From the military area, where all developments are strictly classified, exoskeletons have recently moved to the field of medicine, where both active and passive varieties are used. For all their innovative component, active exoskeletons have a number of disadvantages – high cost, dependence on power sources, high weight, low mobility. Passive exoskeletons use residual muscle strength. To strengthen them, various elements are used (rubber thrusts, springs, etc.), but the latter cease to work or violate the function of the affected limbs even more with abnormal anatomical and mechanical correspondences.

Enrichment of metrological principles in the development of new biotechnological technologies and bioinformatic measuring tools is the application of quantum mechanical methods in biotechnical research. Any process that takes place in a living organism can be modelled with the help of the apparatus of quantum mechanics. In our opinion, this is a very promising direction of preclinical research, which can significantly reduce the number of real, as a rule expensive, experiments. The purpose of this study is to consider the possibility of using quantum mechanical methods for the development of effective osseointegration technology for bone-implant interaction. The external influence of the high-pitched laser on a surface of the material was assessed, and the metrological aspects of the process of an efficient merging of an implant and a bone tissue were taken into account. Described research will form the base for improvement of quality of life of the patient.

The last chapter considers the problem of increasing the efficiency of diagnosis and prevention of the development of nervous, musculoskeletal and cardiovascular diseases, diseases that often lead to disability, especially at a young age. An analysis is made of approaches to solving this problem, associated with the need to process a large pool of unstructured data that requires the use of modern intellectual methods. An integrated approach is proposed which includes the theoretical study of the problem and the practical implementation of research, the creation of methods for finding interdependent factors and the development of special equipment and software. The chapter details the problems associated with the lack of a theoretical study describing the process of biofeedback functioning. A model of biofeedback is presented with elements of the theory of automatic control. A software is developed for the implementation of experimental research of the proposed model of biofeedback. Methodologically, a three-level ontological structure is used to examine analytical decision models of an inclusive process. Based on the ontological description of the process of inclusion, a generalised structure of the information-analytical system was developed, the core of which is the knowledge base, built on the databases on the physical and psychological characteristics of students. A practical implementation of the analysed approach to building an intelligent information system of support for the educational process will allow the creation of individual learning paths for students, which will improve the quality of the educational process and prevent the risk of developing nervous, musculoskeletal and cardiovascular diseases.

S. Uvaysov
MIREA – Russian Technological University, Moscow, Russian Federation

W. Wójcik & A. Smolarz
Lublin University of Technology, Lublin, Poland

CHAPTER 1

Problems of structurability, observability, and measurability in medical measurements

O.A. Avdeyuk & Yu.P. Mukha
Volgograd State Technical University, Volgograd State Medical University, Volgograd, Russian Federation

S.A. Bezborodov
Volgograd State Medical University, Volgograd, Russian Federation

W. Wójcik & M. Chmielewska
Lublin University of Technology, Lublin, Poland

A. Kalizhanova
Institute of Information and Computational Technologies CS MES RK, Almaty, Kazakhstan
University of Power Engineering and Telecommunications, Almaty, Kazakhstan

ABSTRACT: The authors investigate the possibility of the anatomical parameterisation of the EXZAR passive exoskeleton of the upper limb, used for habilitation and rehabilitation of patients with upper flaccid couple (mono) paresis.

1.1 INTRODUCTION

There has been a sharp rise in the development of new technologies in the field of medical practice. At the same time, the technical boom in medicine, biology, and biophysics is accompanied by an increase in specific problems related to the lack of objective criteria for the effectiveness of the implementation of these tools and estimate of this effectiveness. In addition, any medical or experimental technology in medicine, biology, and biophysics is based on using a large number of different instruments, systems, and measuring aids. However, there are no ideas of their joint use from the metrological point of view. There are not even approaches to solving the problems that arose from this. Thus we would like to give some examples from different areas of medical practice.

1.2 MEDICAL MEASUREMENTS

1.2.1 *Blood pressure measuring devices (blood pressure monitors)*

The main sources of errors are: the physical process of air flowing from the cuff bag; the physical process of transformation of the pulse wave of the vessels into a change in the pressure in the space of the bag; diaphragming of the input to the chamber of the measuring transducer; process of formation of indicators of the measuring device. The mentioned sources have a multiparameter character, and the total number of factors causing the measurement error reaches several tens in this case.

1.2.2 *Cardiographic measurement complex*

The main sources of error are: a non-spot area of a tap electrode, which leads to the integration of potentials; the process of positioning the tap electrode, which significantly changes the level of the input signal; the final conductivity of the gel between the skin and the metal (and on a bowl without using of a contact composition); the final conductivity of the conductors connecting the electrodes to the inputs to the cardiographic measuring system; measuring procedure on an electronic elementary medium of a cardiograph. The total number of errors is several dozen.

1.2.3 *Hematologic analysis*

The hematological analysis is an analytical measurement technology with the simplest review of sources of errors formalised in the form of limitations in the measurement technique demonstrated about 50 causes of errors, including such exotic like the length of the smear on the glass and the distribution of thickness along the length of the smear.

1.2.4 *Orthopaedic techniques and technologies for surgical correction of upper and lower extremities*

Such techniques (e.g. The Ilizarov apparatus) uses equipment that does not (from the measuring point of view) have correct means of adjustment. As a result, the reason for the errors is the lack of equipment for determining the exact distance between bone fragments, accurate tension on the spokes, etc. The source of errors is the impossibility of accurately determining the angles of bone fragments for fixing them.

1.3 MEDICAL TECHNOLOGIES

1.3.1 *Evaluation of hemodynamics in glaucoma*

It is generally recognised that one of the most important signs of glaucoma is an increase in intraocular pressure (IOP) above the upper limit of the average statistical rate. However, many authors show insufficient reliability of the tonometric method of investigation, not only in diagnostics but also in monitoring the effectiveness of glaucoma treatment. In 1975 A.M. Vodovozov introduced the concepts of tolerant and intolerant intraocular pressure (IOP) to overcome those difficulties in connection with the orientation toward the average statistical standards of the ophthalmotonus.

Tolerant IOP indicated an individually tolerated pressure that does not cause any functional changes in the optic neural apparatus of the eye. An intolerant IOP indicated that the patient has a characteristic visual impairment, regardless of is this pressure higher or lower, than the average statistical rate of IOP. The disadvantages of the well-known methods of determining the tolerant pressure include a significant element of subjectivity, a long time of the examination of patients, the lack of automatic quality control of sphygmograms, and the level of tolerant IOP inspected manually. All these factors reduce the accuracy of the obtained results and limit the scope of the practical application of these methods. There are a lot of questions about the relationship between tolerant intraocular pressure and the state of general and regional hemodynamics of the eye in patients with glaucoma and its criterial (metrological) evaluation which are still unexplored.

1.3.2 *Diagnosis of the pathology of organs of motion*

The main role of legs are the support and movement of the body in space, which is ensured by the functional unity of all its elements. Legs can perform three functions: to give the body a stable position; work statically, lengthen and shorten the longitudinal axis of the body and rotate it in different directions, and, finally, act independently. The indicator of the distribution of static loads on the knee joint is the mechanical axis of the lower limb, which is normally projected on to the centre of the knee joint. It is important in practical terms to restore the anatomical axis of the thigh and lower limb as the main condition for the projection of the mechanical axis of the lower limb to the centre of the knee joint for normalising of the load on the knee joint during the operative correction of the frontal curvatures of the knee.

To solve these problems, we developed a new system of biomechanical assessments of the human body and methods for determining them and also the creation of a tool for determining biomechanical estimates of human movement organs that are distinguished by high metrological qualities.

We presented a lot of examples. And all of them will testify to the relevance of metrological aspects in medical measurements and in medical technologies in general.

1.4 FORMULATION OF THE PROBLEM

The analysis of all the cited examples were reduced to one: we can build a reliable strategy for therapeutic or surgical methods of treatment on reliable diagnosis and veracious monitoring. This strategy will be realised with the use of reliable measuring tools. Generally, we will understand reliability like a prior confidence in the feasibility of appearance of concrete phenomenon excluding any doubt.

Reliability characterises the feasibility of an event, noting its highest probability value (Vinogradov 1977). The derivative concept of reliability is the concept of accuracy, and the numerical, estimative concept is the error. We will make the highest level of the accuracy to get less level of error. In other words, it turns out that a reliable diagnosis is a diagnosis with a small error; a reliable measurement is a measurement with a small error; a reliable therapeutic or surgical technology is a technology implemented with a small error. The error is a numerical value. Thus, we need to form the notion of an error: medical measurements, medical diagnostics, and medical technology.

Metrological assessments in the solution of a variety of modern medical problems: monitoring, therapy, diagnosis, rehabilitation, etc. are either faintly developed or not examined at all in many cases. We explain this situation by the multidimensionality and systemic complexity of medical tasks. Lately, the problem always arises: "What to measure?" Hence as a consequence: "How to measure?"

1.5 PROBLEMS OF STRUCTURABILITY, OBSERVABILITY AND MEASURABILITY

Professor Akhutin V.M. (Akhutin 1976) defined the biotechnical system (BTS), which is the subject of this work: "Biotechnical system is a combination of biological and technical elements, combined in a single functional system of purposeful behaviour." At the same time, a class of biotechnical measuring and computing systems (BTMCS) was singled out within a variety of options for creating and using biotechnical systems (Popechitelev 2006). Measurements must be executed with the subsequent processing of the experimental data with the use of the BTMCS (Popechitelev 2006). However, it is necessary to concentrate attention on the peculiarities of medical measurements, which are connected with the use of plot images (images containing information) as the main kind of impact on the person on whom his reaction arises. This circumstance determines that the BTMCS is always a specialised measurement tool that allows you to adapt it to the object of measurement.

Thus, the problem of biomedical measurements is associated with the solution of successive problems, which can be named in the following order: the structuring problem, the observability problem, the measurability problem, the controllability problem (Mukha et al. 2017).

There is a very large number of definitions of a structure (Mesarovic & Takahara 1978, Nikolayev & Brooks 1985, Volkova & Denisov 2013). Let us dwell on the fact that a structure is a composition of certain functional elements and connections between them. The function of the structure as a whole is completely determined in this case by the set of the functional elements and their interrelationships.

Structurability is the ability to define a set of functional elements in the system and assign relations between them in such a way that the external function of the system remains unchanged, i.e. it must be independent of the choice of sets of elements and connections between them. Obviously, the choice of the system parameter is essentially determined by the effective procedure for designating of the structure.

So we understood that observability is the possibility of isolating in a multicomponent system a multiply-connected type of certain fundamental parameters. Parameters included in all displays of input quantities at the output. Thus, if such a condition is not met, then the system becomes not completely observable for the selected set of fundamental parameters. We solve the problem of choice of a system parameter by the structurability of a multicomponent multiply connected system, so the observability turns into a criterion for selecting a system parameter. It allows us to correct, direct the process of structurability within the framework of a kind of feedback.

The choice of the system parameter in the solution of the structurability problem, corrected at the stage of solving the observability problem, creates a basis for solving the measurement problem. So we solve all tasks of choosing a system of measured standards for a system parameter (most often a vector) and constructing a scale for the measuring system. In other words, we synthesise a set of algorithms for processing measurement information that allows a metrological analysis process to be performed and to estimate of the reliability of the obtained measurement results.

Finally, the measuring process should differ in controllability. Controllability means the possibility of transferring a representative point from any area of the state space to the origin if the system is characterised by a certain state represented by the position of the representing point in the state space (Besekersky & Popov 1977). Thus, the controllability problem is the basis for carrying out the measurement tests, the measuring experiment, for creating a measuring experimental setup.

Then we analyzed how issues of structuring, observability and measurability were considered within the metrological aspects of biomedical measurements.

1.6 STRUCTURISATION OF COMPLEX MEDICAL SYSTEMS

Measurements in medical practice occupy one of the leading places, and they have a diverse character: from the metabolic level to the level of individual functional physiological systems (FUS) and the whole organism as a whole. However the more complex the technology of the experiment is, the more metrological idea is obscured. The estimated and measured components of the experiment are lost. In addition, there is no systemic focus of measurements: the therapeutic effect is the evaluation of the reaction of the organism, that is, the one-dimensional study of the "impact-response" connection. The existing technology of medical measurements connects the measured signal with the process of detecting a signal of artefact origin and it's clustering in order to determine the connection of the signal with the disease. This technology does not involve the processes associated with the physiological state since it does not take into account the structural relationships of complex medical subsystems. In this case, the physiological state of the body should be understood as an integral set of coordinated physiological systems defined on a system-wide metabolism and existing on a system-wide set of goals. However, it should be noted that it is difficult to use structural relations at the content level of their description, as it is at the moment (Cardman & Vogt 1977). At the same time, the application of formalisation is possible here and its principles are in our following conclusions.

The semantic relation is valid within the framework of any medical technology: (state or result Re) = (therapeutic impact or TI) (state of subject Sb), or from a formal point of view: $Re = TI\ (Sb)$. All elements of the relation are sets. Thus, the set of results of the technology *Re* is equivalent (with confidence 0.99) to the set of mapping of therapeutic effects TI of the set of states of the subject Sb itself. Then the technology as a whole can be represented by combining all the *i*-results in to set of results *Re*:

$$\mathrm{Re} \equiv \mathrm{TI_m}\ (\mathrm{TI_{m-1}} \cdots (\mathrm{TI_1}(\mathrm{Sb}) \cdots)) \tag{1.1}$$

where $TI_{i(i \in \overline{1,m})} \subset Z_v$ is the set of therapeutic effects. At the same time, an effective technological medical process satisfies the condition that the result at each step of Re_i with high reliability (for example, $D > 0.9$) belongs to the family of nominal states of the subject $SSbN$: $D[\mathrm{Re}_i \in SSbN] \geq 0.9$, where S is a set of states; Sb is a subject, and N is a nominal.

The main difference of the considered inequality is the introduction of structural formalisms (through sets and their elements) representing a generalised medical technological operation. We used an algebraic topology as the apparatus of system formalisation in this case (Speneur 1971). The multiple-theoretic apparatus evidently transform a meaningful description of the medical object into the language of the formal representation: the main objects of formalisation, the set and the complex of sets, admit this. At the same time, the adequacy between the formal systems and the material systems of the world, including medical systems (for example, physiological systems), consists in the presence of a structure, its elements with certain functions and connections between them. Thus, the first step in determining the medical system is its structuring, which is the isolation of certain functional elements and the links between them. This forms the basis for determining the functions of the system as a whole and assigning a system formal parameter. It is the exit of the output element: the assignment element assigns the output parameter. Then the system function becomes the one that is formed due to the consecutive transmission of the input action, the action of the medium from the input side, to the dedicated output. Obviously, it is advisable to consider the place of environmental impact as input.

The proposed scheme of sequential formalisation makes it possible to make the transition from a meaningful description to a formal description at levels of considerably greater complexity, and then to simplify stepwise by the adoption of analytic-algorithmic descriptions preceding metrological analysis with using of natural formal transformations of category-functor and graph schemes. In a broad sense, we mean that the information about the process is changing of a certain parameter (IP_i), which is adequate to the changes in the process itself. Under the information flow (IPt_j) we mean the movement of information about a certain process through the environment in which this process is realised, including in the measuring system. Under the information network (IN) we mean a special organisation of the environment in which the information process develops and any information flows exist. The above statements can be illustrated formally:

$$\left.\begin{aligned} (IP'_1 \cup \ldots \cup IP'_n) &= IPt_1 \\ (IP''_1 \cup \ldots \cup IP''_n) &= IPt_2 \\ (IP''_1 \cup \ldots \cup IP''_n) &= IPt_2 \\ \ldots\ldots\ldots\ldots\ldots \\ (IP^k_1 \cup \ldots \cup IPt^k_n) &= IPt_k \end{aligned}\right\} \Rightarrow IPt_1 \cup IPt_2 \cup \cdots \cup IPt_k = IN. \quad (1.2)$$

In this case, one can distinguish the observed process in the environment:

$$A \to B \Rightarrow F:\ (A, B)\&B = F(A)\&A = F^{-1}(B)$$

Then the information process can be represented as follows: μ: $F(A) \to F(B)$. In this case, $F(A)$ and $F(B)$ are the adequate changes of the objects A at the input of the process F and B at the output of the process, which in the pair characterise the changes occurring adequately to the process F, that is μ: $[F(A),\ F(B)]$. In other words, μ is a parametric copy of process F, information copy. The category of the measuring parameter of a certain measurement process is the homology $H = [F(A),\ F(B);\ \mu]$. It is a construction, which mapping a synthesised process in the form of consecutive images (modules, groups, concepts, add-ons, and so on) for any process. The distinctive quality of the marked process should be the "simplicity" of the analysis. That means, that the structure of such a process is easily formalised with the use of the developed apparatus.

The formal links in accordance with the physiological structure is represented by a graph:

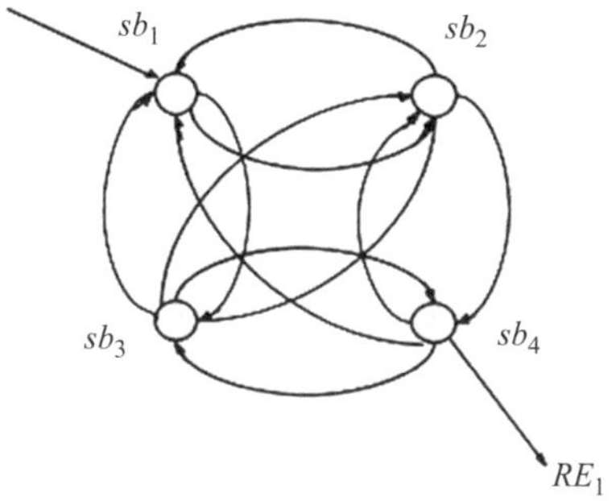

(1.3)

Here (sb_i) are the elements of the physiological structure; LV_i – i-th medical effect; RE_i – is the result of the response of the physiological structure.

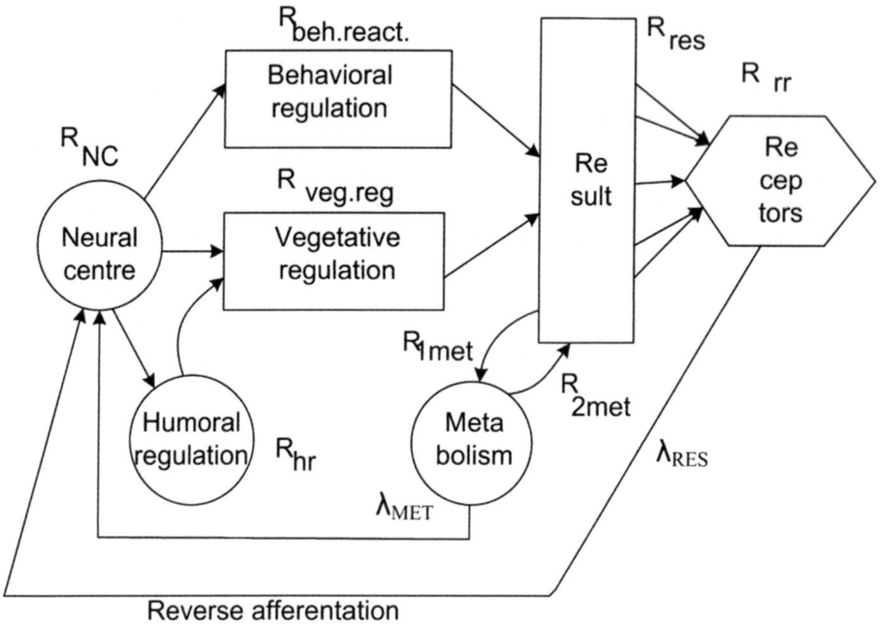

Figure 1.1. Block-diagram of the functional physiological system.

Then the operational form of the treatment effect sequence can be written as follows:

$$\begin{cases} TI_1(Sb_1, Sb_2, Sb_3, Sb_4) \equiv RE_1 \\ TI_2(RE_1) \equiv RE_2 \\ \ldots \\ TI_m(RE_{m-1}) \equiv RE_2 \equiv RE \end{cases} \tag{1.4}$$

An example of the effective determination of interrelated elements in the form of physiological systems is the functional physiological systems (FUS) of Anokhin-Sudakov (Sudakova 1999) (Figure 1.1):

Here the following notations are accepted: R_{RES} – the operation of obtaining the results; R_{VA} is a vegetative adjustment operation; R_{1MET} – metabolism operation in the RES channel; R_{2MET} – metabolic operation in the λ_{MET} channel; R_{PREG} – an operation of behavioural regulation; R_{HR} is the humoral regulation operation; R_{NC} – operation of the functioning of the nerve centre; $\lambda_{MET}(t)$ is the output parameter in the metabolic canal; $\lambda_{res}(t)$ is the output parameter in the result channel of the functionally physiological system; $<R_{RES} \cup R_{1MET}>$ – specific of the joint value of the operations R_{RES} and R_{1MET}.

The operational formalisation of TI on the basis of the structure of the physiological system must be presented in the following equations:

$$R_{\text{CMET}} \begin{cases} \lambda(t)_{\text{MET}} = R_{\text{2MET}} < R_{RES} \cup R_{\text{1MET}} > \\ \lambda(t)_{RES1} = ||R_{\text{PP}}||R_{\text{KPP}}||R_{RES}||R^1_{\text{K}RES} \begin{Bmatrix} R_{\text{PREG}} \\ R_{\text{BPET}} \end{Bmatrix} R_{\text{KHLI}} R_{\text{HLI}}(LV_1) \\ \lambda(t)_{RES2} = ||R_{\text{PP}}||R_{\text{KPP}}||R_{\text{PE3}}||R^2_{\text{K}RES}||R_{\text{BPE3}}||R_{\text{KTPET}} R_{\text{TPET}} R_{\text{HLI}}(LV_1) \end{cases} \tag{1.5}$$

Here R_{CMET} is the operation of commutating the outputs of the results receptors; R_{CRES} – the operation of commutating the results; R_{CR} – operation of commutation in channels of vegetative regulation; R_{CNC} is a switching operation for controlling of the nerve centre.

An important feature of the apparatus of structural formalisation is the lack of the necessity of any analytical description for the function, which was reproduced because the functional ligaments are given in the form of mappings. However, while all other attributes of the function will remain: the domain of definition and existence, the features of their task, the conditions for the existence of mappings, and the ways of their transformation. The most effective representation of the structure is way through the consideration of information flows and nodes of the transformation of the information parameter by sort, form, intensity, character (deterministic/random), places of multiplication and de-multiplication, rings of iteration (Tsvetkov 2005, Ferreira et al. 2016).

Structural formalisation contributes as a basis for the formation of metrological concepts in medical technologies. The main principles of structuring are as follows:

- Metrological assessments are of a structural nature (evaluation principle);
- Measurement is the model of the observed process (the principle of identifying a system parameter);
- A measuring instrument is an identical converter (basic principle).

Structural formalisation becomes more efficient in the framework of the system-technical approach when the system S is considered a subset of the quadruple of the form $S \subset <X, Y, F, Z>$, and the input objects X and output objects Y are formed as Cartesian products of arbitrary objects,

$$\begin{matrix} V_i : X \subset V_1 \times V_2 \times \ldots \times V_k \\ Y \subset V_{k+1} \times V_{k+2} \times \ldots \times V_n \end{matrix} \quad \textit{and}$$

which are used to describe all knowledge about the system. Moreover, it is assumed, that the pair $(x, y) \in S$ forms a system element if an element c of the state space of a system $c \in C$ exists (known from its meaningful descriptions) when there is an equality $Y = R(c, X)$. Here $R \subset F$ is the operating principle of the system, which makes it possible to realize the necessary complex F of system actions (for example, medical technology) under the conditions of implementation of Z.

We formalized the measurement situation with all the stated assumptions within the framework of medical technology as follows:

$$\begin{aligned} &M_{measur.sit.} = \{RE = Lv(C, v_{sz}); \\ &M_{fus} \subset Z;\ M_y \subset v_{medium} \equiv X; \\ &Lv \subset LV_m \ldots V_1(v_{medium}) \Rightarrow \\ &\Delta RE \subset RE_R - RE_{NOM} \in C_{NOM}\} \end{aligned}$$

Here v_{medium} is the effect of the medium; RE_{NOM} – the response of the physiological system in a healthy state C_{NOM}.

Summarising, we note that the structuring process includes the following steps:

1. We defined the set-theoretic formalism of the phase space (state space): a set of elements that determine the state of the object was established. Then we got the set of operations on the set of the state elements (set-theoretical maps of any kind, including various algebras), and the set of rules for realising mappings in the state space.
2. We analyzed the phase space in order to establish possible set-theoretic structures of mapping operations defined earlier.
3. Information flows were formed, admissible essential set-theoretic mapping structures were established.

Thus, structuring from a formal point of view is the establishment of successive transformations in the phase space in the form specialised categories. All the considerations on structuring are well illustrated by the definition of systemic physiological functions within the framework of multidimensional measurement technology. The general architecture of the functional system (Vinogradov 1977) contains information flows associated with the activity of the nerve centre (NC) within the framework of behavioural regulation (BR), vegetative regulation (VR), and humoral regulation (HR). Information was demonstrated in the results (RE) of this activity, in the results of the metabolisms accompanying all kinds of regulation (RRE) and activity. This information was obtained in the feedback channels in the form of humoral influences and reverse afferentation. The graph of general architectonics by P. K. Anokhin looks like this:

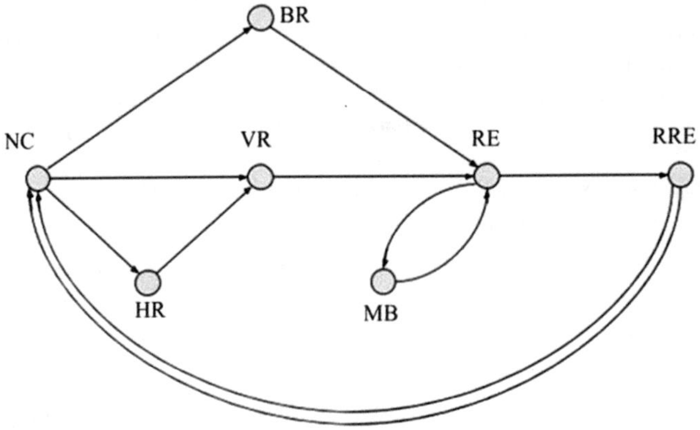

(1.6)

Each of the mappings of the graph (1.6) is associated with the transfer of information, each of the vertices of the graph is conjugated with the processing of information. We took into account that both of the processing of information and its transmission are performed in synchronous and asynchronous modes, and the functioning of the functional system takes place under conditions of the constant influence of the external environment. Then it became clear for us why the problem of integral measurements of the system parameters of biomedical objects requires the detailed elaboration for the possible formalisation of measurement technology. The formalisation of the behavioural space of the object (organism) plays a significant role in this case. It was possible for us to determine the structure of information flows that form the information portrait of a complex system based on the structure of the functional system (1.6) and the concepts of the metabolic process. This structure includes information vectors for all types of regulation (BR and VR) along the channel of reverse afferentation and the loop of metabolisms.

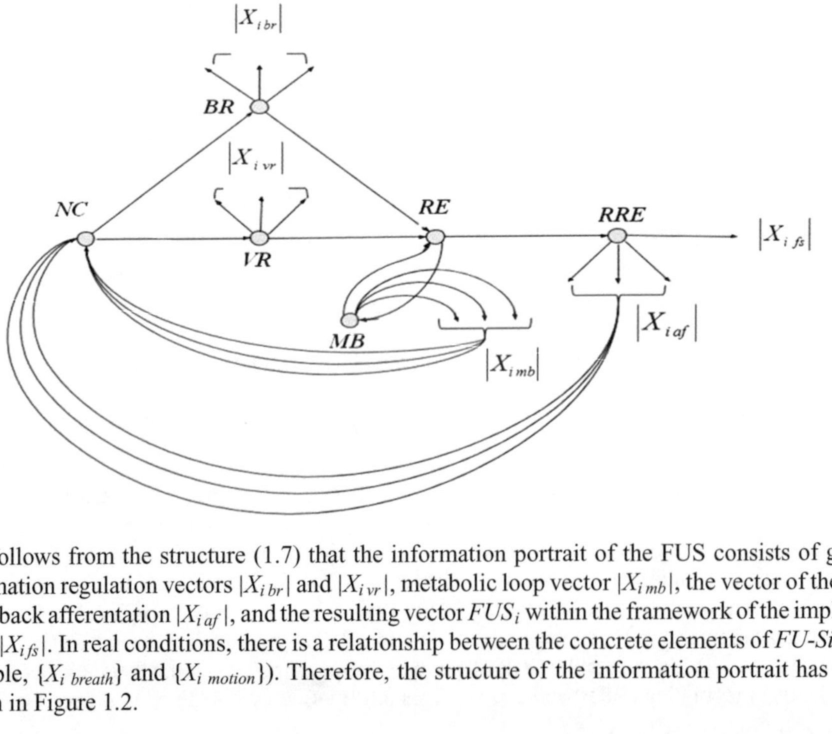

(1.7)

It follows from the structure (1.7) that the information portrait of the FUS consists of groups of information regulation vectors $|X_{i\,br}|$ and $|X_{i\,vr}|$, metabolic loop vector $|X_{i\,mb}|$, the vector of the channel of the back afferentation $|X_{i\,af}|$, and the resulting vector FUS_i within the framework of the implemented stasis $|X_{i\,fs}|$. In real conditions, there is a relationship between the concrete elements of *FU-Sistem* (for example, $\{X_{i\ breath}\}$ and $\{X_{i\ motion}\}$). Therefore, the structure of the information portrait has the form shown in Figure 1.2.

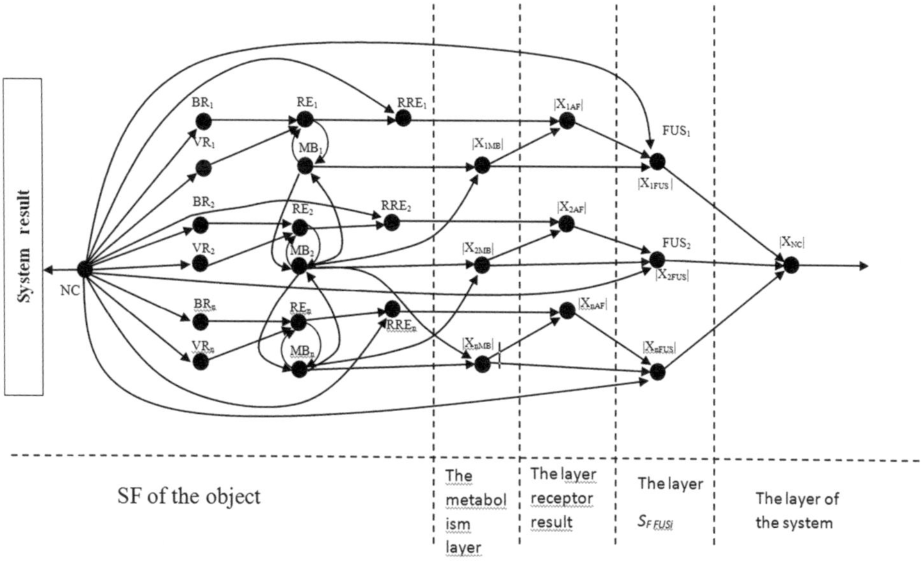

Figure 1.2. Structure of the information portrait.

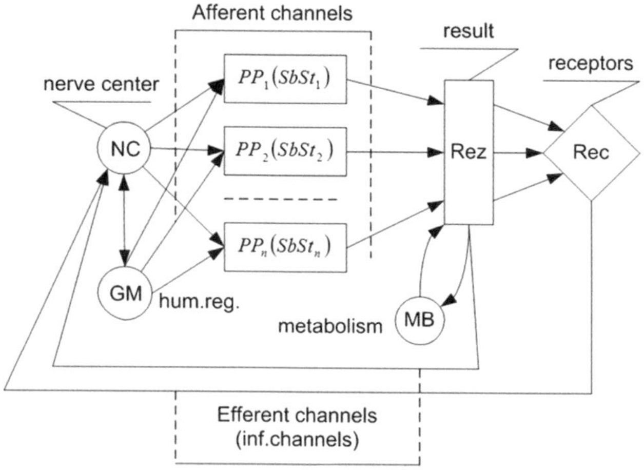

Figure 1.3. General structure of the FUS.

1.7 THE OBSERVABILITY PROCEDURE

"Physiological functional systems in an organism are dynamic centrally peripheral organisations, selectively united in self-regulating by the corresponding needs" in accordance with (Sudakova 1999). Thus, it is extremely important to establish the features of the formal representation of physiological stagnations and their hierarchical relationship. Physiological stasis is always adequate for concrete FUS. It is also connected by a constant function with realisation. The structure of any FUS (Fly 2011) includes a management centre, attracted sub processes, information channels, receptors (sensors), control channels, a subsystem of metabolisms, a subsystem for determining the result of the FUS (Figure 1.3).

The involved sub processes form the result space, and the subsystem of metabolisms is the cellular sub processes in this case. Therefore, any FUS is a set of processes that differ in their own stasis,

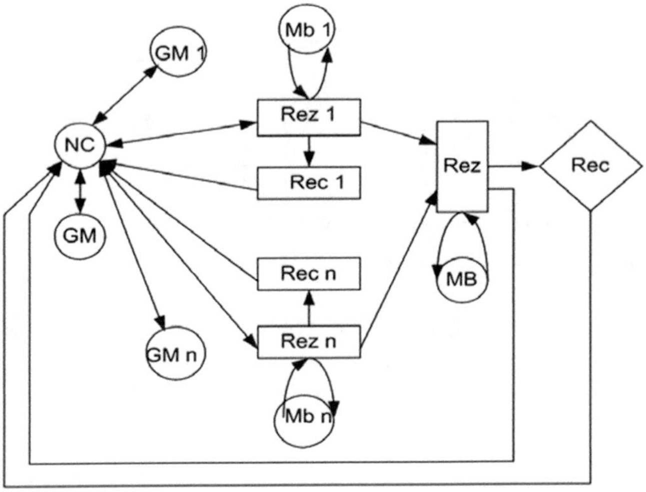

Figure 1.4. Structure of the FUS with the involved processes.

the output parameter of which is used to form the result space (Figure 1.4). In this case, the system parameter of the FUS can be represented by the following relation:

$$\lambda_{FUS}(St) = NCU\{PP_i(SbSt_i) \cup INFC_{EF} \cup CUP_{AF} \cup REZ \cup MB \cup REC, \tag{1.8}$$

where *St* is the stasis state of the FUS; $\lambda_{FUS}(St)$ is the system parameter of the stasis state; PP_i is the system parameter of the *i*-th involved process $SbSt_i$; $INFC_{pF}$ –the state of an effective information channel; CUP_{AF} – the state of the afferent control channel; *NC* – the state of the nervous centre; *Rez* – the state of the FUS for the elements of the preparation of results; *MB* – state of the FUS for the organisation of the metabolic processes; *Rec* – the state of the receptors for the elements of the FUS.

The operational mapping for the functions of the system signal transmission is in the follows equation (1.9) in accordance with the relation (1.8) and the structure of the FUS (Fly 2011), shown in Figure 1.4.

$$\lambda_{NC}(t) = (REC_9)\,(REZ_8)\,K_2 \left\{ \begin{array}{l} K_1' \left\{ \begin{array}{l} (REC_6')\,(REZ_5')\,(NC_3', GM_4') \\ MB_7' \end{array} \right. \\ K_1'' \left\{ \begin{array}{l} (REC_6'')\,(REZ_5'')\,(NC_3'', GM_4'') \\ MB_7'' \end{array} \right. \\ (MB_7) \end{array} \right\} K_0(NC_1, GM_2) \tag{1.9}$$

In this equation, all *K* are commuting operators realising the hierarchical order of transmission. So K_0 is an activation operator for the channels of the involved processes (′) and (″) through the departments of the brain NC_3' and NC_3'' respectively. The operator K_0 works with the involvement of the humoral control operations GM_3' and GM_3' respectively. K_1' – the commuting operator for activating the system signal of the involved process $\varphi_{NC}'(t) = (REC_6')\,(REZ_5')\,(NC_3', GM_4')$ and $\varphi_{MB}'(t) = MB_7''$. Similarly to all that, the activation of another involved channel occurs: $\varphi_{NC}''(t) = (REC_6'')\,(REZ_5'')\,(NC_3'', GM_4'')$ and $\varphi_{MB}''(t) = MB_7''$, using the commutative operator K_1'. Finally, the operator K_2 form out the hierarchical ordering in forming of the system signal $\lambda_{NC}^*(t)$ among all the signals:

$$\varphi_{NC}'(t), \quad \varphi_{NC}''(t), \quad \varphi_{MB}'(t), \quad and \quad \varphi_{MB}(t) = MB_B.$$

Thus, the equation of transformation of physiological dimensions (1.9) is a model of the hierarchical interrelation between the physiological stasis of the basic physiological system and the involved physiological systems. At the same time, the law of the specific interrelation between the FUS, FUS′ and FUS″ is determined by the law of commutation in this case:

$$K(t) = K_2(K_1')(K_0) \cup K_2(K_2'')(K_0). \tag{1.10}$$

We took into account the relationship between physiological processes through their synchronisation using the commutation law (1.10).

1.8 SYNCHRONIZATION OF PHYSIOLOGICAL PROCESSES

The complete set of physiological systems are organised so that their structures contain components that work in several physiological systems at once. We made that conclusion based on the definition of the physiological state. Then we formulated the following thesis: systemic physiological stasis is a state of dynamic equilibrium, the effectiveness of which is higher the greater the coordination of dynamic processes in the physiological system. We executed an assessment of the level of coherence of these dynamic processes only within the framework of the formalisation of the interaction for the dynamic physiological systems (Mukha et al. 2010). We set the following definition to formalise the interaction: the physiological situation is the set:

$$M_{FPS} = \{M_{\text{FUS}}, M_{\text{DDEF}}, M_{PC}, M_{COS}, M_{\text{SP}},\},$$

where M_{FUS} is a categorical model of the functional physiological system; M_{DDEF} is a model of the domain of the definition of a functional physiological system; M_{PC} is the set of physiological constants; M_{COS} – a set of conditions for the functioning of the FUS; M_{SP} is a model of the system parameter.

In accordance with the definition of the formal-physiological situation, the dynamic synchronisation method of the FUS can be represented in the form of the following set of steps (Mukha 2006).

Step 1. We construct the categorical models of the FUS, $M_{\text{FUS}\ i}$, which are considered in the task of dynamic synchronisation.

Step 2. The dynamic components are distinguished and their domains of definition and existence are determined among the $M_{\text{FUS}\ i} \subset M_{FPS}$.

We consider such subcategories that realise their mappings within the framework of periodic or periodised processes in this case. The argument parameters and the boundaries of their changes are determined for these processes, as well as the kind of parameters for the results of subcategory mappings and the boundaries of their changes. It corresponds to the construction of the sets and M_{DDEF} and M_{SP}.

Step 3. We identify the components that are complex or common for the under consideration for $M_{\text{FUS}\ i} \subset M_{FPS}$. The representation of these components is realised through the parameters of metabolism, nervous and hormonal regulation of physiological parameters in this case.

Step 4. The task of dynamic characteristics is realised by performing the presentation of components at the previous stage at the biophysical and biochemical level. We consider a physical description of metabolic reactions and their construction in a mathematical form on this step. We determine the physical nature of periodic or periodised processes (biophysical description) and specify a formal representation of dynamic characteristics using the consideration of the $\text{M}_{\text{FUS}i}$. In addition, we make it possible to determine physiological constants and conditions for the realisation of metabolic processes using the examination of biochemical reactions that exist within the complex of the periodised processes (and so to form a set of and M_{PC} and M_{COS}.

Step 5. We make an experiment to form the set for adjacent physiological functional systems and perform a spectral analysis to identify the boundaries of the norm.

Step 6. Then we use a method for controlling dynamic characteristics, find the correspondence between the experimental characteristics and optimal characteristics, and, if necessary, assign a correction.

Thus, the observability procedure consists of the following steps (Mukha et al. 2003):

1. Graph structures are constructed in correspondence to the full space of states (a complete state graph).

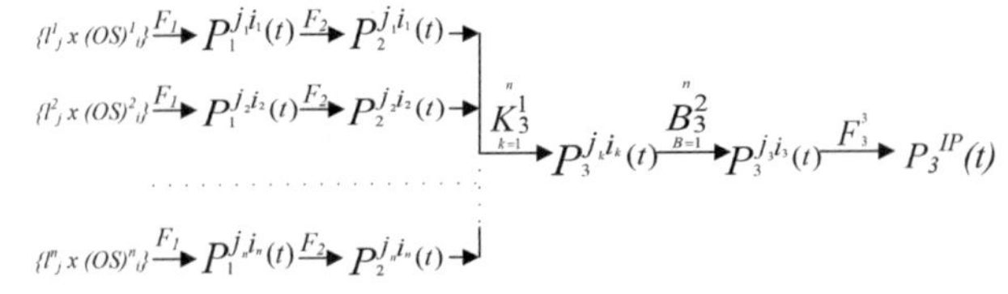

Figure 1.5. Structure of measurement of integral parameters.

2. If it is necessary, the set of least external stability of the complete state graph is determined.
3. The replacement state graph (the second-order graph of the complete state graph) is restored.
4. Many observable system parameters are formed on the basis of substitution complexes.
5. The set of the parameters-complexes for replacement are unconditionally significant observable parameters: they depend on all state parameters and cover all sets of the state elements.

We should take into consideration that it is possible for the complete space of states to be a FUS (or a set of FUS: $\{FUS_i\}$) according to the definition of physiological states. The section of FUS (spatio-temporal) fixes a concrete state. We represent information flows by categories of FUS on the basis of the object by its state parameters.

1.9 MEASURING PROCEDURE

A method of observation is important in this procedure. An ideology of systemic measurements is a base for it (Fly 2011). The concept of system measurements or measurements of the integral parameter were mentioned in the introduction. The heterogeneous information flows exist in the observed object. They are distinguished by an individual measure, have different information conversion channels and individual numerical transformations. However they are combined into the common algorithm at the stage of forming the result of the measurement by the system measurements of the integral parameter. This leads to the synthesis of the combined output system parameter. So, multidimensional studies of assessing the physiological state of the body require a specific organisation of the measurement procedure (Mukha 2003).

All well-known methods of measurement are represented by the apparatus of variable structures. Such structures are obtained from the most complex structures by the switching (changing) of the component parts-mappings.

We used the fundamental cybernetic principle of object representation, the "black box", in constructing of the structures for measurement methods: the initial set of parameters – the function of the input-output connection – the resulting set of parameters.

We concluded that many structures of measurement methods are not investigated. This sphere is open to the formation of new structures. Thus, we make all measurements with subsequent processing of the experimental data using the BTMCS (Popechitelev 2006). However, it is necessary to concentrate attention on the peculiarities of medical measurements, which are connected with the use of plot images (images containing information) as the main kind of impact on the person on whom his reaction arises.

We can determine with the final circumstance that the BTMCS are always specialised measuring tools. It will be adjusted to the object of measurement. We represented such a measurement process in the most complete form using the category of integral measurements (Mukha 2003).

We used a principle of measuring the integral parameters for the subset $P_2^{ik\,jk}(t)$ form the intermediate values of the parameters $i_k j_k$, which are used for a calculation of a generalised parameter for full characteristics of the technological process at an object. So, we added the mappings, K_3^1, B_3^2, F_3^3 that compress the object information (see Figure 1.5). $P_3^{IP}(t)$

Here K_3^1 is the sub-operator of the operator F3 ($K_3^1 \subset F_3$), switching the subsets $P_2^{jn\ in}(t)$; the number of switches is determined by the content of the operator K_3^1, therefore j and i have been obtained the indices k; B_3^2 is the sub-operator of $F_3(B_3^2 \subset F_3)$, the analytic or numerical maps of the subsets $P_2^{jk\ ik}(t)$; the number of the mapping is determined by the content of the operator B_3^2, therefore j and i have been obtained the indices B, F_3^3– the sub-operator of the operator $F_3(F_3^3 \subset F_3)$, which maps the subsets $P_2^{jB\, jB}(t)$ to the set of indication of the integral parameter.

The operators, K_3^1, B_3^2, F_3^3 satisfy an equation:

$$K_3^1 \cup B_3^2 \cup F_3^3 = F_3 \tag{1.11}$$

The formation of a systemic parameter will be considered using the example of the joint work of a functional physiological system that maintains blood pressure (*BP*) in the body at the optimal level for metabolism, and a functional system that determines the volume of circulating blood (*VB*) at the optimal for tissue metabolism.

Then we gave an example of our previous consideration. Here is an organisation, which may be well illustrated by this measurement category (Mukha & Slugin 2008):

$$\left\{\begin{array}{l} BP_1(t) = WH(t) \times \|l_1\| \\ BP_2(t) = DB(t) \times \|l_2\| \\ VB_1(t) = BD(t) \times \|l_3\| \\ VB_2(t) = BF(t) \times \|l_4\| \end{array}\right\} \rightarrow \left|\begin{array}{l} \xrightarrow{F_1^{WH}} \mathrm{P}_1^{\mathrm{PC}}\|l_1\|(t) \xrightarrow{F_2^{WH}} \\ \xrightarrow{F_1^{DB}} \mathrm{P}_1^{DB}\|l_2\|(t) \xrightarrow{F_2^{DB}} \\ \xrightarrow{F_1^{BD}} \mathrm{P}_1^{BD}\|l_3\|(t) \xrightarrow{F_2^{BD}} \\ \xrightarrow{F_1^{BF}} \mathrm{P}_1^{BF}\|l_4\|(t) \xrightarrow{F_2^{BF}} \end{array}\right|$$

$$\times \left\{\mathrm{P}_{2|\|l_1\||}^{WH}(t) \times \mathrm{P}_{2|\|l_2\||}^{DB}(t) \times \mathrm{P}_{2|\|l_3\||}^{BD}(t) \times \times \mathrm{P}_{2|\|l_4\||}^{BF}(t)\right\}$$

$$\rightarrow \times \times \rightarrow p_3^{j_k i_k} \rightarrow p_3^{j_B i_B} \xrightarrow{F_3^3} p_3^{IP}(t) \tag{1.12}$$

$\|l_1\|$, $\|l_2\|$, $\|l_3\|$, $\|l_4\|$ – measures of the parameters of the heart, blood depositing, blood loss and blood formation, respectively; F_1^{WH} – initial mapping for the parameters of the work of the heart in a convenient form for measuring transformations; $F_{1\|l_1\|}^{WH}$(t) is the set of results for the initial mapping of the work of the heart, F_1^{DB} – the initial mapping of the parameters estimating the mass of the deposited blood into a form, which is suitable to implement measurements; $F_{1\|l_2\|}^{DB}$(t) is the set of results of the initial mapping for the parameters of the volumes of the deposited blood; F_1^{BD} – the initial mapping of the parameters evaluating the characteristics of the process of blood destruction; $F_{1\|l_3\|}^{BD}$(t) is the set of results of the initial mapping for the characteristics of the process of blood destruction; $F_{1\|l_4\|}^{BD}$(t) – the initial mapping of parameters evaluating the characteristics of the process of blood formation; $F_{1\|l_4\|}^{BF}$(t) is the set of the results of the initial mapping for the characteristics of the process of blood formation; F_1^{WH} is an intermediate mapping for the result set $\mathrm{P}_{1\|l_1\|}^{WH}$(t) in form, which is the same to uniform of the measurement standard; F_2^{DK} – is an intermediate mapping of the result set $\mathrm{P}_{1\|l_2\|}^{DB}$(t) into a form of the same type as the measurement standard; F_2^{BD} – the intermediate mapping of the result set $\mathrm{P}_{1\|l_3\|}^{BD}$(t) to a form of the same type as the measurement standard; F_2^{BF} is an intermediate mapping of the result set $\mathrm{P}_{1\|l_4\|}^{BF}$(t) to a form of the same form as the measurement standard; $\mathrm{P}_{2\|l_1\|}^{WH}$(t) is the set of results of the intermediate map for parameters of the heart; $\mathrm{P}_{2\|l_2\|}^{DB}$(t) is the set of results for the intermediate map of blood deposition parameters; $\mathrm{P}_{2\|l_3\|}^{BD}$(t) is the set of results for the intermediate map of the parameters of the blood destruction process; $\mathrm{P}_{2\|l_4\|}^{BF}$(t) is the set of results for the intermediate mapping of the parameters of the blood formation process; $\overset{4}{\underset{k=1}{K_3^1}}$ – a mapping that determines the hierarchical commutation of the results of $\mathrm{P}_{2\|l_i\|}^{M}$(t) depending on the organization of the algorithm for the process of forming the integral parameter (IP); $\mathrm{p}_3^{j_k i_k}(t)$ is the set of results of the commuting mapping in the database management form; $\overset{4}{\underset{B=1}{B_3^2}}$ – display of the results $P_{2\|l_i\|}^{M}$(t) in the form of numerical values of the integral parameter placed in the database under the control of the map k_1^3; $\mathrm{p}_3^{j_B i_B}(t)$ is the set of results of the numerical map B_3^2; F_3^3– the mapping of the results $\mathrm{p}_3^{j_B i_B}(t)$ in a form, which is suitable for documenting the values of the integral parameter; $p_3^{IP}(t)$ – the set of the results for the integral parameter in the documented form: magnetic, paper, video.

Category (1.12) has a structure that is the initial both for the organisation of the measurement experiment and for the synthesis of the structure of the measuring and computing complex. Thus, we solve the problem of polygraphic (i.e., multiparameter) studies to assess the physiological state of the organism in accordance with the definition given earlier.

Our purpose of synthesising IIS-structure was to construct an operator for the converting input information for any number of inputs (sources of measured information parameters) into output values for any number of outputs, which were equal to the number of receivers-consumers of the output information. Such an operator was called a measuring convolution.

1.10 CONCLUSIONS

We summarised all our results and note that the science of complexly organised systemic medical dimensions is experiencing a period of rapid development. We consider medical technology systematically with the application of structural formal ideology. So, we got an advance in the right direction when solving metrological problems in medicine. Our main principle was to determine the elements of a system and rules of their interaction. Such way of the investigation allows us to get an algebraic system and represent any technology, any object in the form of a structure, on which it is possible to formulate the necessary estimates and declare synthesis processes, including metrological ones.

REFERENCES

Akhutin, V.M. 1976. Biotechnical aspects of synthesis of biotechnical systems. *Cybernetics* 4: 3–26.

Besekersky, V.A. & Popov, E.P. 1977. *The theory of automatic control*. Moscow: Science.

Cardman, J. J. & Vogt, R. 1977. *Homotopy invariant algebraic structures on topological spaces*. Moscow: Mir.

Ferreira, A., Novotny, A., & Sokołowski, J. 2016. Topological derivative method for electrical impedance tomography problems. *Informatyka, Automatyka, Pomiary w Gospodarce i Ochronie Środowiska* 6(2): 4–8. https://doi.org/10.5604/20830157.1201308

Mesarovic M. & Takahara, Ya. 1978. *General theory of systems: mathematical foundations*. Moscow: Mir.

Mukha, Yu. P. 2006. Structural synthesis of the IS / NS system function for a complex measurement situation at a medical facility. *Biomedical Technologies and Radioelectronics* 4: 26–32.

Mukha, Yu. P. 2011. Systemic medical measurements of the state of the organism. *Millimeter waves in biology and medicine* 1: 2–31.

Mukha, Yu. P., Akulov, L.G. & Naumov, V. Yu. 2010. System organization of experiments for the study of the dynamics of functional systems in biology and medicine. *Biomedical radioelectronics* 6: 43–52.

Mukha, Yu. P., Avdeyuk, O.A. & Koroleva, I. Yu. 2003. *Algebraic theory of synthesis of complex systems*. Volgograd: VolgGTU, 2003.

Mukha, Yu. P., Bezborodov, S.A. & Guschin, A.V. 2017. *Metrological aspects of medical measurements*. Volgograd: Publishing house VolgGMU.

Mukha, Yu. P. & Slugin, V.I. 2008. Metrological analysis in assessing the functional state of the cardiovascular system of man. *Biomedical technologies and radio electronics* 4: 52–58.

Nikolayev, V.N. & Brooks, V.M. 1985. *System engineering: methods and applications*. Moscow: Mechanical engineering.

Popechitelev, E.P. 2006. *Man in the Biotechnical System: Proc. allowance*. Sankt-Petersburg: LETI.

Speneur, E. 1971. *Algebraic topology*. Moscow: Mir.

Sudakova, K.V. (Ed.) 1999. *Normal physiology: course of physiology of functional systems*. Moscow: Medical information agency.

Tsvetkov, E.I. 2005. *Fundamentals of mathematical metrology*. Sankt-Petersburg: The Polytechnic.

Vinogradov, I. M. (Ed.) 1977. *Matematicheskaya entsiklopediya*. Moscow: Sov. Entsiklopediya.

Volkova, V.N. & Denisov, A.A. 2013. *Theory of systems and systems analysis*. Moscow: Yurait.

CHAPTER 2

Metrological features of a pathospecific device for the diagnostic of glaucoma

A. Guschin
Volgograd State Medical University, Volgograd, Russian Federation

Yu.P. Mukha
Volgograd State Medical University, Volgograd, Russian Federation
Volgograd State Technical University, Volgograd, Russian Federation

K. Gromaszek & E. Łukasik
Lublin University of Technology, Lublin, Poland

O. Mamyrbayev
Institute of Information and Computational Technologies CS MES RK, Almaty, Kazakhstan

ABSTRACT: The chapter describes the structure of the pathospecific device for the diagnosis of glaucoma. Performed a description of the phase space is given and a metrological analysis of the errors possible with the use of such an installation. Using of such devices can improve the quality of glaucoma diagnostics and increase the productivity of diagnostic physicians.

2.1 INTRODUCTION

Glaucoma is a pathology of intraocular pressure (IOP), which causes irreversible neurodegenerative changes in the structures of the retina and optic nerve. IOP consists of "fast" and "slow" components. "Slow" IOP components are associated with the balance of production and drainage of intraocular fluid and the dynamics of these indicators is relatively slow. Determining the "fast" components of IOP by the volume and velocity characteristics of the blood flow in the vascular system of the eye. Both these factors of IOP formation, but especially the "fast" one, are associated with the state of systemic hemodynamic, largely determined by the tone of various parts of the autonomic nervous system.

Traditionally, the most widely used method of investigating IOP is tonometry, which is an indirect measurement of IOP in terms of the degree of deformation of the shells of the eye under the influence of external pressure of known force. In this way, we can measure only "slow" IOP components, whereas the dynamics of neurodegenerative changes that determine the functional damage from glaucoma significantly associated with the "fast" IOP components.

Thus, the significant spread of the disease and the degree of disability due to it, are due not only to the shortcomings of therapy, but also to the inadequacy of diagnosis including the terminal ("painful") stage of the disease and the absence in the arsenal of a practical doctor of an accessible and sufficiently accurate automated method for assessing the state of compensation for hydro- and hemodynamic parameters of the eye. This leads to untimely and inadequate administration of treatment and, as a consequence, to the progression of the disease.

The issues of distinguishing between the concepts of "health" and "norm" as applied to glaucoma is widely discussed in the scientific literature. There is a very widespread opinion about the state of "norm" as a single state, "the best of really possible homogeneous states". At the same time, studies on adult healthy people have shown that the "norm" in one age population can be heterogeneous and should be evaluated taking into account individual and typological properties and the peculiarities of the organization of the systemic activity of the organism (Fokin et al. 2006; Shiga et al. 2013).

This determines the purpose of this work, which consists in the development of a pathospecific measuring device for the diagnosis of glaucoma.

The achievement of this goal associated with the solution of the following research tasks:

- Formalization of the phase space of the device being developed;
- Determine the data structure with which this installation will work;
- Metrological analysis of the overall structure of the device.

To increase of accuracy of determining the pathological nature of an increase in IOP, it is necessary to take into account the "fast", hemodynamic components of IOP. For this, the use of non-invasive methods such as ophthalmic and sphygmographic is possible. These methods developed to determine, respectively, the speed and volume characteristics of the blood flow in the vascular system of the eye; they in this situation are well complementary.

This determines the high practical importance of metrological analysis of the dynamics of the characteristics of the hydro- and hemodynamic of the eye, as a single system, in phase space.

2.2 PHASE SPACE

The described phase space characterized by the dimension associated with the multidimensional nature of the data obtained from specific studies. Therefore, for the integration within the pathospecific diagnostic installation for the diagnosis of glaucoma, the following measurements are suitable.

Proceeding from the foregoing, the phase space of the projected measuring device generalized in the following form (Figure 2.1).

As can be seen from the presented illustration, at the most general level, the phase space can be described as three-dimensional, which corresponds to the three main measuring channels of the complex pathospecific measuring device for the diagnosis of glaucoma (Balalin & Gushchin 2003).

A number of measured quantities form each of the measurements of the phase space. Their detailed composition is given in Table 2.1.

Hydrodynamic parameters: "P_0" is the true intraocular pressure, "C" is the outflow coefficient of the intraocular fluid, "F" is the minute volume of chamber moisture, and "BQ" is the Becker quotient (P_0/C).

Tonography parameters are as follows: "OPPA" – ocular pulse pressure amplitude; "SIPV" is a systolic increase of the pulse volume; "A/C" is the ratio of the duration of an anacrotic to the duration of a catacrosis; "α" is the angle of the anacrotic surge of the pulse wave; "β" is the angle of decline of the pulse wave; "α/β" is the ratio characterizing the quality of the recording; "PVPM" is a pulse volume per minute, "EOVI" is an elasticity index of the ocular vessels (SPPO/AGPD).

Rheography parameters is: "RQ" – rheographic quotient; "A" – duration of an anacrotic, "C" – duration and cataracts; "A/A" is the ratio of Amplitude/Anacrotic; "MSFF" – the maximum speed of fast filling; "ASSF" is the average speed of slow filling; "AFF" – acceleration of fast filling, "ASF" – acceleration of slow filling; "IT" – the index of tolerance; "RSI" is a rheographic systolic index; "PI" is the "plateau" index.

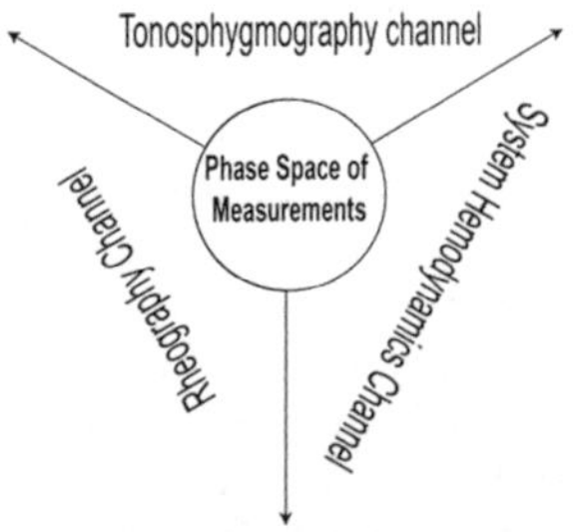

Figure 2.1. Generalized composition of the phase space of the functioning of the pathospecific measuring device.

Table 2.1. Composition of channels in pathospecific measurement device.

Tonosphygmograpy Channel	Rheography Channel	System Hemodynamics Channel
P_0	RQ	HR
C	A	SBP
F	C	DBP
BQ	A/A	
OPPA	MSFF	
SIPV	ASSF	
A/C	AFF	
α	ASF	
β	IT	
α/β	RSI	
PVPM	PI	
EOVI		

Parameters of systemic hemodynamic: "HR" – heart rate; "SBP" – systolic blood pressure; "DBP" – diastolic blood pressure.

Now it is easy to obtain a general formalized representation of the phase information space of the form (2.1):

$$IP = \{I_{ts}, I_r, I_h\}, \tag{2.1}$$

Where I_{ts} is the information of the channel of tonosphygmography; I_r – rheography channel information; I_h – information channel of systemic hemodynamic.

In expanded form, taking into account the data of Table 2.1, the same can be represented in the following detailed form (2.2):

$$IP = \left\{ \begin{array}{l} I_{P0}, I_C, I_F, I_{BQ}, I_{OPPA}, I_{SIPV}, I_{\frac{A}{C}}, I_\alpha, I_\beta, I_{\frac{\alpha}{\beta}}, I_{PVPM}, I_{EOVI} \\ I_{RQ}, I_A, I_K, I_{\frac{A}{A}}, I_{MSFF}, I_{ASFF}, I_{AFF}, I_{ASF}, I_{IT}, I_{RSI}, I_{PI} \\ I_{HR}, I_{SBP}, I_{DBP} \end{array} \right\}. \tag{2.2}$$

In statement (2.2) the designations of the elements of the information phase space correspond to those in Table 2.1.

The review of the phase information space, characterizes its multidimensionality and, as a consequence, complexity. Therefore, when designing such a pathospecific measuring installation, it is expedient to formulate an algorithm for its operation in such a way that when forming the final summarizing results, a specific measuring and diagnostic situation taken into account, the features of which are presented below.

Thus, the physiological prediction of various functional states in the process of adaptation to the effects of various stimuli of various nature is complex and not fully resolved by the medical and biological problem. At the same time, physiological prediction allows not only to anticipate the adverse outcomes of adaptation, but also opens great possibilities for its use in the study of various levels of functioning of the human and animal organism with a quantitative and qualitative assessment of the mechanisms for providing adaptive and compensatory responses.

In response to the intolerant level of IOP, the mechanisms of autoregulation of the tonus of the vessels of the eye occur, which leads to an increase in vascular tone and a decrease in the elasticity of the vessels of the eye fundus. This is reflected in the changes observed in the data of sphygmography (decrease in SPPS and PESG, increase in the AHAP). Changes in the tone of the vascular wall, in turn, lead to a compensatory increase in pressure in *a. ophthalmica* and recovery of reduced perfusion pressure.

The complexity of the information space of hydro- and hemodynamics leads to the need to choose a system parameter of the technology. A diagnostic situation is an algebraic system of the form:

$$M_{DS} = \{M_{SMFS}, M_{SCES}, M_{SMDC}, G(X, G_C)\}. \tag{2.3}$$

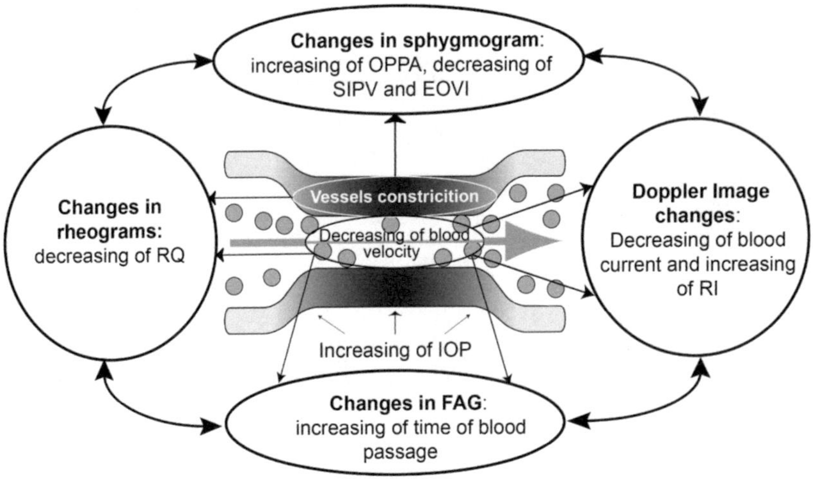

Figure 2.2. Interrelation of the considered methods of the study of ocular hemodynamics.

In statement (2.3) M_{SMFS} is the set of models of the function of the system; M_{SCES} is a set of conditions for the existence of a system; M_{SMDC} – a set of models of diagnostic criteria for assessing the state of the system; G (X, G_c) is a graph model of the structure of the system.

In accordance with this definition, in the structural scheme, which consists of the set of elements of the system X and the set of their interconnections (G_C), the M_{SMFS} is distributed by the set of functions realized by the elements of the system. Each element $m_{j\ SMFS} \in M_{SMFS}$ is accompanied by a subset of M_j M_{SCES} of the function m_{jSMES} and a subset of the criteria for their realization M_{jSMDC}. Thus, in the analysis of the diagnosis with respect to hydro- and hemodynamics, one can consider the efficiency of the implementation of each m_{jSMFS} with the corresponding M_{jSCES} and M_{jSMDC}. This reduces the dimensionality of IP space while maintaining the systemic nature of the task of monitoring technological safety and, therefore, facilitates the choice of a particular observable system parameter. The entire information flow of the pathospecific measuring device used for the adaptive adoption of medical diagnostic solutions. Thus, the developed pathospecific diagnostic device allows evaluating the amplitude and volume parameters of the eye's blood flow and, on this basis, to judge the state of adequacy of intraocular blood flow and the consistency of the mechanisms of autoregulation of the tonus of the vessels of the eye.

The phase space forming data of various methods of investigating the hemodynamics of the eye closely related to the generality of the object of study and its changes. This relationship graphically illustrated as follows (Figure 2.2).

It can be seen on this illustration that the indices depending on the state of the vascular wall (via sphygmo- and rheography data) and the indicators reflecting the characteristics of the blood flow (data of Doppler and FAH), due to their close physical connection, complement each other. For a more accurate interpretation of the changes observed in sphygmography, it is necessary to take into account the results of applying methods based on other physical principles (Odstrcilik et al. 2014). The question of the relationship between the level of tolerant intraocular pressure, the parameters of general hemodynamics and the state of regional eye hemodynamics in patients with glaucoma remains underexplored. This applies both to studies based on the method of sphygmography, and to cases of application of various variants of Doppler and FAG. In addition, in the known works, performed using the method of sphygmograms, the strict quality control of the received records usually not performed, which, in addition to ignoring the effect on the results of sphygmograms of changes in system hemodynamics, in some cases could lead to a decrease in the reliability of the results of the studies.

The form of a graph characterizing information flows in the pathospecific measuring diagnostic device. Such a graph shown in Figure 2.3.

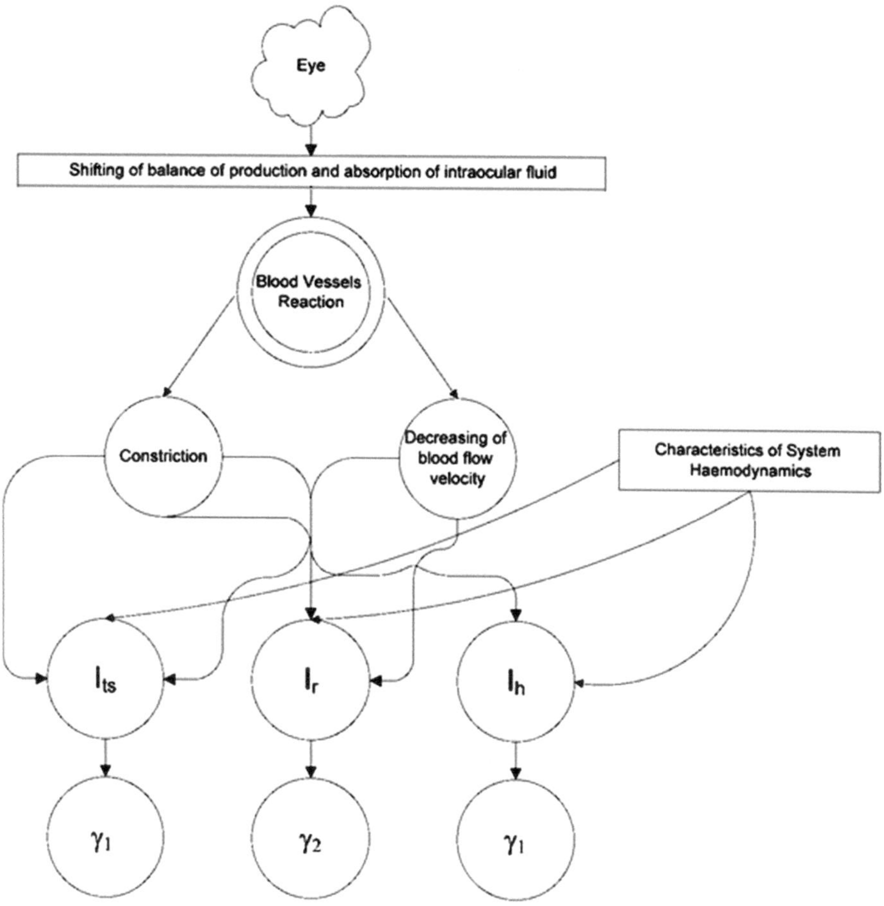

Figure 2.3. Graphic representation of information flows at the input of a pathospecific measuring device.

Figure 2.3 graphically illustrates the relationship of the pathophysiological processes occurring in the eye and the input characteristics of the pathospecific measuring device (γ 1.3).

The presented results make it possible to draw a general conclusion about the expediency of combining the methods of examining ocular hydro- and hemodynamics with methods of investigating systemic hemodynamics within the framework of a single diagnostic measuring device for the diagnosis of glaucoma. Based on these data to indices, the measurement of which is expedient to integrate within such pathospecific the measuring device, may include the following: an intraocular pressure, outflow of intraocular fluid quotient, systolic increment pulse volume of the eyeball, vascular elasticity quotient, systolic and diastolic blood pressure and age patient.

The pathospecific diagnostic unit includes rheography modules, tonosphygmography and measurement of systemic hemodynamics parameters.

The presented data make it possible to carry out synthesis of the general structure of the considered pathospecific diagnostic setup as a multichannel information measuring system. Such a structure shown in Figure 2.4.

The structure of the pathospecific measuring device for the diagnosis of glaucoma, presented in Figure 2.4, consists of 3 structurally identical measuring channels, designed, respectively, to measure the characteristics of tonoglyphograms, ophthalmic rheograms and characteristics of systemic hemodynamics. Each of these channels consists of a primary measuring transducer (an organ-specific sensor), a secondary transducer (an amplifier with characteristics corresponding to the characteristics

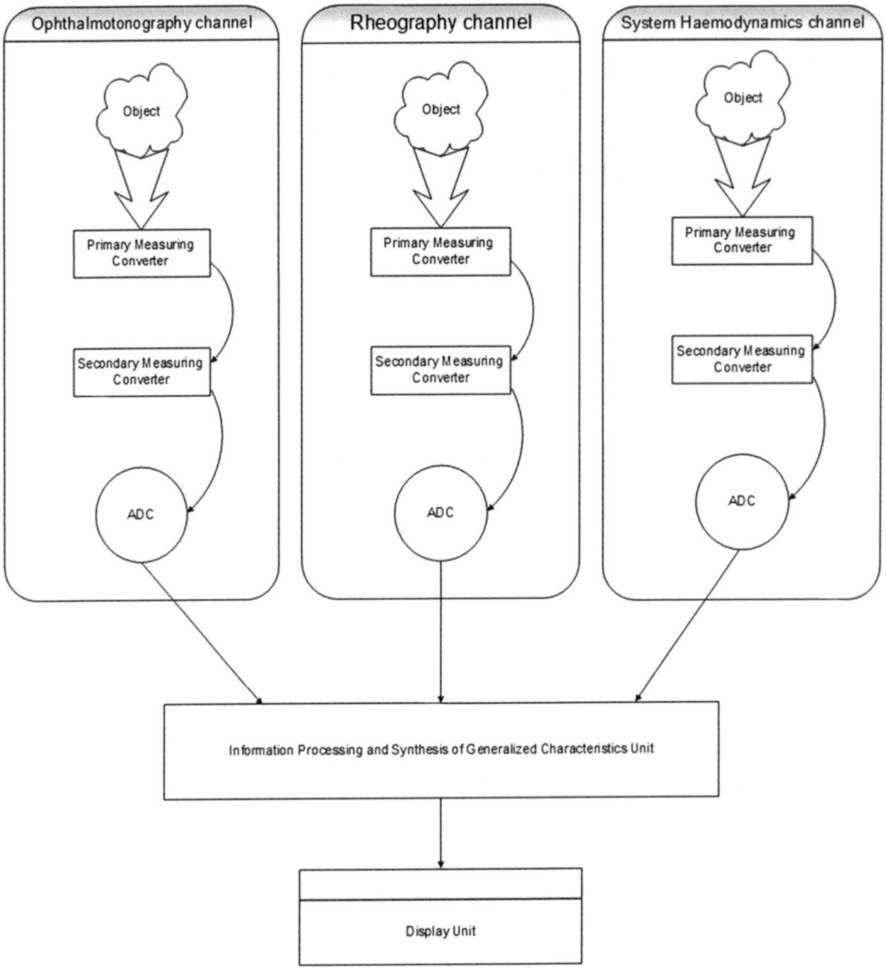

Figure 2.4. General structure of pathospecific measurement device for diagnostic of glaucoma.

of the sensor used in the channel) and an ADC that converts the measurement information into a suitable for digital processing form. Such processing performed in the PC-based hardware-software unit for processing the measurement information and synthesizing generalized indicators. All results of information processing are output in a form convenient for perception to the unit for issuing measurement results. Thus, in its structure, this information measuring system counted as a measuring system of a chain type.

For this information measuring system, it is expedient to study its metrological characteristics, which reflect the properties of the system, which have a determining effect on the result and the accuracy of the measurements. The normalization of metrological characteristics is the establishment of a set of metrological characteristics and methods for their presentation. General principles of rationing, applied to this measuring system:

- Possibility of comparison and selection of measuring instruments,
- The possibility of determining the uncertainty of the measured value, taking into account the normalized metrological characteristics, by practically realizable methods,
- The ability to determine the measurement (measure) of the uncertainty of the measurement results carried out with the help of this measuring instrument.

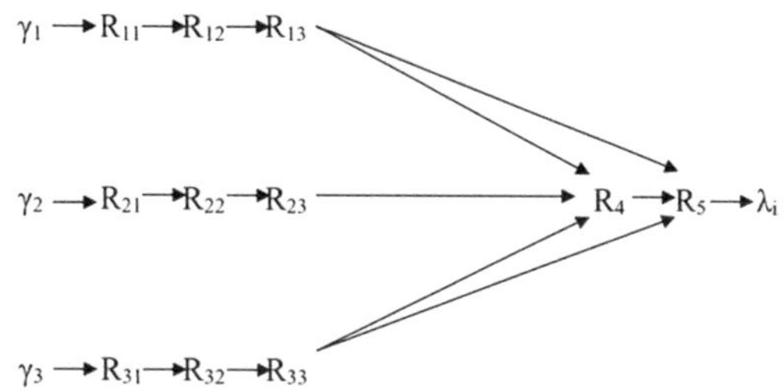

Figure 2.5. Graph of structure of information flows.

2.3 DESCRIPTION OF MEASUREMENTS

The theory of analytical and algorithmic description of measurement processes developed by E.I. Tsvetkov (2010, 2012) is most applicable to the sphere of measurement of eye hydro- and hemodynamics.

As an initial structure based on which it is possible to form a measurement equation suitable for describing a pathospecific measuring device for the complex study of ocular hydro- and hemodynamics, it is advisable to use the structure of information flows, which is illustrated by the graph (Figure 2.5).

These flows are sources of information about the form of the organ of vision and the cardiovascular system of the subject.

R_i – mapping of transformations carried out in the course of research: 1 – ophthalmotonosfigmography; 2 – rheography; 3 – measurements of blood pressure and heart rate.

R_{ij} – graph display of control of the sequence of formation of a set of measurement results, which includes the implementation of the following algorithms of the pathospecific measuring device – obtaining data on the dynamics of intraocular pressure, the dynamics of blood filling of the vessels of the eye, and the functional characteristics of systemic hemodynamics.

Structurally, the described pathospecific measuring device consists of 3 measuring channels, 3 calculation units and a computer data output unit. Below is a detailed description of the vertices of the graph (2.9) that make up the set R_{ij}.

R_{11} – location of the object in the measurement space, its preparation (packing, application of local anesthesia);

R_{12} – the imposition of a tonographer and the acquisition of data on the dynamics of IOP, the mechanical characteristics of the eye pulse and the index of elasticity of the cornea;

R_{13} – automatic processing of the obtained data with the calculation of generalizing indices characterizing the dynamics of IOP, eye pulse and elasticity of the cornea of the eye;

R_{21} – location of the object in the measurement space, its preparation (packing, application of local anesthesia);

R_{22} – imposition of the ophthalmic image sensor and data collection on the dynamics of volume and velocity characteristics of the eye pulse;

R_{23} – automatic processing of the obtained data with the calculation of generalizing indices characterizing the dynamics of volume and velocity characteristics of the eye pulse;

R_{31} – location of the object in the measurement space, its preparation;

R_{32} – superimposition of the tonometer sensor and data collection of blood pressure and heart rate;

R_{33} – input of the obtained data into a pathospecific measuring device;

R_4 – unit for calculating the generalized individualized IOP tolerance index;

R_5 – the block of a conclusion of results on the computer monitor, representing a part of the user interface of the path-specific measuring installation.

λ_i – a set of output information flows of a path-specific measuring device consisting of:

λ_1 – output information flow of tonosphygmography;

λ_2 – output information flow of ophthalmography;

λ_3 – output information flow of characteristics of systemic hemodynamics;

λ_4 – output information flow, which is an array of data containing information about finding the parameters of the hydro- and hemodynamics of the examined eye within the limits of individual tolerant values.

Based on the graph presented above (Figure 2.5), it is possible to compile a system of measurement equations for each measuring channel:

– for the tonosphygmography channel:

$$\lambda_{1j}(t) = R_5 R_{13} R_{12} R_{11} \gamma_{1j}(t) = R_5 \varphi_{1j}(t), \tag{2.4}$$

where

$$\varphi_{1j}(t) = R_{13} R_{12} R_{11} \gamma_{1j}(t) \tag{2.5}$$

is the result of tonosphygmography;

– for the rheography channel:

$$\lambda_{2j}(t) = R_5 R_{23} R_{22} R_{21} \gamma_{2j}(t) = R_5 \varphi_{2j}(t), \tag{2.6}$$

where

$$\varphi_{2j}(t) = R_{23} R_{22} R_{21} \gamma_{2j}(t) \tag{2.7}$$

is the result of rheography;

– for the system hemodynamics channel:

$$\lambda_{3j}(t) = R_5 R_{33} R_{32} R_{31} \gamma_{3j}(t) = R_5 \varphi_{3j}(t), \tag{2.8}$$

where

$$\varphi_{3j}(t) = R_{33} R_{32} R_{31} \gamma_{3j}(t) \tag{2.9}$$

is the result of measurements of HR and BP

– for the tolerant IOP channel

$$\lambda_4(t) = R_5 R_4 R_{k1} \begin{cases} \varphi_{1j}(t) \\ \varphi_{2j}(t) \\ \varphi_{3j}(t) \end{cases} \tag{2.10}$$

is the result of tolerant IOP computation.

From the statements above (2.4–2.10), we can derive general equation of measurements in pathospecific measurement device:

$$\lambda_{ij}(t)_{\overline{i=1,4}} = R_5 R_{k2} \begin{cases} \varphi_{1j}(t) \\ \varphi_{2j}(t) \\ \varphi_{3j}(t) \\ R_4 R_{k1} \begin{cases} \varphi_{1j}(t) \\ \varphi_{2j}(t) \\ \varphi_{3j}(t) \end{cases} \end{cases} \tag{2.11}$$

This equation is convertible in graph (Figure 2.6).

The total measurement error is the difference between the results of the real and hypothetical measurement procedure. This information about the measurement situation makes it is possible to compose the formal expression of the total error of the measuring channel of the tonosphygmography:

$$\lambda_{1j}(t) = R_5 R_{13} R_{12} R_{11} \gamma_{1j}(t) = R_5 \varphi_{1j}(t), \tag{2.12}$$

where

$$\varphi_{1j}(t) = R_{13} R_{12} R_{11} \gamma_{1j}(t). \tag{2.13}$$

From the statements (2.12, 2.13) it is possible to compose the equation for total measurement error in tonosphygmography channel:

$$\Delta\lambda_{1j}(t) = \Delta_5 \lambda_{1j}(t) + \Delta\varphi_{1j}(t), \tag{2.14}$$

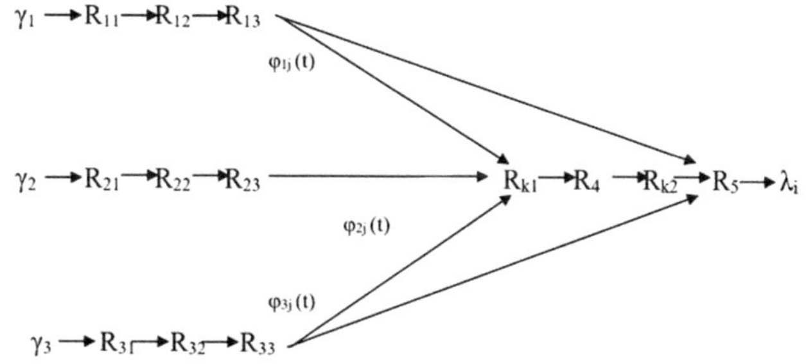

Figure 2.6. General Graph of measurements in pathospecific measurement device.

where

$$\Delta\varphi_{1j}(t) = R_{13}R_{12}R_{11}\gamma_{1j}(t) - R^{\Gamma}_{13}R^{\Gamma}_{12}R^{1}_{11}\gamma_{1j}(t). \tag{2.15}$$

The described total error we can decompose into elements as follows:

$$\Delta_5\lambda_{1j}(t) = R_5\varphi_{1j}(t) - R^{\Gamma}_5\varphi_{1j}(t) \tag{2.16}$$

also

$$\Delta_{\varphi 1j}\lambda_{1j}(t) = R^{\Gamma}_5\varphi_{1j}(t) - R^{\Gamma}_5\varphi^{\Gamma}_{1j}(t). \tag{2.17}$$

Further,

$$\Delta_{13}\varphi_{1j}(t) = R_{13}R_{12}R_{11}\gamma_{1j}(t) - R^{\Gamma}_{13}R_{12}R_{11}\gamma_{1j}(t), \tag{2.18}$$

$$\Delta_{12}\varphi_{1j}(t) = R^{\Gamma}_{13}R_{12}R_{11}\gamma_{1j}(t) - R^{\Gamma}_{13}R^{\Gamma}_{12}R_{11}\gamma_{1j}(t), \tag{2.19}$$

$$\Delta_{11}\varphi_{1j}(t) = R^{\Gamma}_{13}R^{\Gamma}_{12}R_{11}\gamma_{1j}(t) - R^{\Gamma}_{13}R^{\Gamma}_{12}R^{\Gamma}_{11}\gamma_{1j}(t). \tag{2.20}$$

The equation of the total error of the channel of tonosphygmography, which is the sum of the partial ones, can have the form:

$$\Delta\lambda_{1j}(t) = \Delta_5\lambda_{1j}(t) + \Delta_{13}\varphi_{1j}(t) + \Delta_{12}\varphi_{1j}(t) + \Delta_{11}\varphi_{1j}(t). \tag{2.21}$$

with

$$\Delta_{\text{инстр}}\varphi_{1j} = \Delta_{13}\varphi_{1j}(t) + \Delta_{12}\varphi_{1j}(t) \tag{2.22}$$

$$\Delta_{\text{мет}}\varphi_{1j} = \Delta_5\lambda_{1j}(t) + \Delta_{11}\varphi_{1j}(t) \tag{2.23}$$

From the statement (2.11) it is possible to compose the equation for total measurement error in rheography channel:

$$\lambda_{2j}(t) = R_5R_{23}R_{22}R_{21}\gamma_{2j}(t) = R_5\varphi_{2j}(t), \tag{2.24}$$

where

$$\varphi_{2j}(t) = R_{23}R_{22}R_{21}\gamma_{2j}(t). \tag{2.25}$$

From the statements (2.24, 2.25) it is possible to compose the equation for total measurement error in rheography channel:

$$\Delta\lambda_{2j}(t) = \Delta_5\lambda_{2j}(t) + \Delta\varphi_{2j}(t), \tag{2.26}$$

where

$$\Delta\varphi_{2j}(t) = R_{23}R_{22}R_{21}\gamma_{2j}(t) - R^{\Gamma}_{23}R^{\Gamma}_{22}R^{\Gamma}_{21}\gamma_{2j}(t). \tag{2.27}$$

The described total error we can decompose into elements as follows:

$$\Delta_5\lambda_{2j}(t) = R_5\varphi_{2j}(t) - R^{\Gamma}_5\varphi_{2j}(t) \tag{2.28}$$

also

$$\Delta_{\varphi 2j}\lambda_{2j}(t) = R^{\Gamma}_5\varphi_{2j}(t) - R^{\Gamma}_5\varphi^{\Gamma}_{2j}(t). \tag{2.29}$$

Further,

$$\Delta_{23}\varphi_{2j}(t) = R_{23}R_{22}R_{21}\gamma_{2j}(t) - R_{23}^{\Gamma}R_{22}R_{21}\gamma_{2j}(t), \quad (2.30)$$

$$\Delta_{22}\varphi_{2j}(t) = R_{23}^{\Gamma}R_{22}R_{21}\gamma_{2j}(t) - R_{23}^{\Gamma}R_{22}^{\Gamma}R_{21}\gamma_{2j}(t), \quad (2.31)$$

$$\Delta_{21}\varphi_{2j}(t) = R_{23}^{\Gamma}R_{22}^{\Gamma}R_{21}\gamma_{2j}(t) - R_{23}^{\Gamma}R_{22}^{\Gamma}R_{21}^{\Gamma}\gamma_{2j}(t). \quad (2.32)$$

The equation of the total error of the channel of rheography, which is the sum of the partial ones, can have the form:

$$\Delta\lambda_{2j}(t) = \Delta_5\lambda_{2j}(t) + \Delta_{23}\varphi_{2j}(t) + \Delta_{22}\varphi_{2j}(t) + \Delta_{21}\varphi_{2j}(t). \quad (2.33)$$

With,

$$\Delta_{\text{инстр}}\varphi_{2j} = \Delta_{23}\varphi_{2j}(t) + \Delta_{22}\varphi_{2j}(t) \quad (2.34)$$

$$\Delta_{\text{мет}}\varphi_{2j} = \Delta_5\lambda_{2j}(t) + \Delta_{21}\varphi_{2j}(t) \quad (2.35)$$

From the statement (2.11), it is possible to compose the equation for total measurement error in system hemodynamics channel:

$$\lambda_{3j}(t) = R_5R_{33}R_{32}R_{31}\gamma_{3j}(t) = R_5\varphi_{3j}(t), \quad (2.36)$$

where

$$\varphi_{3j}(t) = R_{33}R_{32}R_{31}\gamma_{3j}(t). \quad (2.37)$$

From the statements (2.36, 2.37) it is possible to compose the equation for total measurement error in system hemodynamics channel:

$$\Delta\lambda_{3j}(t) = \Delta_5\lambda_{3j}(t) + \Delta\varphi_{3j}(t), \quad (2.38)$$

where

$$\Delta\varphi_{3j}(t) = R_{33}R_{32}R_{31}\gamma_{3j}(t) - R_{33}^{\Gamma}R_{32}^{\Gamma}R_{31}^{\Gamma}\gamma_{3j}(t). \quad (2.39)$$

The equation of the total error of the channel of system hemodynamics, which is the sum of the partial ones, can have the form:

$$\Delta_5\lambda_{3j}(t) = R_5\varphi_{3j}(t) - R_5^{\Gamma}\varphi_{3j}(t) \quad (2.40)$$

also

$$\Delta_{\varphi 3j}\lambda_{3j}(t) = R_5^{\Gamma}\varphi_{3j}(t) - R_5^{\Gamma}\varphi_{3j}^{\Gamma}(t). \quad (2.41)$$

Further,

$$\Delta_{33}\varphi_{2j}(t) = R_{33}R_{32}R_{31}\gamma_{3j}(t) - R_{33}^{\Gamma}R_{32}R_{31}\gamma_{3j}(t), \quad (2.42)$$

$$\Delta_{32}\varphi_{3j}(t) = R_{33}^{\Gamma}R_{32}R_{31}\gamma_{3j}(t) - R_{33}^{\Gamma}R_{32}^{\Gamma}R_{31}\gamma_{3j}(t), \quad (2.43)$$

$$\Delta_{31}\varphi_{3j}(t) = R_{33}^{\Gamma}R_{32}^{\Gamma}R_{31}\gamma_{3j}(t) - R_{33}^{\Gamma}R_{32}^{\Gamma}R_{31}^{\Gamma}\gamma_{3j}(t). \quad (2.44)$$

The described total error we can decompose into elements as follows:

$$\Delta\lambda_{3j}(t) = \Delta_5\lambda_{3j}(t) + \Delta_{33}\varphi_{3j}(t) + \Delta_{32}\varphi_{3j}(t) + \Delta_{31}\varphi_{3j}(t) \quad (2.45)$$

With,

$$\Delta_{\text{инстр}}\varphi_{3j} = \Delta_{33}\varphi_{3j}(t) + \Delta_{32}\varphi_{3j}(t) \quad (2.46)$$

$$\Delta_{\text{мет}}\varphi_{3j} = \Delta_5\lambda_{3j}(t) + \Delta_{31}\varphi_{3j}(t) \quad (2.47)$$

From statements (2.12–2.47), it is possible to compose the equation for total measurement error in t IOP tolerance channel:

$$\lambda_{4j}(t) = R_5R_4R_{k1}\begin{cases}\varphi_{1j}(t)\\ \varphi_{2j}(t)\\ \varphi_{3j}(t)\end{cases} = R_5\varphi_{4j}(t) \quad (2.48)$$

Where

$$\varphi_{4j}(t) = R_4 R_{k1} \begin{cases} \varphi_{1j}(t) \\ \varphi_{2j}(t) \\ \varphi_{3j}(t) \end{cases}. \tag{2.49}$$

Equation of total measurement error in this channel:

$$\Delta\lambda_{4j}(t) = \Delta_5\lambda_{4j}(t) + \Delta\varphi_{4j}(t) \tag{2.50}$$

The described total error we can decompose into elements as follows:

$$\Delta_5\lambda_{4j}(t) = R_5\varphi_{4j}(t) - R_5^{\Gamma}\varphi_{4j}(t) \tag{2.51}$$

also

$$\Delta_{\varphi 4j}\lambda_{4j}(t) = R_5^{\Gamma}\varphi_{4j}(t) - R_5^{\Gamma}\varphi_{4j}^{\Gamma}(t). \tag{2.52}$$

Thus, the metrological analysis of the pathospecific device for the diagnosis of glaucoma developed within the framework of this study has a number of peculiarities connected with the fact that the errors in the measurement process are formed from the known passport values of the corresponding indices and from the errors associated with the specific implementation of the device's hardware and software.

2.4 CONCLUSIONS

It can be concluded that the developed pathospecific measuring device for the diagnosis of glaucoma is the representative of a new class of medical equipment intended to support the adoption of medical solutions, in particular, related to the problems of glaucoma diagnosis. The use of such an installation will significantly reduce the overall complexity of the diagnostic process for this disease, increase the productivity of medical personnel and, in general, improve the quality of diagnosis of such a socially significant incurable chronic disease as glaucoma.

REFERENCES

Balalin, S.V. & Gushchin, A.V. 2003. New possibilities of research of tolerant IOP in patients with primary open-angle glaucoma with the help of automated ophthalmotonosfigmography. *Glaucoma* 2(3): 15–19.

Fokin VP, et al., 2006. Tonosfigmographic method for the determination of tolerant intraocular pressure in patients with glaucoma, *Volgograd Scientific Medical Journal* 2.

Odstrcilik J., Kolar R., Tornow R. P., Jan J., Budai A., Mayer M., Vodakova M., et al., 2014. Thickness related textural properties of retinal nerve fiber layer in color fundus images, *Comput. Med. Imaging Graph.* 38: 508–516.

Shiga Y., Omodaka K., Kunikata H., Ryu M., Yokoyama Y., Tsuda S., Asano T., Maekawa S., Maruyama K., Nakazawa T., 2013. Waveform analysis of ocular blood flow and the early detection of normal tension glaucoma, *Invest. Ophthalmol. Vis. Sci.* 54: 7699–7706

Tsvetkov, E.I. 2010. *Metrology*. Sankt-Petersburg: KopiServis.

Tsvetkov, E.I. 2012. Calculated metrological analysis of measurement results of the amplitude of local signals. *Bulletin of the North-West Branch of the Metrological Academy* 28: 5–10.

CHAPTER 3

Metrological analysis in haematological research

Yu.P. Mukha & D.N. Avdeyuk
Volgograd State Technical University, Volgograd, Russian Federation
Volgograd State Medical University, Volgograd, Russian Federation

V.Yu. Naumov & I.Yu. Koroleva
Volgograd State Technical University, Volgograd, Russian Federation

P. Komada & J. Smołka
Lublin University of Technology, Lublin, Poland

I. Baglan
Al-Farabi Kazakh National University, Almaty, Kazakhstan

ABSTRACT: The quality of medical care depends on the correctness of the diagnosis, which is based on the results of clinical and diagnostic measurements. Measurements, including haematological ones, can be influenced by many factors in the pre-analytical, analytical and post-analysis stages. We used the concept of bio-instrumental information-measuring systems in our work in order to take into account the changes in the measured parameters due to adaptation processes in a human body. In such a system, the primary transformer of the input action is the investigated biological object, which makes it possible to specify the study of the properties of the bio-object. An analysis of the biological component of such a system is possible within the framework of the general theory of functional systems. It is necessary to use the system analysis to construct an adequate model: the identification of the structure and the indication of the participants of the interrelations and the nature of the interaction, which, within the framework of the theory of functional systems, allowed the mathematical formalisation of the physiological model to be carried out. The authors constructed a diagram of information flows of the bio-instrumental information-measuring system in their work using the mathematical apparatus of categories and functors. Adaptation contours were identified, and an algorithm for processing the measurement result was given.

3.1 INTRODUCTION

Metrological support of laboratory research is one of the most important problems, its solution is relevant, as it can provide high accuracy and reproducibility of the results of the analysis, and, consequently, increase the reliability of diagnostic conclusions formed on the basis of these results.

In many applied problems of medicine at the present stage, the study of the human body as a complex multi-level and multiply connected dynamic object is required. The construction of an analytical model in assessing a person's functional state without using a systemic approach is impossible in principle, since multilevel feedbacks have a complex analytical representation. in many works on physiology the organism is viewed as a complex dynamic system interacting with the external environment, therefore it is necessary to study the connection between the elements of the external environment, the biological object and the measuring system within the framework of a single systemic trip. The study and construction of measuring systems within this direction is relevant in the study of complex biological systems, since it establishes an unambiguous connection between the object and the measurement instrument, provides the necessary accuracy and reliability in the analysis and decision making.

In this work, a class of bio-instrumental information and measurement systems (BIIS) is used that is used in analytical measurements. It is characterised by the fact that it can be used in haematological studies, and in these systems the biological object under investigation is the primary transducer of the input effect, which makes it possible to specify the study of the properties of the bio-object.

3.2 METHODOLOGY

At the present time, laboratory diagnostics is an independent direction of medical science, which can claim objectivity if laboratory research is metrologically correct. The provision of clinical and laboratory research (CLI) at the level of clinical diagnostic laboratory (CDL) is to develop and implement measures to prevent the negative impact of factors:

- Pre-analytical stage (violation of the rules of labelling, storage, primary processing);
- Analytical stage (violation of the rules of the analytical procedure, errors in calibration of the method and adjustment of the measuring device, acquisition and use of reagents and other consumables not allowed for use);
- Post-analytical stage (evaluation of the likelihood and reliability of the obtained results of studies, their preliminary interpretation) of steps that can prevent the receipt of a reliable result of laboratory research.

In modern laboratory medicine, a process aimed at improving the comparability of results is called the harmonisation of laboratory data (Menshikov et al. 2002). Development of an efficient and cost-effective management system for CLI is a modern solution to the issue of harmonisation of results and prompt correction of current clinical and laboratory diagnostic problems (QLD).

The analysis of publications (Verkhovodova 2007; Zaikin et al. 2009), devoted to the problem of the quality of medical care, allows us to say that the use of modern functional diagnostic and laboratory studies and computerisation, the creation of automated control systems in laboratory and preventive institutions improve the quality of medical care, and quality assessment medical service to the population is one of the most urgent issues facing the national healthcare system today and its solution in creating automation workplaces of doctors, laboratory technicians and administrators.

We considered the implementation of a unified approach to the study of the measurement procedure, which would reflect all the factors that may affect the result of the diagnostic study, for example, haematological studies, because the general analysis of bioassay from peripheral blood is performed more often than other bio-fluids and is one of the most important laboratory tests, since it often makes it possible to immediately determine the direction of the diagnostic search.

The analytical stage consists of measuring the necessary parameters of the bioassay and their subsequent analysis. The result of the analysis can be influenced by:

- Statistical errors due to the counting of a small number of cells;
- Distribution errors caused by uneven distribution of cells in the chamber;
- Mechanical errors due to technical imperfection of the computation chamber.

Analysis of this study shows that the structure of information transformations of this method contains the main sequence of operations and several auxiliary chains of operations with reagents.

The main sequence consists of two parts: the main one consists of those operations that involve the transformation of the bioassay and the measurement of its optical characteristics, the auxiliary is associated with the preparation and measurement of the optical characteristics of the blank sample, both of which are carried out in parallel with the analysis of a reagent that is determined in the analysis procedure as a standard solution. The notion that all operations at the analytical stage are informational allows us to use the information theory apparatus (Mukha 2003) to determine and calculate certain metrological parameters.

In the general case, the total error of the analytical stage of the CLI consists of errors in the technological operations of sample preparation and instrumental error of the analyser. The errors in the preparation of preparatory operations are divided into two groups: inaccuracies associated with the initial preparation and storage of the bioassay; accuracies due to the nature of the preparatory technological operations at the analytical stage.

Instrumental error consists of errors introduced by different blocks and cascades of conversion of the measured physical quantity to the output signal, as well as from the errors in the normalisation of the analyser scale in terms of the concentration of the liquid component under study (mass, volume, counting) or the kinetic parameter of the process under study (initial velocity, period duration, activity, etc.).

The error at the output of the complex analyser is a linear combination of the error of the individual blocks performing the transformations $R_1, \ldots, R_m$, with the error of each subsequent block independent of the results transformation functions obtained in the previous blocks, but only of their derivatives in the vicinity of the points of nominal values.

The synthesis of bio-instrumental information and measurement system for analytical measurements will help in improving the quality of medical care, for assessing the quality of haematological clinical and diagnostic studies conducted, using successive metrological analysis, the general theory of functional systems, and the mathematical apparatus of categories and functors.

When classifying the errors that occurred during the pre-analytical stage of the study, it was said that the blood test could be affected by the state of the digestive system, the patient's physical or emotional tension, biological rhythms, drug or drug use, alcohol use, physiotherapy, x-ray exposure, etc. Thus, the haemopoietic system of the patient's body is inextricably linked with the process of haematological research and it makes sense to talk about the bio-instrumental information-measuring system (BIMS) (Mukha 2004).

In BIMS, the primary transformer of the multi-parameter input action on the organism is the biological object itself, while it contains the mathematical model of the object under investigation, based on the initial parameters of the biological model.

The construction of a rigorous mathematical model of the biological system under investigation is most often difficult or even impossible, due to the lack of a priori information about the actual mechanisms of the functioning of the object of study, or because of the complexity of the representation of the object itself and information about it.

The analysis of the biological component of such a system is possible within the framework of the general theory of functional systems (Sudakov 2011), which allows to explore different manifestations of a living organism from new positions, from its homeostatic functions to active purposeful activity in the external environment. The theory is based on several postulates:

- The result of the activity is the leading system-forming factor;
- The general principle of the organisation of functional systems;
- Self-regulation;
- Functional systems of different levels are isomorphic;
- Individual organs and tissues are selectively mobilised into functional systems of different levels;
- Functional systems are hierarchically linked;
- Functional systems are multi-parametrically regulated by final results.

In analysing the physiological model of the haematopoietic system of the organism, a large number of deep inverse relationships are revealed within the framework of the bio-cybernetic approach of the theory of functional systems of Anokhin-Sudakov (Sudakov 2011). The analytical representation of the model with such a quantity of only explicit feedbacks is impossible in principle, otherwise the simplifications that will inevitably arise will lead to an inadequate mathematical representation. Therefore, in order to construct an adequate model, it is necessary to use the system analysis: the identification of the structure and the indication of the participants of the interrelations and the nature of the interaction, which, within the framework of the theory of functional systems, will allow the mathematical formalisation of the physiological model. The revealed structure in the framework of a certain mathematical formalisation apparatus, in our case, the theory of categories and functors, can be written down analytically, if necessary, however, the main purpose of the formalisation apparatus used is the correct representation of the structure and the systematisation of the acquired knowledge, which ensures the simplicity and convenience of understanding by researchers and users.

The definition of the structure of information flows is a fundamental moment in the process of designing an information and measuring system (IMS), as it defines the composition of functional blocks and the direction of functional connections between them (Mukha 2003). As in the design of any IMS using structural methods, the design of the structure of information flows of the system for diagnosing the functional state of the haematopoietic system of the body consists of the following stages:

- Setting the structure of information flows of the IMS and the object of observation (OO);
- Definition of the structure of interacting objects;
- Identification of the structure of links;
- Determination of the nature of the information composition of the elements of the structure.

In turn, the chosen structure of information flows allows to determine the errors in the presentation of information by each IMS unit, the block-structural relationship, the degree of adequacy of the entire measuring system. We formalised below the model of the haematopoietic system of the organism, within the framework of the set-theoretic representation and the categorical-functorial approach, we will indicate the properties of the objects participating in the haematopoiesis process and describe the scope of their determination. The end result of the functioning of the circulatory system of a person, regulating its condition, is a set of uniform blood elements (SUEB), adequate to external and internal conditions of the organism's existence. In its morphological structure, the haematopoietic system is a complex of selectively involved components, in which interaction and mutual relations, despite their opposite nature, take the form of interaction in obtaining a focused beneficial result – SUEB, which ensures the preservation of the SUEB within the limits of the norm. This complex includes: (1) central organs, (2) peripheral formations, (3) local and (4) central regulators, these components differ in structure, tissue identity and chemical specificity.

The optimal level of SUEB is programmed in the central nervous system by an action acceptor based on afferent synthesis. The main internal contradiction in the development of the regulation of the aggregate state of the blood lies in the fact that the very magnitude of the deviation of the aggregate state of the blood from the necessary optimal level triggers regulating devices that ensure a reduction in this deviation.

The actual material accumulated to date by haematology indicates that the circulatory system is mosaic, i.e., SUEB in different parts of the blood flow and organs is not the same. It must be emphasised that this is a natural, normal state of the circulatory system. Different parts of it in different ways and at different levels determine the necessary SUEB in the circulating blood.

As already we mentioned above, SUEB is adequate to internal and external influences. The external influence acting on the body is processed by the central control loop, which in turn carries out regulatory control on the internal environment of the organism. External action, in general, has an enumerable set of diverse manifestations and is a form of stress tests and/or a set of conditions surrounding the object of the environment (Mucha 2004; Wajman et al. 2013). Thus, by carrying out the same combinations of external influences on different organisms or on the same organism, but in different manifestations of the functional state, we have the opportunity to investigate the change in the body's SUEB, as a response to external influences.

We denote the entire variety of manifestations of external influences as the space of external influences as:

$$Q = \left\{ Q^{\langle k_1 \rangle} \right\} \tag{3.1}$$

where $k_1 = 1, 2, \ldots, N$ – the serial number of a certain set of external actions established and regulated by the researcher, N is the total number of sets of external influences that organise the space Q.

The haemopoietic system of the organism is represented by four levels, on which regulatory control is carried out. Each level is a set of states of the control action, so we will represent the control level space in a general way:

$$X = \left\{ X^{\langle K_2 \rangle} \right\} \tag{3.2}$$

where $k_2 = 1, 2, \ldots, M$ – uniquely characterises the set of states of a particular control level, M – the number of levels of management of the haemopoietic system.

The internal environment of the body is all internal organs that exert both direct and indirect control over a multitude of shaped elements of the body's blood. In this case, the objects of the internal environment are in direct subordination of the control objects. Let's formally represent the space of the internal environment without indicating the relationships and their nature:

$$I = \{I^{\langle k_3 \rangle}\} \tag{3.3}$$

where $k_3 = 1, 2, \ldots, L$, characterises a specific set of objects of the internal environment, L is the number of analysed objects of the internal environment of the organism.

The result of the control of the circulatory system by the organs of haemopoiesis and the internal environment of the body is unambiguously manifested in the SUEB, that is, the result of management, characterising the external impact, can be represented by a discrete mapping from a set of uniform blood elements:

$$F = \{F^{\langle k_4 \rangle}\} \tag{3.4}$$

where $k_4 = 1, 2, \ldots, P$, a specific implementation of the control process on a set of blood elements, and P is their total number.

All objects and mappings exist in a strictly defined space of laws. The space of laws consists of a set of rules and laws of normal physiology that uniquely determine the functioning and interaction of objects. That is, you can represent in the form:

$$V = \{V^{\langle k_5 \rangle}\} \tag{3.5}$$

where $k_5 = 1, 2, \ldots, O$ – characterises a specific provision of the code of laws, O – total number of analysed provisions.

Under the influence of internal and external factors on the haematopoietic system, according to the laws of normal physiology, a set of blood elements is established in the human body, the condition of which can be estimated as a result of a blood test.

The further measuring procedure depends on the method of analysis.

There are two main classes of instruments for measuring blood parameters (Korenevsky et al. 2009). The first shows the change in electrical resistance of the solution at the moment of passage of the shaped element of blood through the aperture. The second, when changing, records the deviations of the light rays caused by the passage through them of the formed elements of the blood. A very common first-class device is the Coatler blood analyser. In this instrument, the analysed blood sample is examined together with an anticoagulant that interferes with the process of normal blood clotting and prevents the clumping of blood cells counted in the compartments of the count.

Let us consider the operational transformations R of the measured quantities, starting with the blood sample entering the haematoanalyser $\gamma_j(t)$ and ending with the registration of indications on the PC.

The blood sample is divided into two parts, then one of them enters the second mixing chamber and the lysis CML_2 without changes (R_T – identical transmission of the information flow), and the second to the dilution chamber DC_1, where it is diluted R_{P1} in relation to 1:224 a solution that is close in its optical characteristics to plasma. This solution is divided into two parts. One enters the first mixing chamber and the CML_1 lysis, and the second enters the second dilution chamber DC_2, in which the solution is further diluted R_{P2} in relation to 1:250.

The lysis agent destroys the membrane of erythrocytes in CML_2, releasing the solution contained in the haemoglobin. In addition, in CML_1 with Drabkin's solution, haemoglobin is converted into cyan-haemoglobin R_L in accordance with the requirements of the analysis methodology.

Then the solution is sent to the OCLKC, made in the form of a cuvette and an aperture tube, through the calibration hole of which, matched to the size of the shaped elements, a solution is drawn through the vacuum pump.

Further analysis is associated with the application of an electric current from both sides of the wall separating the liquid, then when the blood cells are filtered through the aperture tube, the electrical stress of the circuit will vary, and accordingly the electric current will change. Pulse value R_I will characterise the particle size, and the number of pulses R_K – the number of particles passing through the hole with electrical conductivity, other than the electrical conductivity of the solution.

In order to increase the reliability of the measurement, the system uses in parallel three counting devices R_C^i ($i = 1,..,6$), having one common electrode in the OCLKC cuvette and three independent electrodes in the aperture tubes. The output signal from each of the gratings is fed to the pre-amplifier R_U, the amplified voltage pulses are passed through an analog discriminator whose threshold voltages are set during calibration.

During the suction through the fluid aperture, besides the useful pulses, there are background pulses created by particles of foreign inclusions. The size of the background pulses is much smaller in magnitude than the information pulses, so using amplitude discriminators can be filtered out R_{FR} unnecessary information impulses.

The received signal is averaged R_{US} using the methods of statistical analysis, is formed by the final scheme R_{FORM} and enters the interface block IB R_{IB}, where it is converted into a digital code R_{ADC}, which is transmitted R_S to PC for processing R_{DP} and mapping R_R.

Counting of erythrocytes is similar, with the difference that the concentration of red blood cells is higher, so they must be further diluted in DC_2. The camera CML_2 is working for differential counting of leukocytes. To illustrate the way to formalise the hardware of BIMS, the transformations described above are sufficient.

Thus, the measuring procedure has the form:

$$\lambda_j^* = R_R R_{DP} R_S R_{ADC} R_{IB} R_{FORM} R_{US} R_{FR} R_{KK} R_U R_C^i R_K R_I R_L R_{P2} R_{P1} \gamma_j(t) \tag{3.6}$$

where $\gamma_j(t)$– analysed sample, j – analysis number, R_{P1} – dilution operator, R_{P2} – additional dilution operator, R_L – operator of solution and treatment with Drabkin's solution, R_I – pulse recording operator, R_K – pulse counting operator, R_C^i – counting operation, where i = 1, . . . , 6 is the number of the counting chamber, R_{KK} – calibration operator, R_{FR} – filtering operator, R_{US} – averaging operator, R_{FORM} – output statement operator, R_{IB} – interface processing operator, R_{ADC} – analog-to-digital conversion operator, R_S – commutation operator, R_{DP} – end-processing operator, R_R – mapping operator.

As a result of the first stage of the formalisation of BIMS, based on the physiological model, it is possible to represent the structure of information flows (Figure 3.1).

In the appendix to the task for the development of the BIMS of research, there are a lot of blood elements, we will examine in more detail the component composition of the above described sets, characterise the objects and give their domains of definition.

As a result of external influences: the environment, psycho-emotional situation, physical activity, etc. the living organism passes through some stressful conditions and, accordingly, adapts to the changed conditions. This process functions according to certain laws, is continuous and does not have the property of periodicity (Sudakov 2011).

Despite the fact that the blood for analysis is usually taken in the morning, nevertheless many patients are not aware of the influence of adaptation processes on the blood system. As a result, the obtained data may be unreliable, due to the fact that the human body is in a state of stress. Such situations can be monitored using questionnaires, which will indicate the main factors affecting the blood system, and this introduction will play a dual role, since in addition to its main function – determining the reliability of the results obtained, will also perform an educational function, since patients, answering questions, will learn about the factors that affect haematopoiesis.

We will formalise the management and adaptation process, construct a structure and indicate all the relationships.

According to the definition of a topological space (Goldblatt 1983; Johnston 1986), a topology must be defined on the functioning space of the system. That is, there must be some set $\Im$ subsets of S that have the following properties (called axioms of topological structures):

- Every union of sets in $\Im$ is a set from $\Im$;
- The intersection of every finite family of sets from $\Im$ is a set from $\Im$.

Under the elements of the state space of the control process, we mean the set of sets of responses of the organism that characterise the effectiveness of the control process.

According to works (Sudakov 2011), the space X, is represented by the following subsets $X^k = \{X_1^k, X_2^k, X_3^k, X_4^k\}$: $X_1^k = \{X_1^j\}$ – a set of states of the genomic-nuclear control level, where $j = 1, 2 \ldots N_{X1}$ – the number of states of transcription factors – DNA-binding proteins of different

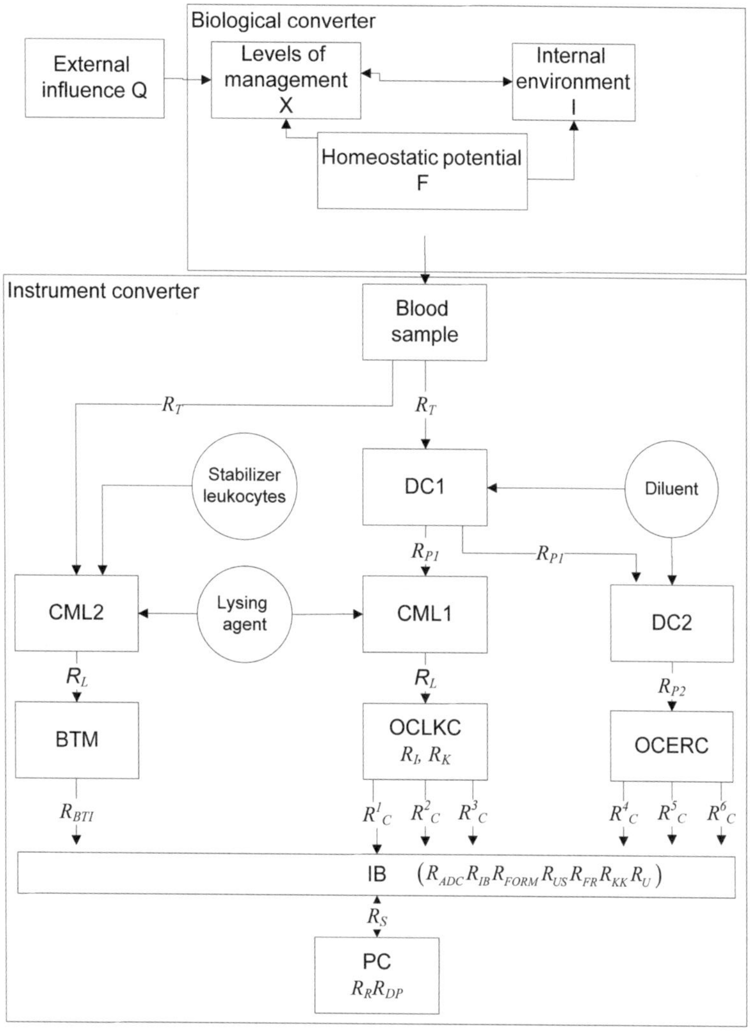

Figure 3.1. Structure of BIMS.

families, functioning from early stages of development and regulating the expression of haematopoietic cell genes; $X_2^k = \{X_2^j\}$ – a number of states of the intracellular control level, where $j = 1, 2 \ldots N_{X2}$ – the number of states that are reduced to the production of haematopoietic cells in the cytoplasm of special trigger proteins that affect the genome of these cells; $X_3^k = \{X_3^j\}$ – multiple states of the intercellular control level, where $j = 1, 2 \ldots N_{X3}$ – the number of actions of the caylions, haemopoietins, interleukins produced by differentiated blood or stroma cells and affecting the differentiation of the stem haematopoietic cell; $X_4^k = \{X_4^1, X_4^2, X_4^3, X_4^4\}$ – a lot of states of the organismic level of management, consisting in the regulation of haematopoiesis by the integrating systems of the organism, where $X_4^1 = \{X_4^{1_j}\}$ – a set of mechanisms of nervous regulation, $X_4^2 = \{X_4^{2_j}\}$ – set of conditions of the endocrine system, $X_4^3 = \{X_4^{3_j}\}$ – many mechanisms of immune regulation, $X_4^4 = \{X_4^{4_j}\}$ – set of states of control mechanisms of the circulatory system.

The sets considered form a subset $\Im$ topological space X They satisfy the axioms of topology, since they characterise a single space representing the control system of a biological object.

Consider the topology of the space of external influences represented by subsets $Q^k = \{Q_1^k, Q_2^k, .., Q_m^k\}$, where m – number of included in the study sets of external influences on the organism under study. Under the elements of set Q_j^k we will understand the diversity of external influences – psycho-emotional state, physical loads, geomagnetic state, weather manifestations at the time of the study, etc. The formalisable space Q is closed, and the sets Q_j^k enumerable. The formation of space and its elements is carried out directly by the researcher himself, which in turn allows for more specific diagnostics. In this case, the sets that form the space are defined and described, and the order of their occurrence and the conditions of interaction are indicated.

In this chapter, the space consists of seven closed sets, the choice of which is due to the classification of errors in the haematological analysis (Mukha 2007). The elemental composition of the sets and their number can be changed depending on the method of blood analysis, provided that the recording is correct and the nature of the interactions is indicated.

Let us list the analysed objects of the space of external influences on the organism: $Q_1^k = \{q_1^j\}$ – represents the set of temperatures at which registration takes place. Accordingly, within the framework of the study, the choice of temperature is chosen in the interval most comfortable for the organism $-25°\text{C}$, i.e. $q_1^1 = 20°\text{C}, q_1^2 = 21°\text{C}, \ldots, q_1^8 = 27°\text{C}$. $Q_2^k = \{q_2^j\}$. – multiple levels of geomagnetic situation at the time of recording the signal, respectively: $q_2^1 =$ "*below the norm*", $q_2^2 =$ "*the norm*", $q_2^3 =$ "*above the norm*". $Q_3^k = \{q_3^j\}$ – set of moments of the time of the day, represents intervals close to the moment of balance of the parasympathetic and sympathetic parts of the higher nervous system, as a rule this value is in the interval from nine to eleven hours, that is, $q_3^1 = 8\,h, q_3^2 = 8\,1/2\,h, q_3^3 = 9\,h, \ldots, q_3^9 = 12\,h$. $Q_4^k = \{q_4^j\}$ – a lot of psycho-emotional states of the body, where $j = 1, 2 \ldots N$ – ordinal number of the regulated state. $Q_5^k = \{q_5^j\}$ – Many loads on the body, where $j = 1, 2 \ldots N$ – ordinal number of the load regulated by the researcher. Load can have both physical and mental character. $Q_6^k = \{q_6^j\}$ – a set characterising the number of full years of the organism, respectively, the elements of the set characterise the age group of the study, $Q_7^k = \{q_7^j\}$ – a set characterising the constitution of the body, a physiological parameter that is a function of weight and anthropometric indicators.

We formalise the structural interrelation between the space of external influences and the space of control levels: each element of external influence $Q^k \in Q$ corresponds to a single state of regulatory management $X^k \in X$. Mutual uniqueness is determined by the physiology of the organism, since under arbitrarily close experimental conditions Q^k and Q^{k+1} we will not get the same state of regulatory management X^k, due to changes in the body, as well as in external influences. That is, there is a one-to-one mapping $\mathbf{R}: Q \to X$, aligning $Q^k \in Q$ a single object $X^k \in X$. The absence of restrictions on continuity allows us to assert that the mapping $\mathbf{R}: Q \to X$ – homomorphically.

$$\mathbf{R}: Q \to X \tag{3.7}$$

In this mathematical model, an informative parameter that uniquely characterises the operation of all levels of management is the set of blood elements, represented by the set $F = \{F^{\langle k \rangle}\}$.

The control process is analysed on a specific area of the circulatory system by an invasive or non-invasive method, therefore, the element of the set F^k is the specific state of a plurality of blood cells. Thus, there is a unique mapping of the space X on a multitude of realisations of the control process in the haematopoietic system $F = \{F^k\}: \mathbf{Y}: X \to F$, which unambiguously corresponds to a particular state of the management level $X^k \in X$ object $F^k \in F$. The absence of restrictions on the continuity of the mapping allows us to speak of a homomorphic map:

$$\mathbf{Y}: X \to F \tag{3.8}$$

The implementation of regulatory management of the haematopoietic system of the body can be investigated and classified. The condition of a plurality of blood cells, obtained from the body, $F^k \in F$ is displayed in qualitative and quantitative indicators by means of a family of mathematical transformations (3.6) within the framework of the categorical-functorial representation of the set of uniform elements of blood. In the future, these indicators are modified by a family of classification transformations into a concrete conclusion. As a result of successive mappings of mathematical and classification transformations to the object $F^k \in F$ one-to-one correspondence of an object $O^k \in O$ – a concrete conclusion, that is:

$$O^k = CL\left(MT\left(F^k\right)\right) \tag{3.9}$$

The change in the functional state of the system is characterised by a combination of a large number of processes taking place in this system. As a result of external influence, the organism experiences stress and adapts in a certain way to the changed conditions. In full accordance with the physiological model presented in the first chapter, the adaptation process is under the complete control of the controls of the haemopoiesis. The process of control is performed by a neuro-humoral action, both on the internal environment of the organism, and on the haematopoietic system itself, while it is a process with deep feedback.

The internal environment of the organism in the physiological model under consideration with respect to the effect on the set of blood elements is formalised as follows: we represent the space of the internal environment of the organism by subsets – $I^k = \{I_1^k, I_2^k, I_3^k, I_4^k, I_5^k, I_6^k, I_7^k, I_8^k\}$. The internal environment of the body is determined by glands of internal and external secretion, internal organs that are in direct subordination to the parasympathetic and sympathetic parts of the autonomic nervous system, and also to the hypothalamic-pituitary level of the central contour of control. Let us imagine a multitude of states of endocrine glands, innervated by the sympathetic department of the higher nervous system: $I_1^k = \{I_1^j\}$, where $j = 1, 2 \ldots N$ – uniquely identifies a specific gland that has a direct control effect on a multitude of shaped blood elements. A number of states of endocrine glands, innervated by the sympathetic department of the higher nervous system: $I_2^k = \{I_2^j\}$, where $j = 1, 2 \ldots N$ – uniquely determines a specific gland, which has an indirect control effect on a multitude of shaped elements of the blood. A number of states of endocrine glands, innervated by the parasympathetic department of the higher nervous system: $I_3^k = \{I_3^j\}$, where $j = 1, 2 \ldots N$ – uniquely identifies a specific gland that has a direct control effect on a multitude of shaped blood elements. Many states of endocrine glands, innervated by the parasympathetic department of the higher nervous system: $I_4^k = \{I_4^j\}$, where $j = 1, 2 \ldots N$ – uniquely determines a specific gland, which has an indirect control effect on a multitude of shaped elements of the blood. A variety of conditions of internal organs innervated by the sympathetic department of the higher nervous system: $I_5^k = \{I_5^j\}$, where $j = 1, 2 \ldots N$ – uniquely determines the state of a particular body that has an indirect control effect on a multitude of blood cells. Multiple states of internal organs innervated by the parasympathetic department of the higher nervous system: $I_6^k = \{I_6^j\}$, where $j = 1, 2 \ldots N$ – uniquely determines the state of a particular body that has an indirect control effect on a multitude of blood cells. Many states of receptor responses (baroreceptors, chemoreceptors, etc.): $I_7^k = \{I_7^j\}$, where $j = 1, 2 \ldots N$ – uniquely determines the state of a particular group of receptors. The complete complex response of the body to external influences is built on the basis of primary metabolic changes in tissues, in addition, the source of energy occurring in the body processes are the processes of metabolism. Therefore, it is necessary to define in the space of the internal environment of the body a lot of metabolic states of the organism as a whole: $I_8^k = \{I_8^j\}$, where $j = 1, 2 \ldots N$ – uniquely determines the metabolic state.

The sets $I^k \in I$ form a subset $\Im$ topological space I and satisfy the axioms of topology, since they characterise a single space of the internal environment of the organism.

Direct interaction of the organism's level of control and the internal environment of the body is due to the innervation of the internal organs and glands by the autonomic nervous system. In addition, the direct control of the hypothalamic-pituitary level is realised, which has a dual nature of regulation: nervous and humoral. That is, a homomorphic mapping takes place:

$$P : X \to I \tag{3.10}$$

Feedback of the internal environment and haematopoiesis control levels is ensured by the receptors' response (changes in blood pressure-baroreceptors, chemical composition of blood-chemoreceptors, etc.) to the autonomic nervous system on the one hand, and direct analysis of the hypothalamic-pituitary metabolic rate, on the other. That is, a homomorphic mapping is defined:

$$W : I \to X \tag{3.11}$$

The internal environment of the body carries out a modulating effect on SUEB release of hormones into the blood, thereby increasing or decreasing it. Feedback is provided by changing the metabolic state under the changed conditions of SUEB. That is, the following homomorphic maps are realised: (3.11) is a direct map and (3.12) is the inverse.

$$P : I \to F \quad (3.12)$$

$$L : F \to I \quad (3.13)$$

Let us represent the spaces and their interactions discussed above by the diagram of the regulatory control process (3.14):

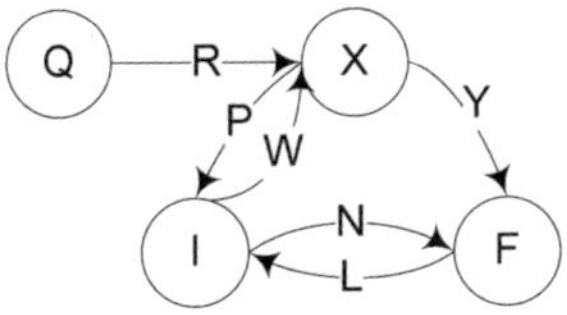

(3.14)

We examined the general nature of the interactions of the process of neuro-humoral regulation when the organism adapts to the changing environmental conditions without taking into account the quantitative contribution of each of the subsystems. Since each individual organism is individual, it is impossible in principle to construct a rigorous mathematical model to describe this process, since it reduces to solving a set of parametric differential equations with a set of unknowns. At the same time, the processes taking place in the body pass through certain scenarios common to all and fully represented by the laws of normal physiology.

Next, consider the space of laws of normal physiology V, we indicate the nature of the interaction of each of the participants in the process and construct a general structure of information flows.

A living organism is a multiply connected multilevel complex system, functioning according to its strictly defined laws of physiology. Therefore, in the further description, it is necessary to formalise and form a structural description of these laws and rules that establish the participants, the nature and sequence of the relationships.

We consider the topological space (3.2) and describe the interactions between objects X^k, F^k and I^k. The set X_1^k – determines a set of states of the genomic-nuclear level of management of the haemopoietic system that implements a variety of blood elements F, that is, a homomorphic mapping $\chi_1^1 : X_1 \to F$. In this χ_1^1 and in subsequent morphisms the notation is accepted: the lower index defines the object from which the mapping occurs, the upper index is the serial number of this mapping. Accordingly, this entry means that from the object X_1 the first order is displayed (3.15).

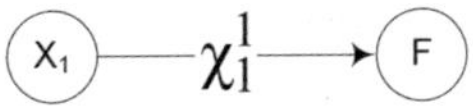

$$X_1 \xrightarrow{\chi_1^1} F \quad (3.15)$$

At the intracellular level X_2^k in the cytoplasm of haematopoietic cells, a number of special trigger proteins are produced that affect the genome of these cells $\chi_2^1 : X_2 \to X_1$ (3.16).

$$\begin{array}{c} X_1 \xrightarrow{\chi_1^1} F \\ \uparrow \chi_2^1 \\ X_2 \end{array} \quad (3.16)$$

The intercellular level includes the action of the ceylons, haemopoietins, and interleukins produced by differentiated blood or stroma cells and affecting the differentiation of the haematopoietic stem cell. Elements of haemopoiesis-inducing microenvironment control the processes of haematopoiesis both

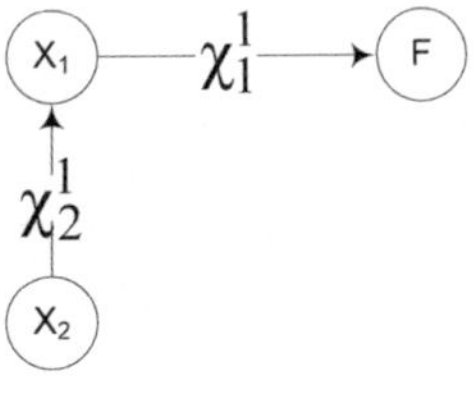

through the produced cytokines $\chi_3^1 : X_3 \rightarrow X_1$, and due to direct contacts with haematopoietic cells $\chi_3^2 : X_3 \rightarrow F$ (3.17).

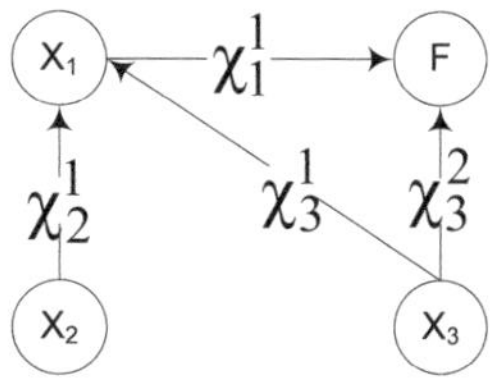

(3.17)

The anterior part of the hypothalamus participates in the regulation of the constancy of the composition of blood lymphocytes, whereas the posterior part of the hypothalamus stimulates the development of neutrophilic leukocytosis to lymphopenia. The nuclear structures of the posterior hypothalamic region exert a tonic effect on erythropoiesis, whereas the anterior hypothalamus is the center of inhibitory effects on the regeneration of the erythron. However, under normal physiological conditions, the activity of all parts of the hypothalamus proceeds consistently as a single functional whole. Indeed, although the differential, unequal influence of individual nuclear structures is experimentally revealed, the entire multifaceted activity of the hypothalamus acts integrally and is integrated with the activity of the cortex of the cerebral hemispheres and other parts of the central nervous system. Despite all these facts, to connect certain functions of the blood system with a certain nuclear structure, as well as outline the ways of neuro-humoral influences of the hypothalamus on the blood system is not yet possible.

It is believed that the influence of the hypothalamus on the executive mechanisms of the blood system is realised through the vegetative department of the nervous system and through hormonal and specific humoral factors. We define structurally the homomorphic mapping of the whole regulatory control of the object by the haematopoietic system: $\chi_4^1 : X_4 \rightarrow F$ (3.18).

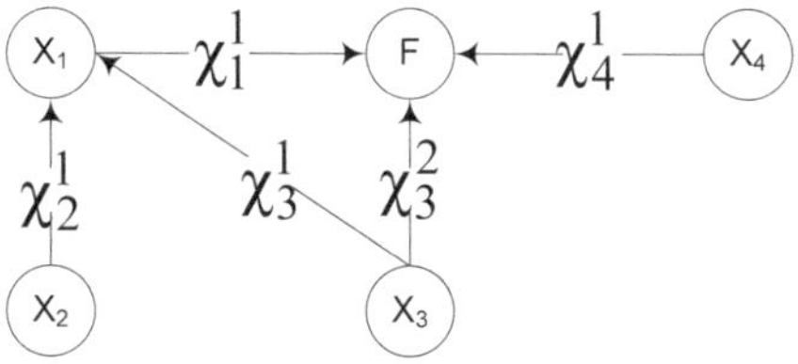

(3.18)

Define for the study of the gland of internal secretion, having both parasympathetic and sympathetic innervation, in the form $I_1 \cap I_3$. That is, there is a direct homomorphic map of the object X_4^1 into the object $I_1 \cap I_3 : \chi_4^2 : X_4^1 \rightarrow I_1 \cap I_3$. Similarly, we represent homomorphic mappings on the glands of external secretion and internal organs: $\chi_4^3 : X_4^1 \rightarrow I_2 \cap I_4$ and correspondingly, $\chi_4^4 : X_4^1 \rightarrow I_5 \cap I_6$ (3.19).

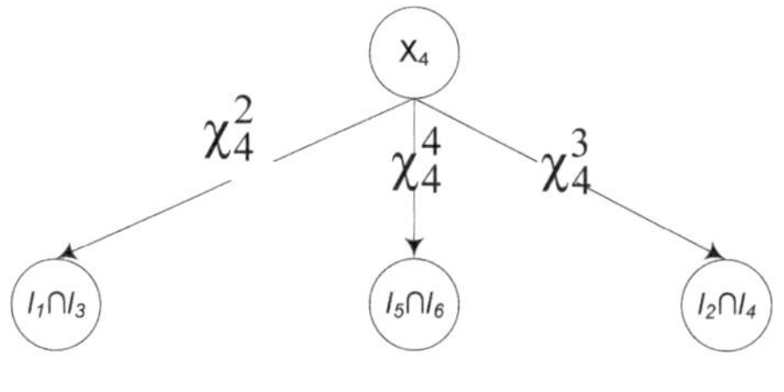

(3.19)

The number of blood elements is perceived by the interceptors of the bone marrow, spleen, and lymph nodes, which was shown by numerous experiments with perfusion of these organs with solutions containing various number of shaped elements.

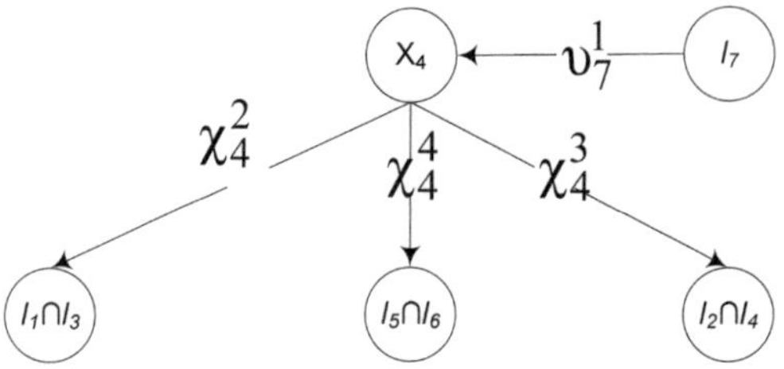

(3.20)

Deviation of the number of elements from the level providing normal metabolism through receptor apparatuses includes a set of processes that ensure the return of the given index to the optimal level by the principle of self-regulation, thus, a constant homomorphic mapping of the set of receptor states to the object X_4^1: $\upsilon_7^1 : I_7 \rightarrow X_4^1$ (3.20).

The vegetative level carries out a direct continuous reciprocal exchange of information with the hypothalamic-pituitary level, since the latter represents the level of integration of the vegetative and endocrine systems. That is, there are two continuous homomorphic mappings between objects: χ_4^5 : $X_4^1 \rightarrow X_4^2$ and $\chi_4^6 : X_4^2 \rightarrow X_4^1$.

The most important factor that stimulates the formation of erythrocytes by the bone marrow are erythropoietins –hormones of a helicoproteinic nature containing sialic acid. Erythropoietins regulate the intensity of proliferation and the direction of differentiation of stem progenitor cells, affect the maturation of erythrocytes (accelerate the synthesis of haemoglobin, facilitate the release of reticulocytes from the bone marrow). The main place of production of erythropoietins is the juxtaglomerular apparatus of the kidney, an inactive form of the substance is formed in it, which is activated by interaction with blood proteins. Hence, there is a homomorphic mapping objects $I_1 \cap I_3$ in the object $X_3 : \upsilon_1^1 : I_1 \cap I_3 \rightarrow X_3$ (3.21).

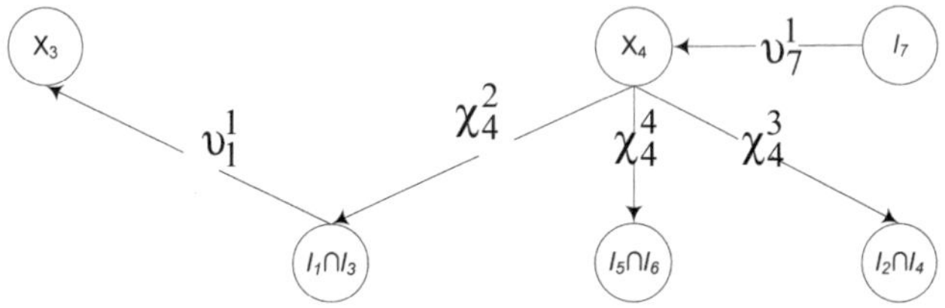

(3.21)

The hypothalamic-pituitary regulation level due to its dual nature (neuro-humoral regulation) also has a direct and reverse homomorphic mapping to the internal environment of the organism, that is: $\chi_4^4 : X_4^1 \rightarrow I_5 \cap I_6$ and $\chi_4^5 : X_4^1 \rightarrow X_3$ – direct and $\upsilon_8^1 : I_8 \rightarrow X_3$ and $\upsilon_8^2 : I_8 \rightarrow X_4^1$ – reverse (3.22).

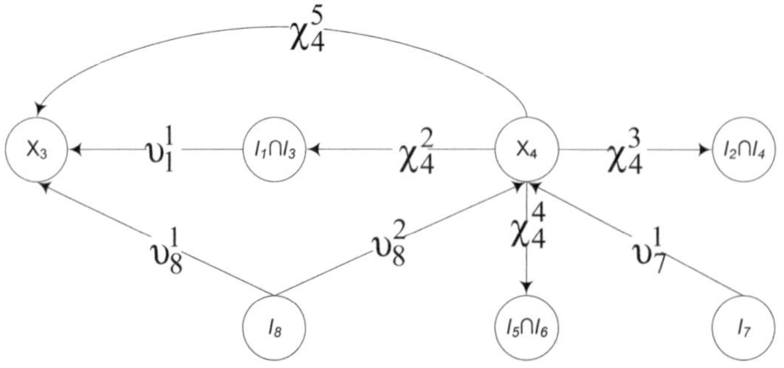

(3.22)

The internal environment of the body has a modulating effect on the haematopoietic system by changing the metabolic state of the whole organism. This process is associated with the successive changes in functioning regimes in the internal organs and glands of internal and external secretion. With variations in external influences, for example physical exertion, the operating modes of the body systems (endocrine, excretory, etc.) and internal organs (kidneys, liver, etc.) change. Then, by feedback, the operation mode of all systems and subsystems of the whole organism is controlled for transition to the most efficient functional state. Mathematically, these processes can be expressed by direct and inverse homomorphic mappings: $\upsilon_8^6 = \upsilon_1^1 \circ \upsilon_8^1$ and $\varphi_1^1 : F \to I_5 \cap I_6$ respectively.

According to the laws of normal physiology, changing the regimes of glands functioning both internal and external secretion has a direct effect on internal organs. These interactions between the components of the internal environment of the body are represented by the following homomorphic mappings $\upsilon_1^2 : I_1 \cap I_3 \to I_5 \cap I_6$ and $\upsilon_2^1 : I_2 \cap I_4 \to I_5 \cap I_6$. All internal organs have receptor innervation, which provides feedback to the nervous system. In the model under consideration, an object is distinguished, representing the entire variety of receptor responses, which can be expressed by the following homomorphic mapping between objects: $\upsilon_5^2 : I_5 \cap I_6 \to I_7$ (3.23).

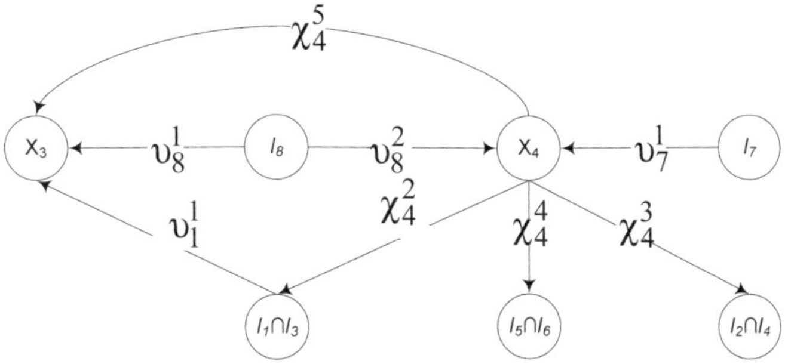

(3.23)

Each external effect on the body causes a chain of regulatory processes aimed at effective interaction at the most basic, cellular level. The source of energy of these processes and vital activity in general are metabolic reactions. The organism, as a highly complex self-organising dynamic system, operates according to the principle of the least energy consumption. Consequently, the whole process of adaptation can be defined as the achievement of optimal metabolism in general. Rhythmic activity of the heart reflects not only the transfer of the substance necessary for the functioning of various cells, but also the transmission of information, since the pulse wave is a universal synchroniser of the processes of energy and substance exchange in internal organs and in cells that do not have direct innervation of the central nervous system. In this case, the metabolism of the body as a whole depends on the work and affects the work of all types of glands and internal organs. This interaction can be represented in the form of the following direct homomorphic mappings: $\upsilon_5^1 : I_5 \cap I_6 \to I_8$ – impact of internal organs, $\upsilon_1^2 : I_1 \cap I_3 \to I_8$ – influence of endocrine glands and $\upsilon_2^2 : I_2 \cap I_4 \to I_8$ – the effect of endocrine glands on the metabolic state of the body. The inverse homomorphic maps have the form: $\upsilon_8^3 : I_8 \to I_1 \cap I_3$ – the influence of the metabolic state on the functioning of the glands of external secretion, $\upsilon_8^4 : I_8 \to I_2 \cap I_4$ – impact on the functioning of endocrine glands, $\upsilon_8^5 : I_8 \to I_5 \cap I_6$ – influence on the work of internal organs. Due to the peculiarities of hypothalamic-pituitary functioning, there is a direct transmission of information: $\upsilon_8^2 : I_8 \to X_4^1$ – the inverse homomorphic mapping (3.24).

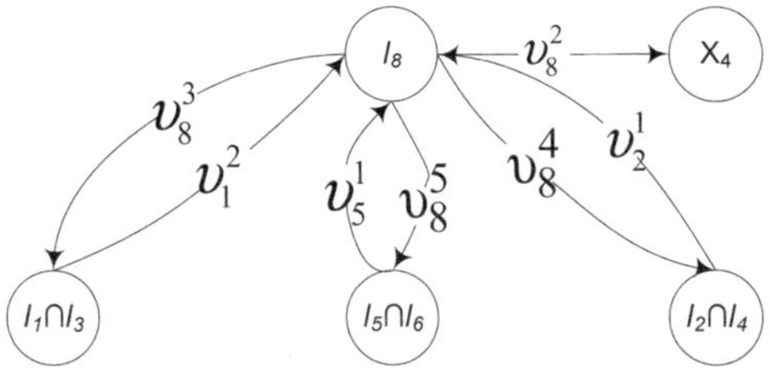

(3.24)

External effects on the body affect different levels of regulation of haematopoiesis and a specific type of external influence can, for example, fully activate the vegetative and only partially hypothalamic-pituitary. Activation and its degree depend on the amount of external influence and individual characteristics of the organism, which in turn is of particular interest to the researcher.

Thus, the formal impact can be represented by the following homomorphic mappings: $\tau_1^1 : Q \to X_2$ – influence, leading to changes in the intercellular level of management; $\tau_1^2 : Q \to X_3$ – influence, leading to changes in the intracellular level of management; $\tau_1^3 : Q \to X_4^1$ – effect on the nervous system, $\tau_1^4 : Q \to X_4^2$ – impact on the endocrine system $\tau_1^5 : Q \to X_4^3$ – influence on mechanisms of immune regulation, influence on mechanisms of regulation of circulatory system (3.25).

As a result of a more detailed description of the functioning of the model within the framework of the formalised space of laws, we present an extended diagram of the information flows of the haematopoietic regulation process made up of the morphisms (3.18), (3.22), (3.23), (3.24) considered above.

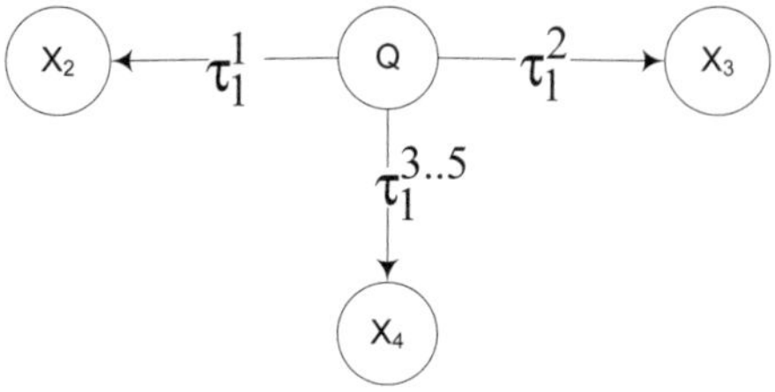

(3.25)

The following is an extended diagram of the haematopoiesis regulation process (3.26), the topological structure of each participant is described, the interrelations are both instantaneous and permanent, in order to trace the dynamics of information flows, further formalisation will be carried out within the framework of the theory of categories and functors. On this structure we indicate and describe the categories, morphisms, represent the rules of transitions within each category and between categories.

Each morphism represented on the diagram is a complex process of dynamic interaction of various functional systems of the organism and, if necessary, can be presented in more detail.

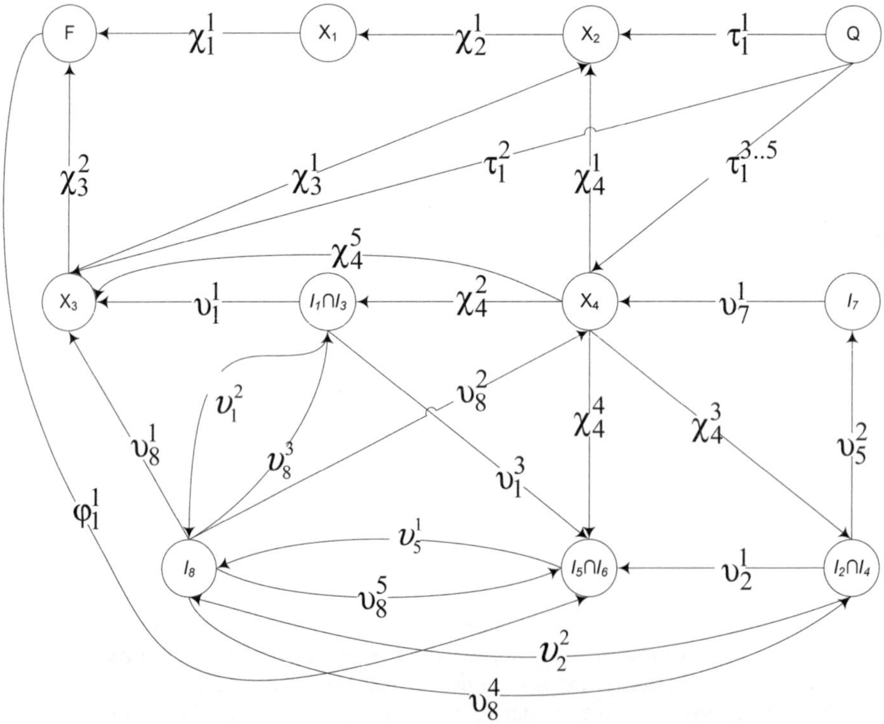

(3.26)

3.3 RESULTS

The structure of information flows (3.26) we obtained is a description of the state of the measurement object at an arbitrarily given time. Its functionality is determined by the rules of its transitions from one state to another, given by functorial and category maps. Thus, the synthesised structure makes the analysis of the regulation of the haematopoiesis process more complete and visual, and the possibility of decomposition allows the researcher to carry out more detailed research, visually displays the processes of adaptation of the organism under external influences and naturally lends itself to the construction of automated systems.

The one-to-one correspondence of categories and functors to real objects and their relations determines the reliability of the model being compared.

Define the categorical diagram of the information flows of the haematopoietic system control process (Mukha 2004) as an "imposed" structure of the information-measuring system of the diagnostic profile. That is, we will represent the system parameter, the number of blood elements, within the framework of a formalised structure. This will ensure, on the one hand, an unambiguous study of the properties specified by the model from the original signal, and, on the other hand, the detailed model of the object and the transition to the design of an automated measuring system.

Let us magine an external effect, determined by a combination of specific elements $Q^k = \{Q_1^k, Q_2^k, .., Q_m^k\} \in Q$ space of external influences on the organism, that is, forming elements $Q_j^k = \{q_j^l\}$, we set the conditions for the study. At the same time, in accordance with normal physiology, the adaptive contour is activated, the diagram (3.1). Synthesis of the categorical model of information flows BIMS was described in detail earlier (Mukha 2004). The following indications have been used: Q – the space of external influences, X – the space of control levels, I – the space of the internal environment of the body, F – the set of blood elements, R, Y, Z, W, S – functorial mapping from category to category; morphisms between categories objects are represented by arrows with small Greek letters, the lower index of the morphism indicates the direction from which the information flow begins, the upper index indicates the serial number of the information flow from the object.

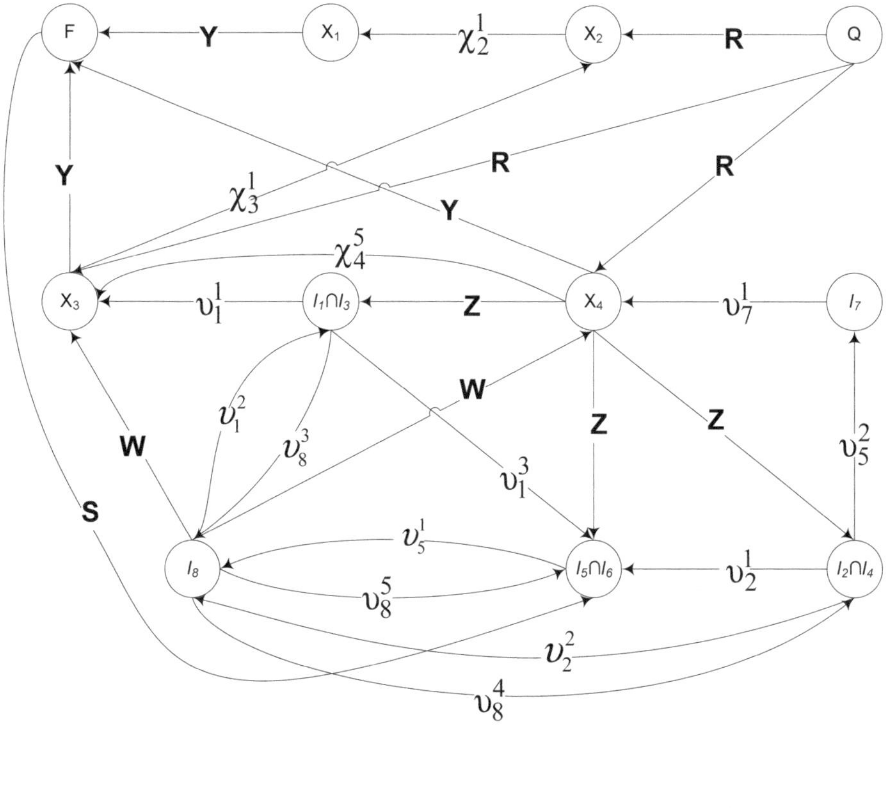

(3.27)

Adaptation circuit is an integral level of management of the body's haematopoietic system, aimed at optimal maintenance of the body's metabolism as a whole. In response to external influences, local and distant mechanisms of regulation of category X are included, which allow maintaining a multitude of blood elements F within the limits corresponding to the norm.

For example, external impact $Q^k = \{q_j^i\} \in Q$ can be formed as follows: $Q^k = \{q_1^5, q_2^2, q_3^5, q_4^1, q_5^1, q_6^3, q_7^1\}$, where the subscript indicates a set of previously defined values that affect the human body, and the superscript indicates a specific object of this set, that is, in this case, the external impact indicators can be as follows: a study is conducted at a temperature comfortable for the patient $q_1^5 = 22°\text{C} \in Q_1$, normal geomagnetic situation $q_2^2 =$ «the norm» $\in Q_2$, during the physiological balance of both departments VNS $q_3^5 =$ «10» $\in Q_3$, when the psycho-emotional state corresponds to the first regulated type $q_4^1 =$ «1» $\in Q_4$ and at the first standard load $q_5^1 =$ «1» $\in Q_5$, the age of the patient and the constitution of the body are determined by anthropometric characteristics and recorded: $q_6^3 =$ «18» $\in Q_6$ and $q_7^1 =$ «1» $\in Q_7$ respectively.

In addition, it is possible to determine the control action so that one of the objects $q_j^i \in Q$ are constants, according to the task of the researcher, while others vary: $Q^k = \{q_j^i, q_l^i\} \in Q$, where j – number of variable parameters, l – numbers of constants $j \neq l$.

Approaching the process of haematological research in this way, we can analyse the adaptive response of the haematopoietic system of the body to external influences of a different nature and intensity. Within the framework of this approach, the human body is a biological part of the bio-instrumental information and measurement system (BIMS), which transforms the input information represented by external influence into the output information – the state of a plurality of blood elements expressed in the number of blood elements that is directly transmitted to the input instrumental part of the system – haematological analyser.

Consider the functor mapping R of the category of external influences on the objects of control levels: the mapping $Q^k \mapsto \mathbf{R}(Q^k)$, matching each object Q^k of category Q with object $\mathbf{R}(Q^k)$ of X; the mapping $\mathbf{R}(Q_j^k, Q_l^k): Hom_Q(Q_j^k, Q_l^k) \to Hom_X(\mathbf{R}(Q_j^k), \mathbf{R}(Q_l^k)), j \neq l$. In this case, the object is displayed $Q^k \in Q$ in objects of category X, which can be represented as: $\mathbf{R}: Hom(Q^k, h), h \in X = \{X_2, X_3, X_4\}$. This display characterises the adaptive response of levels of management of the haematopoietic functional system to a variety of external influences.

Let us consider the functor map Y of the haematopoietic management category into the MFC category: the mapping $X_j^l \mapsto \mathbf{Y}(X_j^l)$, matching each object X_j^l from X the object $\mathbf{Y}(X_j^l)$ from F, where l, j – indices that uniquely determine the object; display $\mathbf{Y}(X_j^l, X_p^k): Hom_X(X_j^l, X_p^k) \to Hom_F(\mathbf{Y}(X_j^l), \mathbf{Y}(X_p^k))$.

Within the framework of the adaptive contour model under consideration, the above-defined functor Y maps objects $X_1, X_3, X_4 \in X$ in a monoid F: $\mathbf{Y}: Hom(X, F)$.

That is, $X_4 \mapsto \mathbf{Y}(X_4)$ reflects the organisms' level of impact on SUEB, $X_3 \mapsto \mathbf{Y}(X_3)$ – intercellular level of influence, $X_1 \mapsto \mathbf{Y}(X_1)$ – genomic-nuclear exposure, a $\mathbf{Y}: Hom_X(h) \to Hom_F(Y(h)), h \in \{X_2, X_3, X_4\}$ – reflects the balance of organism, intercellular and genomic-nuclear influences on SUEB.

The change in the SUEB leads to a change in the state of the internal environment of the organism, which can be represented by the functor mapping S of the monoid F into the category I: the mapping $F^k \mapsto \mathbf{S}(I_5 \cap I_6)$, matching each object $F^k \in F$ an object $\mathbf{S}(F^k)$ from I; the mapping $\mathbf{S}(F^k, F^k): Hom_F(F^k, F^k) \to Hom_I(\mathbf{S}(F^k), \mathbf{S}(F^k))$.

That is, the whole category F, one object, is mapped to category I, which can be represented as: $\mathbf{S}: Hom(h, I), h \in F$.

In accordance with the laws of normal physiology, the body's level of control acts on the IFTC both directly and through the stimulation of endocrine glands that have both sympathetic and parasympathetic innervation and are responsible for haemopoiesis-inducing microenvironment. That is, the functor mapping of the object Z X_4 on the object $I_1 \cap I_3$ of the category I: the mapping $X_4 \mapsto \mathbf{Z}(X_4)$, matching each object $X_4 = \{X_4^1, X_4^2, X_4^3, X_4^4\} \in X$ an object $\mathbf{Z}(X_4)$ from I; the mapping $\mathbf{Z}: Hom_X(h) \to Hom_I(\mathbf{Z}(h)), h \in X_4^j$.

In accordance with the laws of normal physiology, mappings describing the innervation control, which describes the mapping of the Z object X_4^1 on the object $I_5 \cap I_6$ of the category I: the mapping $X_4^1 \mapsto \mathbf{Z}(X_4^1)$, matching each object X_4^1 an object $\mathbf{Z}(X_4^1)$ from I; the mapping $\mathbf{Z}: Hom(X_4^1, I_5 \cap I_6)$.

This mapping characterises the balance of sympathetic and parasympathetic influences aimed at changing the metabolic state of the organism as a whole: $\mathbf{Z}: Hom(X_2, I_5 \cap I_6)$.

Homomorphic mapping $\upsilon_5^2 : I_5 \cap I_6 \to I_8$ category of the internal environment of the body is a mapping of all parameters of the state of the organism into receptor responses, then information from a set of receptors is transferred to the nervous system, thereby closing the adaptive contour: mapping $I_8 \mapsto \mathbf{W}(I_8)$, matching each object I_8 from I an object $\mathbf{W}(I_8)$ in X_4; mapping $\mathbf{W}(I_8, I_8) : Hom_I(I_8, I_8) \to Hom_X(\mathbf{W}(I_8), \mathbf{W}(I_8))$.

The functional mapping of the set of receptor responses from category I to category X is represented as: $\mathbf{W} : Hom(I_8, X_4)$.

Sequential mappings are possible by the SUEB reaction to follow and evaluate the input effect of the external environment, describe the degree of tension in the adaptive processes of the haematopoietic system of the organism and the corresponding functional state.

Multi-parameter input action $\gamma_j(t) = Q^j \in Q$ influences the levels of management of the haematopoietic system, in particular the organism level, which, depending on the intensity of the exposure, forms a control signal and selects the control path, that is, it also performs a commutative function. The control influence spreads through several sub-contours of adaptation and is transformed into IFEC.

In the accepted physiological model, four levels of management are defined, which can be distinguished from the categorical diagram of information flows (3.27). Let us analyse the structure of the management model of the haematopoietic functional system of the organism in various physiological situations in which the activity of a certain adaptive contour characterising the functional state is activated. In the absence of pathologies, the activation of each of the contours is determined by external influences on the body in full accordance with the laws of normal physiology.

Depending on the type of external influence, only certain levels of management that are responsible for the adaptation processes in the body can be included. In normal physiology, there is the following classification of states according to the degree of stress of the body's regulatory systems (Sudakov 2011): I state – borderline with the norm with minimum voltage of regulatory mechanisms, caused by complete or partial adaptation of the organism to inadequate environmental factors; II state – tension, manifested by the mobilisation of protective mechanisms, including an increase in the activity of the sympathetic-adrenal system, in which adaptation to inadequate environmental conditions can only be a short-term one; III state – overstrain, which is characterised by the inadequacy of adaptive protective adaptive mechanisms, their inability to provide the optimal adequate response of the organism to the influence of environmental factors; IV state – failure of adaptation mechanisms, or the state of pre-illness.

Let us consider the first state and the adaptive sub-contour that is included in the work of the functional haematopoietic system of the organism. Imagine such an external effect, in which the basic adaptation processes take place at the intracellular level. Regulation in this case occurs without a substantial inclusion of deep feedback mechanisms.

Such external impact is determined by a specific element $Q^k = \{Q_1^k, Q_2^k, .., Q_m^k\} \in Q$ the space of external influences on the body, while in full accordance with normal physiology the first adaptive contour is activated, the diagram (3.28).

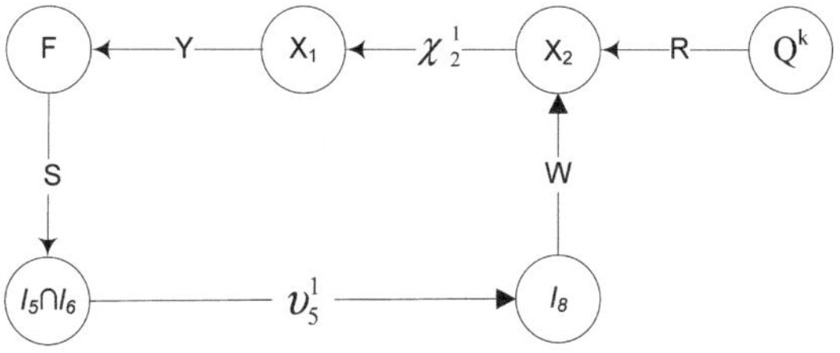

(3.28)

The contour is the lowest level of management that implements adaptation processes that include the management of the haematopoietic system at the intracellular and genomic-nuclear level that affect the composition of the peripheral blood, which, through the system of internal organs and the metabolic reactions of the organism, closes the adaptation contour.

The external influence is formed in such a way that the regulation by the adaptation of the organism does not pass under the control of a more complex intercellular or organismic level. The activation of the first circuit can be determined by small variations in the number of cells in the peripheral blood, changes in the constitution of the organism, or age-related changes.

Let us analyse the diagram (28). Consider the functor mapping R of the category of external influences on the cellular control level: the mapping $Q^k \mapsto \mathbf{R}(Q^k)$, matching to each object Q^k from category Q an object $\mathbf{R}(Q^k)$ from X; the mapping $\mathbf{R}(Q_j^k, Q_l^k): Hom_Q(Q_j^k, Q_l^k) \to Hom_X(\mathbf{R}(Q_j^k), \mathbf{R}(Q_l^k)), j \neq l$.

In this case, the object is displayed $Q^k \in Q$ into one object X_2 category X, which can be represented as: $\mathbf{R}: Hom(Q^k, h), h \in X = \{X_2\}$

Homomorphic mapping $\chi_2^1: X_2 \to X_1$ the category of control levels is the mapping of control actions from the intracellular to the genomic-nuclear control level. Consider the functor mapping $\mathbf{Y}$ management level categories X on SUEB F: the mapping $X_j^l \mapsto \mathbf{Y}(X_j^l)$, matching each object X_j^l из X object $\mathbf{Y}(X_j^l)$ from F, where l, j – indices, uniquely defining the object; display $\mathbf{Y}(X_j^l, X_p^k)$: $Hom_X(X_j^l, X_p^k) \to Hom_F(\mathbf{Y}(X_j^l), \mathbf{Y}(X_p^k))$.

Within the framework of the adaptive contour model under consideration, the above-defined functor $\mathbf{Y}$ displays objects $X_1 \in X$ in a monoid F: $\mathbf{Y}: Hom(X_1, F)$.

So, $X_1 \mapsto \mathbf{Y}(X_1)$ reflects the impact of the genomic nuclear SUEB, a $\mathbf{Y}(X_1^1, X_2^1): Hom_X(X_1^1, X_2^1) \to Hom_F(Y(X_1^1), Y(X_2^1))$ – reflects the balance of the effects of genomic-nuclear and intracellular levels of control on the composition of peripheral blood.

Changing the heart rhythm leads to a change in the state of the internal environment of the body, which can be represented by the functorial mapping S of the monoid F into category I: the mapping $F^k \mapsto \mathbf{S}(I_5 \cap I_6)$, matching each object $F^k \in F$ the object $\mathbf{S}(F^k)$ from I; mapping $\mathbf{S}(F^k, F^k): Hom_F(F^k, F^k) \to Hom_I(\mathbf{S}(F^k)\mathbf{S}(F^k))$.

That is, the whole category F, one object, is mapped to category I, which can be represented as: $\mathbf{S}: Hom(h, I), h \in F$.

In accordance with the laws of normal physiology, simultaneously with the impact on IFEC, there is an effect on internal organs having direct innervation. Homomorphic mapping $\upsilon_5^1: I_5 \cap I_6 \to I_8$ the category of the internal environment of the body is given in the second chapter and represents the mapping of all parameters of the state of the organism into metabolism. Metabolism closes the control loop, that is, the functor mapping W of the object I_8 on the object X_2 categories X: the mapping $I_8 \mapsto W(X_2)$, matching each object $I_8^j \in I_8$ an object $\mathbf{W}(I_8^j)$ from X; mappings $\mathbf{W}(I_8^j, I_8^k)$: $Hom_I(I_8^j, I_8^k) \to Hom_X(\mathbf{W}(I_8^j, I_8^k), \mathbf{W}(I_8^j, I_8^k))$

Summarising the presented mappings, we write down the structural equation of the adaptation of the first circuit:

$$AD^I = \mathbf{W}\left(\upsilon_5^1\left(\mathbf{S}\left(\mathbf{Y}\left(\chi_2^1\left(\mathbf{R}\left(Q^k\right)\right)\right)\right)\right)\right), \; Q^k \in Q \tag{3.29}$$

where k is the number of complex external influence.

Consider the physiological meaning of the mappings of the structural Equation 3.3. On the right-hand side of $\mathbf{R}(Q^k)$ – adaptive response of the intracellular level of control to external influence; $\chi_2^1(\mathbf{R}(Q^k))$ – transfer of control actions from the intracellular to the genomic-nuclear level of control; $\mathbf{Y}(\chi_2^1(\mathbf{R}(Q^k))) = F$ – the state of peripheral blood, the system parameter to be removed.

The adaptation Equation 3.29 is compiled for a hypothetical model of controlling the adaptation of the organism. In the model being implemented, a number of discrepancies with hypothetical realisation arise related to deviations from the ideal parameters of functioning: the autonomic nervous system, the internal environment of the organism, the metabolic state, and the processes of transferring control actions. All these deviations affect the IFEC implementation.

Due to the fact that for a living organism there is no need to strictly achieve a certain state, but it is important that the state of the dynamic system does not come out of a certain area that determines the variety of admissible values of existence, we can write the equation of realisable adaptation for Equation 3.29 in the following form:

$$\begin{aligned} AD^I &= \mathbf{W}\left(\upsilon_5^1\left(\mathbf{S}\left(\mathbf{Y}\left(\chi_2^1\left(\mathbf{R}\left(Q^k\right)\right)\right)\right)\right)\right) + \Delta\mathbf{W} + \Delta\upsilon_5^1 + \Delta\mathbf{S} + \Delta\mathbf{Y} + \Delta\chi_2^1 + \Delta\mathbf{R} + \\ &+ \Delta Q = \mathbf{W}\left(\upsilon_5^1\left(\mathbf{S}\left(\mathbf{Y}\left(\chi_2^1\left(\mathbf{R}\left(Q^k\right)\right)\right)\right)\right)\right) + b_j^k, \quad b_j^k \in B, \end{aligned} \tag{3.30}$$

where

$$B = \begin{cases} \Delta\mathbf{W} = \Delta\mathbf{W}\left(\upsilon_5^1\left(\mathbf{S}\left(\mathbf{Y}\left(\chi_2^1\left(\mathbf{R}\left(Q^k\right)\right)\right)\right)\right)\right) \\ \Delta\upsilon_5^1 = \mathbf{W}\left(\Delta\upsilon_5^1\left(\mathbf{S}\left(\mathbf{Y}\left(\chi_2^1\left(\mathbf{R}\left(Q^k\right)\right)\right)\right)\right)\right) \\ \Delta\mathbf{S} = \mathbf{W}\left(\upsilon_5^1\left(\Delta\mathbf{S}\left(\mathbf{Y}\left(\chi_2^1\left(\mathbf{R}\left(Q^k\right)\right)\right)\right)\right)\right) \\ \Delta\mathbf{Y} = \mathbf{W}\left(\upsilon_5^1\left(\mathbf{S}\left(\Delta\mathbf{Y}\left(\chi_2^1\left(\mathbf{R}\left(Q^k\right)\right)\right)\right)\right)\right) \\ \Delta\chi_2^1 = \mathbf{W}\left(\upsilon_5^1\left(\mathbf{S}\left(\mathbf{Y}\left(\Delta\chi_2^1\left(\mathbf{R}\left(Q^k\right)\right)\right)\right)\right)\right) \\ \Delta\mathbf{R} = \mathbf{W}\left(\upsilon_5^1\left(\mathbf{S}\left(\mathbf{Y}\left(\chi_2^1\left(\Delta\mathbf{R}\left(Q^k\right)\right)\right)\right)\right)\right) \\ \Delta Q = \mathbf{W}\left(\upsilon_5^1\left(\mathbf{S}\left(\mathbf{Y}\left(\chi_2^1\left(\mathbf{R}\left(\Delta Q^k\right)\right)\right)\right)\right)\right) \end{cases} \tag{3.31}$$

The expressions on the right-hand side of Equations 3.31 denote physiological deviations from the nominal values for a given organism, with the nominal values of the remaining parameters. The first equation, for example, denotes deviations in the transmission of metabolic information, the second – deviations from the nominal value of the reaction of internal organs, the last – deviation of the actual external impact from the nominal, etc. In this case, everything functions in the space of internal interconnected compensatory circuits so that the total deviation for a given external effect on the body is minimal, that is, $\Delta\mathbf{W} + \Delta\upsilon_5^1 + \Delta\mathbf{S} + \Delta\mathbf{Y} + \Delta\chi_2^1 + \Delta\mathbf{R} = b_j^I \to \min$. The control law is not arbitrary, but is chosen from some finite set $B \equiv \{b_j^k\},\ k = 1, 2, 3;\ j = 1..n$. Thus, the optimal self-regulation of the organism can be determined using the procedure for minimising the functional$B = (\Delta\mathbf{W}, \Delta\upsilon_5^1, \Delta\mathbf{S}, \Delta\mathbf{Y}, \Delta\chi_2^1, \Delta\mathbf{R}, \Delta Q, t) = \min$.

In the role of functional B is a set of functions of the body, and the construction and description of it is beyond the scope of this work. We note that it is possible to determine its quantitative value.

As a result, the adaptation Equation 3.31 can be written in the form:

$$AD^{IP} = AD^I\big|_{Q^k} + b_k^I \tag{3.32}$$

where $Q^k \in Q, b_k^I \in B$. That is, the realised equation can be represented as the sum of a hypothetical and additional term from the set of realisations of the functional B. Structural Equation 3.32 is a realisable record of the diagram (3.27).

Since during the formalisation of structural equations their physiological interpretation was given in accordance with normal physiology, this allows one to judge the reliability of the mathematical model of the measurement object; and certain interrelations between external influences and system parameters, given in the form of successive functorial mappings, make it possible to specify clinical and diagnostic studies and, as a consequence, to increase the efficiency of diagnostics.

The used mathematical apparatus of categories and functors allows to pass to construction of the automated diagnostic system and to conduct the metrological analysis.

The imposed structure of management of the haemopoietic functional system, built in strict accordance with the normal physiology and bio-cybernetic approach of Anokhin-Sudakov, made it possible to identify the adaptive control contours, record structural and analytical equations and give them a physiological meaning.

The structural-analytical record of the adaptation equations within the mathematical apparatus of categories and functors allowed us to take into account and formalise all the connections arising in the process of adaptation, including deep inverse ones.

3.4 CONCLUSIONS AND RECOMMENDATIONS

In the case when the peripheral blood indices are on the verge of the norm, it is necessary to take into account the measurement error, which consists of the error of the haematoanalyser and the errors due to the biological part of the BIMS: ignoring the age indices of the patient, the inherent individual features of the blood composition, psycho-physiological loads before taking the sample and.

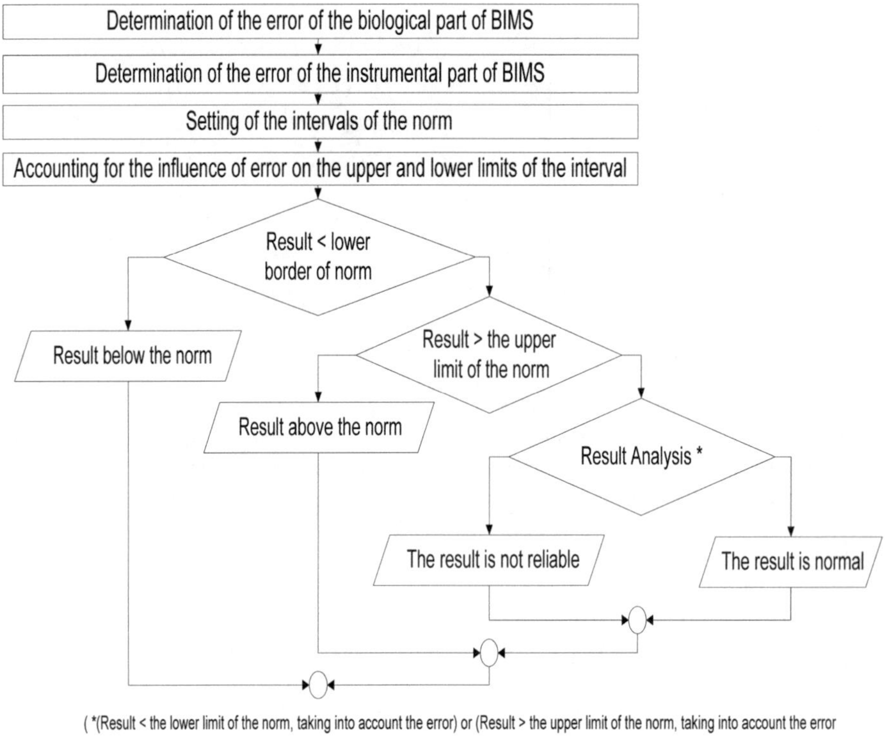

Figure 3.2. Result-processing algorithm.

The software complex, created on the basis of the algorithm proposed in Figure 3.3, allows to take into account these parameters, in accordance with the dependencies obtained earlier, thereby reducing the probability of setting a false-positive or false-negative diagnosis.

Taking into account the dependencies mentioned above and the structural estimation of the error in the instrumental part of the BIMS, we developed an algorithm (Figure 3.2), which makes it possible to implement a software package for the error in analysing the results of clinical and diagnostic measurements in haematological studies.

The software package developed on the basis of the proposed algorithm will allow you to analyse the result of haematological measurements taking into account the measurement error and to display on the screen the message characterising the result was within the limits of the norm, was higher or lower than the norm, or is unreliable because it hit the boundary between the normal and pathological state, and the exact value cannot be determined, since the error is taken into account.

Method of making a decision about the reliability of the result of the study:

- Results of the research result;
- In accordance with the patient's personal data, the criteria influencing the measurement result are exposed;
- If the mark "error counting" is not used, the result is analysed in the interval of the norm with the output of the corresponding message;
- if there is a mark, then the limits of the norm are "blurred" by the appearance of the zone of uncertainty and when a result comes into it, a message is given that it cannot be considered reliable (reanalysis is recommended).

REFERENCES

Goldblatt R. Toposes. 1983. *Categorical analysis of logic*. Moscow: Mir.

Korenevsky N. A., Popevichitel E. P., Philist S. A. 2009. Devices and technical means of functional diagnostics: *Proc. allowance: in 2 hours Part 1*. Kursk: Kursk State University of Technology.

Mac Lane S. 2004. *Categories for a working mathematician*. Moscow: Fizmatlit.

Menshikov, V.V. et al. 2002. *Management in the laboratory clinical diagnostic service*. Moscow: Mir.

Mukha, Yu. P. 2004. Categorical synthesis of the information flow control structure in the transmission of measurement information in telemedicine measuring systems. *Biomedical technologies and radio electronics* 4: 23–29.

Mukha, Yu. P. 2007. Metrological aspects of medical measurements. *Proc. 14 Russian symposium with international participation "Millimeter waves in medicine and biology*: 258–259.

Mukha, Yu. P., Avdeyuk O.A. & Queen, I.Yu. 2003. *Algebraic theory of synthesis of complex systems: monograph*. Volgograd: Publishing house VolgGTU.

Sudakov K. V., 2011. *Functional systems*. Moscow: Publishing house RAMS.

Verkhovodova, O.V. 2007. Quality control of laboratory diagnostics in public health institutions. *Issues of expertise and quality of medical care* 6.

Wajman, R., Fidos, H., Fiderek, P., Jaworski, T., Nowakowski, J., Sankowski, D., & Banasiak, R. 2013. Metrological evaluation of measurement system for two-phase flow fractions determination using 3D electrical capacitance tomography. *Informatyka, Automatyka, Pomiary w Gospodarce i Ochronie Środowiska* 3(3): 49–54. https://doi.org/10.35784/iapgos.1463.

Zaikin E. V., Malakhov V. N., Karinova I. N. 2009. Dynamics of quality indices of biochemical blood tests in clinical diagnostic laboratories participating in the Federal System for External Quality Assessment of Clinical Laboratory Research (FSVOK). *Quality management in the field of health and social development* 5: 81–88.

CHAPTER 4

Increasing the accuracy of laboratory studies of haemoglobin level in blood

I.P. Rudenok
Volgograd State Technical University, Volgograd, Russian Federation

Yu.P. Mukha
Volgograd State Medical University, Volgograd, Russian Federation
Volgograd State Technical University, Volgograd, Russian Federation

A.I. Kireeva
Volgograd State Technical University, Volgograd, Russian Federation

P. Komada & J. Smołka
Lublin University of Technology, Lublin, Poland

S. Amirgaliyeva
Institute of Information and Computational Technologies CS MES RK, Almaty, Kazakhstan
Kazakh Academy of Transport & Communication, Almaty, Kazakhstan

ABSTRACT: The determination of the magnitude of the uniaxial anisotropy arising in the electromagnetic field under the influence of the electromagnetic field in haemoglobin solutions is relevant in the study of its chemical composition. The results, which were obtained in the work, establish a strict interrelation of the parameters of the guided hybrid modes of optical radiation with the tensor of material characteristics of haemoglobin. This allows us to characterize its composition by the magneto-optical response with a very high degree of accuracy.

4.1 INTRODUCTION

Our work was devoted to the synthesis of biological materials, which have previously unknown properties. Our scientific team was able to investigate bianisotropic and bihyrotropic media in a fairly wide frequency range. As an example, we investigated a gradient anisotropic magneto and in particular gyromagnetic haemoglobin solute. The natural consequence of this development technology allows us to analyse the latest diagnostic techniques with the help of optical methods. Many doctors consider in their scientific works on the use of lasers in medicine the development of optoelectronic components and next-generation nodes, which have a number of fundamentally new properties compared to the conventional homogeneous and anisotropic medium. They realized that the issues of metrology in these studies are very acute (Arce-Diego et al. 2004; Kalvach & Szabó 2015; Rao et al. 2004; Weiglhofer 1998). In our final result, we proved the possibility of obtaining new various waveguide properties of monochromatic light waves, light beams and pulses in biological fluids.

Such type of magnetodielectric waveguide structures may have no anisotropy, for example, bi-isotropic medium. If we add this to limited reciprocity, the guide structure becomes chiral (Jagard & Sun 1992). We can include in this concept various biological objects (proteins and DNA collagens) with molecules, which were oriented in helical chains. Strict and correct electrodynamic investigation of compositional structures for optoelectronics based on artificial media of this class and is of great interest (Ivanov 2010). Developing of nanostructures is also popular in recent years (Chernozatonsky et al. 2014).

Electrical properties of the exotic medium allow us to further replace elements and nodes on the silicon optoelectronic nanostructures (Fan et al. 2010). In the pharm analysis, the following compounds of carbon, silicon, tin and lead are used: ammonium carbonate (ammonium carbonate $(NH_4)_2CO_3$ crystalline and solution); potassium bicarbonate (potassium bicarbonate potassium $KHCO_3$) crystal and solution; potassium carbonate (potassium carbonate K_2CO_3) crystalline and solution; sodium bicarbonate (sodium bicarbonate $NaHCO_3$) crystal and solution; sodium carbonate anhydrous (sodium carbonate anhydrous Na_2CO_3) crystalline and a solution (10% and 0.05 mol/l). One of the most promising types of carbon allotropes is being a planar monolayer of atoms that are packed in a two-dimensional hexagonal lattice having a large thermal conductivity. It has carrier mobility and mechanical strength under certain conditions (Gonzalez et al. 2009; Labunov et al. 2010).

There are a lot of mathematical and computational difficulties in the investigation of wave propagation and resonance modal interactions in standard and non-hybrid compositional anisotropic nanostructured waveguides. It is important and requires the development of an adequate mathematical apparatus and bringing modern computer technology.

Some attempts are being made using the method of functional changes and perturbation methods (Hanson 2008). This is the most versatile methods suitable for solving of all linear and nonlinear equations in an ordinary and partial differential, integral, integro-differential, functional with deviating argument, which may be stochastic or deterministic at all boundary and initial conditions. There was a huge variety of different special techniques based on solving of equations in this area: different modifications of the perturbation method (well-known methods of first and second settings on the boundary layer), iterative linearization, regular and singular problems and other approximate and analytical methods.

The profound research and physical applications of interactions of different types of waves with the medium are very important. Particularly the most interesting sphere is for complex environments, which may be characterized by the increasing number of methods. Their objective analysis increased because of great applied significance. For the optical range, it comes to considering the structure, the dimensions of the spatial inhomogeneity of which are comparable to the wavelength of the radiation.

4.2 AN INVESTIGATION PART

For the approximate solutions of wave equations in structures of this class, we may use integral methods, which reduce their solution under the given boundary conditions for the integration of equations in common derivatives obtained from the original by averaging them. There are a lot of works in which authors used matrix method "4×4" for homogeneous bianisotropic structures.

However, the so-called matrix material parameters are independent of the longitudinal wave number and frequency. This fact should not be, because first of all the waveguide refractive index is determined by the parameters of the material in matrix form, and secondly the view of the matrix should depend on the frequency of the waves if we take into account the material dispersion of waveguide structures. Analytical solutions of tasks can be carried out using Fourier's method of integral transformations and method of Green's functions, etc. The numerical solution can be obtained by the iterative and direct variational method and difference equations. One of the direct methods is the reduction method, which was called in the literature the direct method of reduction or decomposition.

We proceeded from the fact that the surface and pseudosurface waves in the waveguide compositional structure with a complex internal environment may be found as an expansion in the complete system of waves in mixed spectrum in waveguide structure of comparison which satisfied the given boundary conditions. The success of this approach depended on the right choice of approximating functions of the system cross-section of the structure. Therefore we constantly faced the challenge of informed choice for the representing functions. As one of the ways for solving this problem was to find such type of functions in the same solution of boundary value problems for an easier comparison of the compositional structure. Then we already used the coefficients of the expansion of the system of linear algebraic equations for forming of the wave equation for the electric and magnetic vectors.

We considered an asymmetric planar waveguide, which central waveguide layer has special transverse dimensions and concrete physical characteristics (Ivanov & Shuty 2007). Let the nonzero diagonal elements of the tensor electric and magnetic permeabilities only depend on the transverse coordinate:

$$\begin{aligned}
&\varepsilon_{ij}(q_0, q_1, \ldots, q_n, x),\ i=j, \quad \varepsilon_{ij}(q_0, q_1, \ldots, q_n, x)=0,\ i \neq j;\\
&\mu_{ij}(g_0, g_1, \ldots, g_n, x), i=j,\\
&\mu_{ij}(g_0, g_1, \ldots, g_n, x)=0, i \neq j;
\end{aligned} \tag{4.1}$$

and there is no dependence on the coordinate y, when $\partial/\partial y=0$. The outer layer and the substrate have respectively scalars $\varepsilon_{\theta H}, \mu_{\theta H}, \varepsilon_n, \mu_n$. In this case, Maxwell's equations are divided into two independent systems of equations to determine the H_y, E_x, E_z (E – waves) and H_x, E_y, H_z (H- waves).

Excluding from the resulting system of equations H_x, H_z, E_x, E_z, we obtained quasi-differential equations for the transverse component of the electric and magnetic field (cross-sectional functions):

$$\begin{aligned}
&\mu_{xx}(g_0, g_1, \ldots, g_n, x)\mu_{zz}(g_0, g_1, \ldots, g_n, x)\frac{d^2\overset{v}{E}_y}{dx^2}\\
&-\mu_{xx}(g_0, g_1, \ldots, g_n, x)\cdot\frac{d}{dx}\mu_{zz}(g_0, g_1, \ldots, g_n, x)\cdot\frac{d\overset{v}{E}_y}{dx}\\
&+\mu_{zz}^2(g_0, g_1, \ldots, g_n, x)\left[\omega^2\varepsilon_{yy}(q_0, q_1, \ldots, q_n, x)\cdot\mu_{xx}(g_0, g_1, \ldots, g_n, x)-\beta^2\right]\overset{v}{E}_y=0,
\end{aligned} \tag{4.2}$$

$$\begin{aligned}
&\varepsilon_{xx}(q_0, q_1, \ldots, q_n, x)\cdot\varepsilon_{zz}(q_0, q_1, \ldots, q_n, x)\frac{d^2\overset{v}{H}_y}{dx^2}\\
&-\varepsilon_{xx}(q_0, q_1, \ldots, q_n, x)\frac{d\varepsilon_{zz}}{dx}(q_0, q_1, \ldots, q_n, x)\frac{d\overset{v}{H}_y}{dx}\\
&+\varepsilon_{zz}^2(q_0, q_1, \ldots, q_n, x)\left[\omega^2\mu_{yy}(g_0, g_1, \ldots, g_n, x)\cdot\varepsilon_{xx}(q_0, q_1, \ldots, q_n, x)-\beta^2\right]\overset{v}{H}_y=0.
\end{aligned} \tag{4.3}$$

Then we assumed that the elements of the tensor of permittivity and magnetic permeability are described by generalized species distributions:

$$\varepsilon_{ii}(q_2, q_4, x)=\varepsilon_{ii,m}(1-q_2x^2+q_4x^4), \tag{4.4}$$

$$\mu_{jj}(g_2, g_4, x)=\mu_{jj,m}(1-g_2x^2+g_4x^4). \tag{4.5}$$

The resulting equation with polynomial coefficients is not Fuchsian. However, it is possible to use Frobenius' method of solution in the form of a generalized power series.

So, we investigated first the wave processes in compositional structures with an inner nonlinear anisotropic-gradient medium in the case of falling of optical non-Gaussian beams. We received and solved a non-linear wave equation to the cross-sectional components of functions with anisotropic gradient coefficients from Maxwell's equations for the electric and magnetic vectors: the system of partial differential equations of hyperbolic type. We took into account the effect of dependence between the complexity of the non-linear waveguide medium, and the parameters, and characteristics of the reflected optical beam.

Dependences from the gradient parameters and types of profiles of the dielectric tensor elements for the coupling coefficient, longitudinal wavenumbers, the efficiency of the wave mode conversion were analyzed for a variety of the reduced transverse dimensions of the composite structure. As an example, we used the dependence of the gradient tensor elements of the second term from the magnetization vector in magnetic-gyrotropic gradient haemoglobin sample for the specific case of an extension to the crystallographic axes. The interaction of waves of the discrete and continuous spectrum also was studied. Our results showed that we need to take into account the two modes of coupled-wave discrete spectrum in equations because of the potential existence of a connection with the modes of the continuous spectrumNormalizing the size $x = \overset{v}{x}/x_0$, we can write Equations (4.1) and (4.2) in a more convenient form for analysis:

$$\mu_{xx,m} \cdot \mu_{zz,m}(1 - 2g_2x^2 + \alpha_1 x^4 - 2g_2 \cdot g_4 x^6 + g_4^2 x^8)\frac{d^2\overset{v}{E}_y}{dx^2}$$
$$- \mu_{xx,m} \cdot \mu_{zz,m}(-2g_2 x + \upsilon x^3 - 6g_2 g_4 x^5 + 4g_4^2 x^7)\frac{d\overset{v}{E}_y}{dx}$$
$$+ (b_0 + b_2x^2 + b_4x^4 + b_6x^6 + b_8x^8 + b_{10}x^{10} + b_{12}x^{12} + b_{14}x^{14} + b_{16}x^{16})\overset{v}{E}_y = 0, \quad (4.6)$$

where:

$$\begin{aligned}
\alpha_1 &= g_2^2 + 2g_4, \upsilon = 2g_2^2 + 4g_4, b_0 = \kappa_{yy}^2 \mu_{zz,m}^2 \overset{v}{\mu} - \beta^2 \mu_{zz,m}^2,\\
b_0 &= \kappa_{yy}^2 \overset{v}{\mu} \cdot \mu_{zz,m}^2 - \beta^2 \mu_{zz,m}^2 = \mu_{zz,m}^2(\kappa_{yy}^2 \overset{v}{\mu} - \beta^2), b_2 = 2\beta^2 \mu_{zz,m}^2 g_2 - \delta_1,\\
b_4 &= \delta_2 - \beta^2 \mu_{zz,m}^2 \cdot \alpha_1, \ b_6 = 2\beta^2 \mu_{zz,m}^2 g_2 g_4 - \delta_3,\\
b_8 &= \delta_4 - \beta^2 \mu_{zz,m}^2 g_4^2, b_{10} = -(\alpha_4 q_2 - 3g_2 g_4^2 - \alpha_3 q_4) \cdot \omega^2 \varepsilon_{yy,m} \mu_{zz,m}^2 \cdot \mu_{xx,m},\\
b_{12} &= (3g_2 g_4^2 q_2 + \alpha_4 \cdot q_4) \cdot \omega^2 \varepsilon_{yy,m} \mu_{zz,m}^2 \mu_{xx,m}^2, b_{14} = -(q_2 g_4^3 + 3g_2 g_4^2 q_4)\\
&\cdot \omega^2 \varepsilon_{yy,m} \mu_{zz,m}^2 \mu_{xx,m}, b_{16} = g_4^3 \cdot q_4 \cdot \omega^2 \varepsilon_{yy,m} \mu_{zz,m}^2 \cdot \mu_{xx,m},\\
\delta_1 &= 3g_2 + q_2, \delta_2 = \alpha_2 + 3q_2 \cdot g_2 + q_4,\\
\delta_3 &= \alpha_3 + \alpha_2 q_2 + 3q_4 g_2, \delta_4 = \alpha_4 + \alpha_3 q_2 + \alpha_2 q_4,\\
\alpha_2 &= \alpha_1 + 2g_2^2 + q_4, \alpha_3 = 4g_2 g_4 + \alpha_1 g_2, \alpha_4 = g_4^2 + 2g_2^2 g_4 + \alpha_1 g_4.
\end{aligned} \quad (4.7)$$

$$\varepsilon_{xx,m} \cdot \varepsilon_{zz,m}[1 - 2q_2x^2 + (q_2^2 + 2q_4)x^4 - 2q_2q_4x^6 + q_4x^8] \cdot \frac{\partial^2 \overset{\vee}{H}_y}{\partial x^2}$$
$$- \varepsilon_{xx,m} \cdot \varepsilon_{zz,m}[-2q_2x + (2q_2^2 + 4q_4)x^3 - 6q_2q_4x^5 + 4q_4^2x^7] \cdot \frac{\partial \overset{\vee}{H}_y}{\partial x}$$
$$+ [d_0 + d_2x^2 + d_4x^4 + d_6x^6 + d_8x^8 + d_{10}x^{10} + d_{12}x^{12} + d_{14}x^{14} + d_{16}x^{16}] \cdot \overset{\vee}{H}_y = 0 \quad (4.8)$$

$$\begin{aligned}
d_0 &= k_{yy}^2 \varepsilon_{zz,m}^2 \overset{v}{\varepsilon} - \beta^2 \varepsilon_{zz,m}^2, \ d_2 = 2\beta^2 \varepsilon_{zz,m}^2 q_2 - V_1,\\
d_4 &= V_2 - \beta^2 \varepsilon_{zz,m}^2 \cdot (q_2^2 + 2q_4), \ d_6 = 2q_2 q_4 \beta^2 \varepsilon_{zz,m}^2 - V_3,\\
d_8 &= V_4 - \beta^2 \varepsilon_{zz,m}^2 \cdot q_4^2,\\
d_{10} &= (-t_4 g_2 + 3q_2 q_4^2 + t_3 g_4)\omega^2 \mu_{yy,m} \varepsilon_{zz,,m}^2 \cdot \varepsilon_{xx,m} \qquad (4.9)\\
d_{12} &= (3q_2 q_4^2 g_2 + V_4 g_4) \cdot \omega^2 \mu_{yy,m} \cdot \varepsilon_{zz,m}^2 \cdot \varepsilon_{xx,m},\\
d_{14} &= -(g_2 q_4^3 + 3q_2 q_4^2 g_4)\, \omega^2 \mu_{yy,m} \varepsilon_{zz,m}^2 \varepsilon_{xx,m},\\
d_{16} &= q_4^3 g_4 \omega^2 \mu_{yy,m} \varepsilon_{zz,m}^2 \cdot \varepsilon_{xx,m}, \ V_1 = 3q_2 + g_2,\\
V_2 &= t_2 + 3g_2 q_2 + g_4, \ V_3 = t_3 + t_2 g_2 + 3g_4 q_2,\\
V_4 &= t_4 + t_3 g_2 + t_2 g_4, \ t_2 = t_1 + 2q_2^2 + q_4, \ t_3 = 4q_2 q_4 + t_1 q_2,\\
t_4 &= q_4^2 + 2q_2^2 q_4 + t_1 q_4, \ t_1 = q_2^2 + 2q_4.
\end{aligned}$$

The solution of the transformed Equation (4.6) we used in the form of a series:

$$\overset{v}{E}_y = \sum_{n=0}^{\infty} a_n x^n, \quad (4.10)$$

the coefficients of which are determined by the recurrence relations arising from the differential equation structure.

$$a_n = -\frac{\mathrm{T}_o a_{n-2} + \mathrm{T}_1 a_{n-4} + \mathrm{T}_2 a_{n-6} + \mathrm{T}_3 a_{n-8} + b_8 a_{n-10} + b_{10} a_{n-12} + b_{12} a_{n-14} + b_{14} a_{n-16} + b_{16} a_{n-18}}{n\,(n-1)\,\mu_{xx,m}\,\mu_{zz,m}}, \tag{4.11}$$

$$\begin{aligned}
\mathrm{T}_o &= 2g_2\mu_{xx,m}\mu_{zz,m}\,(n-2) + b_o - 2g_2\,(n-2)\,(n-3)\,\mu_{xx,m}\,\mu_{zz,m}\,,\\
\mathrm{T}_1 &= \alpha_1\mu_{xx,m}\cdot\mu_{zz,m}\cdot(n-4)\,(n-5) - \mu_{xx,m}\cdot\mu_{zz,m}\cdot\upsilon\cdot(n-4) + b_2,\\
\mathrm{T}_2 &= -2g_2g_4\mu_{xx,m}\cdot\mu_{zz,m}\cdot(n-6)\,(n-7) + 6\mu_{xx,m}\mu_{zz,m}g_2g_4\,(n-6) + b_4,\\
\mathrm{T}_3 &= g_4^2\mu_{xx,m}\cdot\mu_{zz,m}\,(n-8)\,(n-9) - 4g_4^2\mu_{xx,m}\mu_{zz,m}\,(n-8) + b_6
\end{aligned}$$

Similarly, we found the transverse component of the magnetic field (a function of the cross-section) from the Equation (4.8) in form of uniformly convergent sequence. The first and second linearly independent solutions are represented as follows (H – waves):

$$\check{\mathrm{E}}_y = \mathrm{A}_1\Psi_1\,(g_2, g_4, q_2, q_4, æ, x) + \mathrm{A}_2\Psi_2\,(g_2, g_4, q_2, q_4, æ, x)\,. \tag{4.12}$$

For E- waves:

$$\check{\mathrm{H}}_y = C_1\Phi_1\,(g_2, g_4, q_2, q_4, æ, x) + C_2\Phi_2\,(g_2, g_4, q_2, q_4, æ, x) \tag{4.13}$$

Within the substrate coating the expression for the cross section of functions, for example H – waves respectively have the following form:

$$\check{\mathrm{E}}_y = D_1\,\exp\left[-\sqrt{\beta^2 - \omega^2\varepsilon_{\mathit{вн}}\mu_{\mathit{вн}}x}\right] \tag{4.14}$$

$$\check{\mathrm{E}}_y = \mathrm{B}_1\,\exp\left[+\sqrt{\beta^2 - \omega^2\varepsilon_n\mu_n x}\right] \tag{4.15}$$

and the longitudinal components of the electric and magnetic fields in the coating, the guiding layer and the substrate were developed as:

$$\check{\mathrm{H}}_z = \frac{1}{j\omega\mu_{\mathit{вн}}}D_1\cdot\gamma\,\exp\,(-\gamma x) \tag{4.16}$$

$$\check{\mathrm{H}}_z = -\frac{1}{j\omega\mu_{zz}\,(g_2, g_4, q_2, q_4, x)}\cdot\left[\mathrm{A}_1\Psi_{1,x}^{/}\,(g_2, g_4, q_2, q_4, æ, x) + \mathrm{A}_2\Psi_{2,x}^{/}\,(g_2, g_4, q_2, q_4, æ, x)\right], \tag{4.17}$$

$$\check{\mathrm{H}}_z = -\frac{\mathrm{B}_1}{j\omega\mu_n}\chi\,\exp\,(\chi x)\,. \tag{4.18}$$

In the case of propagation of the discrete spectrum for the longitudinal component of the electric field can be written in bianisotropic layer we can use the form of:

$$\check{\mathrm{E}}_z = -\frac{1}{j\omega\varepsilon_{zz}\,(g_2, g_4, q_2, q_4, x)}\cdot\left[C_1\Phi_{1,x}^{/}\,(g_2, g_4, q_2, q_4, æ, x) + C_2\Phi_{2,x}^{/}\,(g_2, g_4, q_2, q_4æ, x)\right]. \tag{4.19}$$

The requirement of continuity of the tangential components of the electric and magnetic vectors:

$$\begin{gathered}
\mathrm{E}_{y1} = \mathrm{E}_{y2}, \quad \mathrm{E}_{y3} = \mathrm{E}_{y2},\\
\mathrm{H}_{z1} = \mathrm{H}_{z2},\\
\mathrm{H}_{z3} = \mathrm{H}_{z2}
\end{gathered} \tag{4.20}$$

It allowed us to obtain the dispersion equations for calculating eigen values of the wave numbers of magnetic and electric surface waves discrete spectrum in bianisotropic gradient structure, as well as other basic parameters characterizing its waveguide properties. For example, the dispersion equation can be written for magnetic waves:

$$\nabla_{13}\nabla_1\begin{vmatrix}\nabla_5 & -\nabla_6\\ \nabla_8 & 0\end{vmatrix}-\nabla_{13}\nabla_2\begin{vmatrix}\nabla_4 & -\nabla_6\\ \nabla_7 & 0\end{vmatrix}-\nabla_{13}\nabla_3\begin{vmatrix}\nabla_4 & \nabla_5\\ \nabla_7 & \nabla_8\end{vmatrix}-\nabla_{10}\nabla_1\begin{vmatrix}\nabla_5 & -\nabla_6\\ \nabla_{12} & 0\end{vmatrix}$$

$$+\nabla_{10}\nabla_2\begin{vmatrix}\nabla_4 & -\nabla_6\\ \nabla_{11} & 0\end{vmatrix}+\nabla_{10}\nabla_3\begin{vmatrix}\nabla_4 & \nabla_5\\ \nabla_{11} & \nabla_{12}\end{vmatrix}=0$$

where:

$$\nabla_{1(2)}=\Psi_{1(2)}(g_2,g_4,q_2,q_4,æ,1),\quad \nabla_3=\exp(-\gamma),$$

$$\nabla_{4(5)}=\mu_{zz}^{-1}(g_2,g_4,1)\cdot\Psi'_{x,1(2)}(g_2,g_4,q_2,q_4,æ,1),$$

$$\nabla_6=\frac{\gamma}{\mu_{вн}}\exp(-\gamma),\quad \nabla_{7(8)}=\Psi_{1(2)}(g_2,g_4,q_2,q_4,æ,-1),\nabla_{10}=\exp(-\chi)$$

$$\nabla_{11(12)}=\mu_{zz}^{-1}(g_2,g_4,-1)\cdot\Psi'_{x,1(2)}(g_2,g_4,q_2,q_4,æ,-1),\nabla_{13}=\frac{\chi}{\mu_n}\exp(-\chi),$$

and $\gamma, æ, \chi$ – transverse wave number of waves, respectively, in the coating, the guiding layer and the substrate.

We considered that the propagation of surface and pseudosurface waves in a three-layer planar gradient bianisotropic structure, which included substrate and an outer layer made of a material with scalar properties $\varepsilon_2,\mu_2,\varepsilon_3,\mu_3$. Central waveguide layer was gradient and magnetodielectric. It was characterized by a tensor of permittivity $\overleftrightarrow{\varepsilon}$ and permeability $\overleftrightarrow{\mu}$. All of the elements in these tensors were depend on the transverse coordinate of generalized spatial profiles:

$$\varepsilon_{ij}(q_0,q_1,\ldots,q_n,x),\ \mu_{ij}(g_0,g_1,\ldots,g_n,x),$$

where $q_0,g_0,\ldots,q_n,g_n$ are the parameters of the spatial gradient profiles elements tensors permittivity and permeability.

We expected that there is no dependence on the coordinate y, so used the equality: $\partial/\partial y=0$. We took for comparison an asymmetric planar compositional structure. Its tensors of permittivity and magnetic permeability had non-zero gradient elements only to main diagonals. As an orthonormal system of its own surface waves in waveguide structure, we took the electric and magnetic waves of the mixed spectrum. In accordance with a comparison, we had found new tensors of material characteristics in the waveguide layer in the additive form. One of the components was a tensor with non-zero gradient elements of the principal diagonal. The other was a tensor with nine nonzero gradient elements.

$$\begin{aligned}\overleftrightarrow{\varepsilon}(q_0,q_1,\ldots,q_n,x)&=\overleftrightarrow{\varepsilon}_{cp}(q_0,q_1,\ldots,q_n,x)+\Delta\overleftrightarrow{\varepsilon}(q_0,q_1,\ldots,q_n,x)\\ \overleftrightarrow{\mu}(g_0,g_1,\ldots,g_n,x)&=\overleftrightarrow{\mu}_{cp}(g_0,g_1,\ldots,g_n,x)+\Delta\overleftrightarrow{\mu}\,(g_0,g_1,\ldots,g_n,x)\end{aligned}\quad(4.21)$$

We took in our investigation the electric and magnetic vectors of the natural waves of asymmetrical gradient bianisotropic waveguide in the form of:

$$\begin{aligned}\vec{E}&=\vec{E}_\nu(q_0,g_0,\ldots,q_n,g_n,æ_\nu,x)\,e^{j(\omega t-\beta_\nu z)}\\ \vec{H}&=\vec{H}_\nu(q_0,g_0,\ldots,q_n,g_n,æ_\nu,x)\,e^{j(\omega t-\beta_\nu z)}\end{aligned}\quad(4.22)$$

These vectors satisfied Maxwell's equations:

$$\Delta_t\times\vec{H}_\nu\,(q_0,g_0,\ldots,q_n,g_n,æ_\nu,x)-j\beta_\nu\left[\vec{k}\times\vec{H}_\nu(q_0,g_0,\ldots,q_n,g_n,æ_\nu,x)\right]$$

$$-j\omega\varepsilon_0\overleftrightarrow{\varepsilon}(q_0,q_1,\ldots,q_n,x)\vec{E}_\nu(q_0,g_0,\ldots,q_n,g_n,æ_\nu,x)=0,\quad(4.23)$$

$$\Delta_t\times\vec{E}_\nu(q_0,g_0,\ldots,q_n,g_n,æ_\nu,x)-j\beta_\nu\left[\vec{k}\times\vec{E}_\nu(q_0,g_0,\ldots,q_n,g_n,æ_\nu,x)\right]$$

$$+j\omega\mu_0\,\overleftrightarrow{\mu}(g_0,g_1,\ldots,g_n,x)\vec{H}_\nu(q_0,g_0,\ldots,q_n,g_n,æ_\nu,x)=0.\quad(4.24)$$

The electromagnetic field of the structure in our work was represented by the form of natural waves in the waveguide structure of comparison:

$$\vec{E} = \sum_{\nu=1}^{N} A_\nu\,(q_0, g_0, \ldots, q_n, g_n, z)\,\vec{E}_\nu^{(+)}\,(q_0, g_0, \ldots, q_n, g_n, æ_\nu, x)$$

$$+\sum_{\nu=1}^{N} B_\nu\,(q_0, g_0, \ldots, q_n, g_n, z)\,\vec{E}_\nu^{(-)}(q_0, g_0, \ldots, q_n, g_n, æ_\nu, x)$$

$$+\sum_{+}^{-}\int_0^{\infty} C(q_0, g_1, \ldots, q_n, g_n, \rho, z)\vec{E}(q_0, g_0, \ldots, q_n, g_n, \rho, x)d\rho,$$

$$\vec{H} = \sum_{\nu=1}^{N} A_\nu\,(q_0, g_0, \ldots, q_n, g_n, z)\,\vec{H}_\nu^{(+)}(q_0, g_0, \ldots, q_n, g_n, æ_\nu, x)$$

$$+\sum_{\nu=1}^{N} B_\nu(q_0, g_0, \ldots, q_n, g_n, z)\,\vec{H}_\nu^{(-)}(q_0, g_0, \ldots, q_n, g_n, æ_\nu, x)$$

$$+\sum_{-}^{+}\int_0^{\infty} C\,(q_0, g_0, \ldots, q_n, g_n, \rho, z) \times \vec{H}\,(q_0, g_0, \ldots, q_n, g_n, \rho, x)\,d\rho. \tag{4.25}$$

Natural waves of mixed spectrum in compositional waveguide had a form of magnetic and electric modes. They had respectively components $H_{x\upsilon}, H_{z\upsilon}, E_{y\upsilon}$; $H_{y\upsilon}, E_{x\upsilon}, E_{z\upsilon}$. Transverse and longitudinal wavenumbers (e.g. TE-waves) satisfied the dispersion equation in the form of:

$$\begin{vmatrix} \Theta_1 & \Theta_2 & -\Theta_3 & 0 \\ \Theta_4 & \Theta_5 & -\Theta_6 & 0 \\ \Theta_7 & \Theta_8 & 0 & \Theta_9 \\ \Theta_{10} & \Theta_{11} & 0 & \Theta_{12} \end{vmatrix} = 0, \tag{4.26}$$

where specific components will be:

$$\Theta_1 = Q_1(q_0, g_0, \ldots, q_n, g_n, æ, 1), \quad \Theta_2 = Q_2(q_0, g_0, \ldots, q_n, g_n, æ, 1), \quad \Theta_3 = \exp(-\gamma),$$

$$\Theta_4 = \frac{\psi'_{1,x}(q_0, g_0, \ldots, q_n, g_n, æ, 1)}{\mu_{zz}(g_0, g_1, \ldots, g_n, 1)}, \quad \Theta_5 = \frac{\psi^{|}_{2,x}(q_0, g_0, \ldots, q_n, g_n, æ, 1)}{\mu_{zz}(g_0, g_1, \ldots, g_n, 1)}, \quad \Theta_6 = \frac{\gamma\exp(-\gamma)}{\mu_3},$$

$$\Theta_7 = Q_1(q_0, g_0, \ldots, q_n, g_n, æ, -1), \quad \Theta_8 = Q_2(q_0, g_0, \ldots, q_n, g_n, æ, -1),$$

$$\Theta_9 = \exp(-\chi), \quad Q_{10} = \frac{Q'_{1,x}(q_0, g_0, \ldots, q_n, g_n, æ, -1)}{\mu_{zz}(g_0, g_1, \ldots, g_n, -1)},$$

$$\Theta_{11} = \frac{Q'_{2,x}\,(q_0, g_0, \ldots, q_n, g_n, æ, -1)}{\mu_{zz}(g_0, g_1, \ldots, g_n, -1)}, \quad \Theta_{12} = \frac{\chi\exp(-\chi)}{\mu_2},$$

All functions $Q_{1(2)}(q_0, q_0, \ldots, q_n, q_n, æ, x)$ are special wave solutions of wave equations in the wave guiding layer, and $æ, \gamma, \chi$ – transverse wave numbers covering the central layer and the substrate; $q_0, g_0, \ldots, q_n, g_n$ – the parameters of the spatial gradient profiles elements tensors permittivity and permeability.

To simplify these calculations, we left only the first terms in the Equations (4.25), (4.26). Substitution complete fields (4.25), (4.26) in the Maxwell's equations and the following simple transformation leads to the following equations:

$$\frac{\partial \mathrm{A}_\nu\left(q_0,g_0,\ldots,q_n,g_n,z\right)}{\partial z}\left[\vec{\kappa}\times\vec{\mathrm{H}}_\nu^{(+)}\left(q_0,g_0,\ldots,q_n,g_n,æ_\nu,x\right)\right]$$
$$-j\omega\Delta\vec{\varepsilon}\left(q_0,q_1,\ldots,q_n,x\right)\mathrm{A}_\nu\left(q_0,g_0,\ldots,q_n,g_n,z\right)\vec{\mathrm{E}}_\nu^{(+)}\left(q_0,g_0,\ldots,q_n,g_n,æ_\nu,x\right)$$
$$+\frac{\partial\,\mathrm{B}_\nu\left(q_0,g_0,\ldots,q_n,g_n,z\right)}{\partial z}\left[\vec{\kappa}\times\vec{\mathrm{H}}_\nu^{(-)}\left(q_0,g_0,\ldots,q_n,g_n,æ_\nu,x\right)\right]$$
$$-j\omega\Delta\vec{\varepsilon}\left(q_0,q_1,\ldots,q_n,x\right)\mathrm{B}_\nu\left(q_0,g_0,\ldots,q_n,g_n,z\right)\cdot\vec{\mathrm{E}}_\nu^{(-)}\left(q_0,g_0,\ldots,q_n,g_n,æ_\nu,x\right)=0, \quad (4.27)$$

$$\frac{\partial \mathrm{A}_\nu\left(q_0,g_0,\ldots,q_n,g_n,z\right)}{\partial z}\left[\vec{\kappa}\times\vec{\mathrm{E}}_\nu^{(+)}\left(q_0,g_0,\ldots,q_n,g_n,æ_\nu,x\right)\right]$$
$$+j\omega\Delta\vec{\mu}\left(g_0,g_1,\ldots,g_n,x\right)\mathrm{A}_\nu\left(q_0,g_0,\ldots,q_n,g_n,z\right)\vec{\mathrm{H}}_\nu^{(+)}\left(q_0,g_0,\ldots,q_n,g_n,æ_\nu,x\right)$$
$$+\frac{\partial\,\mathrm{B}_\nu\left(q_0,g_0,\ldots,q_n,g_n,z\right)}{\partial z}\left[\vec{\kappa}\times\vec{\mathrm{E}}_\nu^{(-)}\left(q_0,g_0,\ldots,q_n,g_n,æ_\nu,x\right)\right]$$
$$+j\omega\Delta\vec{\mu}\left(g_0,g_1,\ldots,g_n,x\right)\mathrm{B}_\nu\left(q_0,g_0,\ldots,q_n,g_n,z\right)\cdot\vec{\mathrm{H}}_\nu^{(-)}\left(q_0,g_0,\ldots,q_n,g_n,æ_\nu,x\right)=0. \quad (4.28)$$

Multiplying the Equation (4.27), (4.28) on complex conjugate electric and magnetic fields, subtracting one equation from the other, and then integrating the resulting equation over an infinite cross-section we obtained the following system of coupled equations for the amplitudes of the waves complete orthonormal system of waves of a mixed spectrum of the compositional structure:

$$\frac{\partial \mathrm{A}_\ell\left(q_0,g_0,\ldots,q_n,g_nz\right)}{\partial z}=-j\kappa_0\sum\mathrm{A}_\nu\left(q_0,g_0,\ldots,q_n,g_n,z\right)$$
$$\cdot\,\Phi_{\ell\nu}(q_0,g_0,\ldots,q_n,g_n,æ_\lambda,æ_\nu,x)\exp(j\Delta\beta_{\lambda\nu})z$$
$$-j\kappa_o\sum_\nu\mathrm{A}_\nu(q_0,g_0,\ldots,q_n,g_n,z)\cdot F_{\lambda\nu}(q_0,g_0,\ldots,q_n,g_n,æ_\lambda,æ_\nu,x)\exp(j\Delta\beta_{\lambda\nu}z)$$
$$-j\kappa_o\sum_\nu\mathrm{B}_\nu(q_0,g_0,\ldots,q_n,g_n,z)\cdot\mathrm{P}_{\lambda\nu}(q_0,g_0,\ldots,q_n,g_n,æ_\lambda,æ_\nu,x)\exp(j\tilde{\Delta}\beta_{\lambda\nu}z)$$
$$-j\kappa_o\sum_\nu\mathrm{B}_\nu(q_0,g_0,\ldots,q_n,g_n,z)U_{\lambda\nu}(q_0,g_0,\ldots,q_n,g_n,æ_\lambda,æ_\nu,x)\cdot\exp(j\tilde{\Delta}\beta_\nu z) \quad (4.29)$$

$$\frac{\partial \mathrm{B}_\lambda\left(q_0,g_0,\ldots,q_n,g_n,z\right)}{\partial z}=j\kappa_o\sum_\nu\mathrm{A}_\nu\left(q_0,g_0,\ldots,q_n,g_n,z\right)$$
$$\cdot\,Z_{\lambda\nu}\left(q_0,g_0,\ldots,q_n,g_n,æ_\lambda,æ_\nu,z\right)\exp(-j\tilde{\Delta}\beta_{\lambda\nu}z)+j\kappa_o\sum_\nu\mathrm{A}_\nu\left(q_0,g_0,\ldots,q_n,g_n,z\right)$$
$$\cdot\,L_{\lambda\nu}\left(q_0,g_0,\ldots,q_n,g_n,æ_\lambda,æ_\nu,x\right)\cdot\exp(-j\tilde{\Delta}\beta_{\lambda\nu}z)$$
$$+j\kappa_o\sum_\nu\mathrm{B}_\nu\left(q_0,g_0,\ldots,q_n,g_n,z\right)\cdot V_{\lambda\nu}(q_0,g_0,\ldots,q_n,g_n,æ_\lambda,æ_\nu,x)\exp(-j\Delta\beta_{\lambda\nu},z)$$
$$+j\kappa_o\sum_\nu\mathrm{B}_\nu\left(q_0,g_0,\ldots,q_n,g_n,z\right)\cdot W_{\lambda\nu}(q_0,g_0,\ldots,q_n,g_n,æ_\lambda,æ_\nu,x)\exp(-j\Delta\beta_{\lambda\nu}z),$$

where some of the terms describing the features of the interaction of the discrete spectrum of waves can be represented:

$$\Phi_{\lambda\nu}(q_0, g_0, \ldots, q_n, g_n, æ_\lambda, æ_\nu, x) = \Psi_{\lambda\nu}(q_0, g_0, \ldots, q_n, g_n, æ_\lambda, æ_\nu, x)$$
$$+ G_{\lambda\nu}(q_0, g_0, \ldots, q_n, g_n, æ_\lambda, æ_\nu, x) + R_{\lambda\nu}(q_0, g_0, \ldots, q_n, g_n, æ_\lambda, æ_\nu, x)$$
$$+ S_{\lambda\nu}(q_0, g_0, \ldots, q_n, g_n, æ_\lambda, æ_\nu, x)$$

$$\Phi_{\lambda\nu}(q_0, g_0, \ldots, q_n, g_n, æ_\lambda, æ_\nu, x) = \Psi_{\lambda\nu}(q_0, g_0, \ldots, q_n, g_n, æ_\lambda, æ_\nu, x)$$
$$+ G_{\lambda\nu}(q_0, g_0, \ldots, q_n, g_n, æ_\lambda, æ_\nu, x) + R_{\lambda\nu}(q_0, g_0, \ldots, q_n, g_n, æ_\lambda, æ_\nu, x)$$
$$+ S_{\lambda\nu}(q_0, g_0, \ldots, q_n, g_n, æ_\lambda, æ_\nu, x)$$

$$\Psi_{\ell\nu}(q_0, g_0, \ldots, q_n, g_n, æ_\lambda, æ_\nu, x) = \int \big[\varepsilon_{yy}(q_0, q_1, \ldots, q_n, x) \cdot$$
$$\cdot E_{y\nu}(q_0, g_0, \ldots, q_n, g_n, æ_\nu, x) \cdot \mathrm{E}^*_{y\ell}(q_0, g_0, \ldots, q_n, g_n, æ_\lambda, x)$$
$$+ \varepsilon_{yz}(q_0, q_1, \ldots, q_n, x) \cdot \mathrm{E}_{z\nu}(q_0, g_0, \ldots, q_n, g_n, æ_\nu, x)$$
$$\cdot \mathrm{E}^*_{y\ell}(q_0, g_1, \ldots, q_n, g_n, æ_\lambda, x) + \varepsilon_{zy}(q_0, q_1, \ldots, q_n, x)$$
$$\cdot \mathrm{E}_{y\nu}(q_0, g_1, \ldots, q_n, g_n, æ_\nu, x) \cdot \mathrm{E}^*_{z\ell}(q_0, g_1, \ldots, q_n, g_n, æ_\lambda, x)$$
$$+ \varepsilon_{zz}(q_0, q_1, \ldots, q_n, x)\, \mathrm{E}_{z\nu}(q_0, g_0, \ldots, q_n, g_n, æ_\nu, x)\, \mathrm{E}^*_{z\ell}(q_0, g_0, \ldots, q_n, g_n, æ_\nu, x)\big]\, dx$$

The system of coupled equations is the most common for the case of gradient bianisotropic waveguide structures. As a result, we can investigate the transformation of co- and counter-waves in non-classical discrete and continuous parts of the wave spectrum using (4.29). Further growth of the transverse dimensions leads to an increase in wave reflection and emissivity of the structure. For different values of the thickness of the waveguide layer coefficient of the discrete spectrum of a wave, reflection can be both larger and smaller than the waves reflection coefficient in a uniform structure. When the transverse dimensions of the waveguide layer are taken sufficiently large value, the reflectance of the magnetic and electric waves homogeneous and composite structures tends to Fresnel.

4.3 THE RESEARCH OF HAEMOGLOBIN IN BLOOD

The study of various biological fluids at the moment is a very intensively developing field of medicine. Advanced experimental work is devoted to the study of the dispersion of radiation in the optical range in solutions of haemoglobin and whole blood. Of particular interest are the magnetic properties of haemoglobins. The solution of haemoglobin is a magnetic fluid with a magnetic moment $\mu \sim 5 \div 6\mu_B(\mu_B$ – Bohr magneton). In most papers in this area, there is no account of the appearance of a uniaxial optical activity induced by a magnetic field, which affects the rotation of the plane of polarization of light propagating through the solution (Harris et al. 1999)

The structure of haemoglobin determines the optical activity of the solution, which can be qualitatively estimated by molecular anisotropy. This paper is devoted to theoretical studies of uniaxial optical activity of haemoglobin solutions of certain conformations induced by electromagnetic field.

The induced optical activity is a function of the frequency of the incident electromagnetic wave and two angles that determine the orientation of the molecule with respect to the direction of propagation of the wave. The inhomogeneity of the electromagnetic fields leads to considerable spatial dispersion and gradient anisotropy of the optical properties. The tensors of the dielectric, magnetic, and magneto-electric permeability thus become functions of the coordinates.

The spatial gradient of material characteristics can be caused by a continuous change in one of the physical parameters that determines the nature of the waveguiding medium. In haemoglobin, in this case a functional dependence of the polarization vector on the direction arises; a similar behaviour is observed for the magnetic moment (Kireeva & Rudenok 2017). Individual properties of the interaction of solutions of haemoglobin and whole blood with optical radiation are determined to a greater extent by their band structure, and also impurities, the method of excitation, temperature, etc. play an important role.

The fundamental optical characteristics of the spectra (the generalized tensor of the complex dielectric permittivity) are dictated by the width of the forbidden band, the structure and mutual arrangement in the momentum space of the extrema of the upper valence band and the lower conduction band, and the effective masses of electrons and holes. Also the form of zones and energy levels for solutions with a small number of atoms in the region of extremum.

Despite significant progress in the study of various biological fluids, little work has been devoted to the propagation of hybrid surface waves in them. Analysis of the discrete spectrum of optical waves in haemoglobin samples of the type considered is carried out for its mathematical model in the form of a homogeneous isotropic medium and individual particular cases of orientation of the principal axes of the dielectric permittivity tensor with respect to the x, y, z axes related to the geometry of the waveguiding sample (Harris et al. 1999)

There are also a number of experimental results on the investigation of dielectric and magnetic permeability and optical anisotropy of haemoglobin solutions (Kireeva & Rudenok 2017)

To determine the magnitude of the haemoglobin solution arising under the action of the uniaxial anisotropy field in the present paper, the author analysed the longitudinal wave numbers of surface waves for the general case of an arbitrary orientation of the principal axes of the tensor when the hybrid waves are the own waves of the mixed spectrum. Based on the results obtained, the angular dependence of the discrete spectrum of modes for a number of sample parameters is calculated.

In our work we presented an analysis of the longitudinal wave numbers of surface waves in gradient of haemoglobin for the general case of an arbitrary orientation of the principal axes of the tensor, when the hybrid waves are the own waves of the mixed spectrum. The angular dependence for the discrete spectrum in the haemoglobin was calculated using previous results.

We considered a transparent layer in blood, in which the elements of the dielectric permittivity tensor smoothly vary in thickness along the transverse coordinate x. We assumed that the waveguide layer is surrounded by a coating and a substrate characterized by scalar permittivity and magnetic permeability $\varepsilon_1, \mu_1, \varepsilon_3, \mu_3$. The magnetic permeability of haemoglobin was assumed to be scalar and equal to μ_2.

Then we supposed that the electromagnetic waves of the discrete spectrum propagated along the z coordinate. Amplitudes of electric and magnetic fields did not depend on the transverse coordinate y. We took a gradient anisotropic waveguide with a dielectric constant tensor whose main axes coincide with the coordinate axes $\overleftrightarrow{\varepsilon}_{э}(q_0, q_1, \ldots, q_n, x)$ from (Harris et al. 1999) as a reference waveguide structure and $q_0, q_1, \ldots, q_n$ were the parameters of the gradient of the spatial profiles for its elements.

Then the anisotropy of the dielectric constant of the structure under consideration can be represented as follows:

$$\varepsilon_{ij}(q_0, q_1, \ldots, q_n, x) = \varepsilon_{ii,э}(q_0, q_1, \ldots, q_n, x) + \overset{\vee}{\varepsilon}_{ij}(q_0, q_1, \ldots, q_n, x), \tag{4.30}$$

where $\varepsilon_{ii,э}(q_0, q_1, \ldots, q_n, x)$, $\overset{\vee}{\varepsilon}_{ij}(q_0, q_1, \ldots, q_n, x)$ – components of the permittivity tensors of the reference structure and the additive term. In practical applications we usually use $\overset{\vee}{\varepsilon}_{ij}(q_0, q_1, \ldots, q_n, x)$ by two, three orders of magnitude less than the first term, so that in what follows we shall denote terms of the second order of smallness in correlation with $\varepsilon_{ii,э}(q_0, q_1, \ldots, q_n, x)$.

Taking into account the completeness of the system of electric and magnetic surface waves of the discrete spectrum (without taking into account the pseudosurface waves of the continuous spectrum) of the reference waveguide, we represented the electric and magnetic field vectors of the haemoglobin under consideration as follows:

$$\vec{E} = \sum_{\nu} A_{\nu}(q_0, q_1, \ldots, q_n, z)\, \vec{E}_{\nu}^{(+)}(q_0, q_1, \ldots, q_n, æ_{\nu}, x) \exp\left[j(\omega t - \gamma_{\nu} z)\right]$$
$$+ \sum_{\nu} B_{\nu}(q_0, q_1, \ldots, q_n, z)\, \vec{E}_{\nu}^{(-)}(q_0, q_1, \ldots, q_n, æ_{\nu}, x) \exp\left[j(\omega t - \gamma_{\nu} z)\right]. \quad (4.31)$$

$$\vec{H} = \sum_{\nu} A_{\nu}(q_0, q_1, \ldots, q_n, z)\, \vec{H}_{\nu}^{(+)}(q_0, q_1, \ldots, q_n, æ_{\nu}, x)$$
$$+ \sum_{\nu} B_{\nu}(q_0, q_1, \ldots, q_n, z)\, \vec{H}_{\nu}^{(-)}(q_0, q_1, \ldots, q_n, æ_{\nu}, x)\,. \quad (4.32)$$

where $æ_{\nu}, \gamma_{\nu}$ – transverse and longitudinal wave numbers, ω – circular frequency, $\vec{E}_{\nu}^{(\pm)}(q_0, q_1, \ldots, q_n, æ_{\nu}, x)$, $\vec{H}_{\nu}^{(\pm)}(q_0, q_1, \ldots, q_n, æ_{\nu}, x)$ – electric and magnetic vectors of forward and backward surface waves of the reference structure (Harris et al. 1999), $A_{\nu}(q_0, q_1, \ldots, q_n, z)$, $B_{\nu}(q_0, q_1, \ldots, q_n, z)$ – their amplitude coefficients.

Substituting the representations (4.30)–(4.32) into Maxwell's equations, then multiplying the resulting equations by the complex conjugate expressions for the direct and inverse electric and magnetic waves and subtracting one from the other while integrating over the cross section of the open structure, we obtained a system of coupled integro-differential equations with respect to amplitude coefficients (Ivanov & Shuty 2007).

We took into account the unidirectional electric and magnetic waves of the discrete spectrum of the reference structure with transverse wave numbers $æ_{\nu}$, $æ_{\mu}$. So a characteristic for the hybrid waves in the haemoglobin solution were found in the following form:

$$\vec{E}_{\Gamma}(q_0, q_1, \ldots, q_n, æ_{\Gamma}, z) = \vec{E}_{э\mu\nu}\left(q_0, q_1, \ldots, q_n, æ_{\mu}, æ_{\nu}, z\right) A_{\nu}(q_0, q_1, \ldots, q_n, z)\,, \quad (4.33)$$

where the matrices of the electric and amplitude vectors:

$$\vec{E}_{э\mu\nu}\left(q_0, q_1, \ldots, q_n, æ_{\mu}, æ_{\nu}, z\right) = \vec{E}_{э\mu}\left(q_0, q_1, \ldots, q_n, æ_{\mu}, z\right) \vec{E}_{э\nu}\left(q_0, q_1, \ldots, q_n, æ_{\mu}, æ_{\nu}, z\right), \quad (4.34)$$

$$A_{\nu}(q_0, q_1, \ldots, q_n, z) = \begin{bmatrix} T_0(q_0, q_1, \ldots, q_n, z) \\ T_1(q_0, q_1, \ldots, q_n, z) \end{bmatrix}. \quad (4.35)$$

$\vec{E}_{э\mu}\left(q_0, q_1, \ldots, q_n, æ_{\mu}, z\right)$, $\vec{E}_{э\nu}\left(q_0, q_1, \ldots, q_n, æ_{\mu}, æ_{\nu}, z\right)$ – electric fields and electric waves of the reference structure. In this case for the amplitude vector-row we used an expression $A_{\nu}(q_0, q_1, \ldots, q_n, z)$. From the system of integro-differential equations (Hanson 2008) we obtained equations of the form:

$$\frac{d\vec{A}(q_0, q_1, \ldots, q_n, z)}{dz}$$
$$= -j \begin{bmatrix} \gamma_{\mu} + \Delta\gamma_{\mu}(q_0, q_1, \ldots, q_n) & K_{\mu\nu}(q_0, q_1, \ldots, q_n) \\ K_{\mu\nu}^{*}(q_0, q_1, \ldots, q_n) & \gamma_{\nu} + \Delta\gamma_{\nu}(q_0, q_1, \ldots, q_n) \end{bmatrix} \vec{A}(q_0, q_1, \ldots, q_n, z). \quad (4.36)$$

Its general solution in the simplest form consists of vectors with exponential factors of the form:

$$\vec{A}_0 \exp\left\{-j\left[\overset{\vee}{\gamma}_{\mu\nu} - \theta_{\mu\nu}(q_0, q_1, \ldots, q_n)\right]\right\}, \quad (4.37)$$

$$\vec{A}_0 \exp\left\{-j\left[\overset{\vee}{\gamma}_{\mu\nu} - \theta_{\mu\nu}(q_0, q_1, \ldots, q_n)\right]\right\}, \quad (4.38)$$

and

$$\vec{A}_0 = \begin{bmatrix} \dfrac{K_{\mu\nu}(q_0, q_1, \ldots, q_n)}{\theta_{\mu\nu}(q_0, q_1, \ldots, q_n) + \Delta_{\mu\nu}(q_0, q_1, \ldots, q_n)} \\ 1 \end{bmatrix}, \quad (4.39)$$

$$\vec{A}_1 = \begin{bmatrix} 1 \\ \dfrac{K^*_{\mu\nu}(q_0, q_1, \ldots, q_n)}{\theta_{\mu\nu}(q_0, q_1, \ldots, q_n) + \Delta_{\mu\nu}(q_0, q_1, \ldots, q_n)} \end{bmatrix}. \tag{4.40}$$

Using the equality (4.33), we obtained the electric vector for the hybrid modes in the following form:

$$\vec{E}_\alpha(q_0, q_1, \ldots, q_n, \gamma_\alpha, x, z) = \left\{ \frac{\vec{E}_\nu(q_0,q_1,\ldots,q_n,æ_\nu,x)\left[\theta_{\mu\nu}(q_0,q_1,\ldots,q_n)+\Delta_{\mu\nu}(q_0,q_1,\ldots,q_n)-K_{\mu\nu}(q_0,q_1,\ldots,q_n)\right]-K_{\mu\nu}(q_0,q_1,\ldots,q_n)\vec{E}_\mu(q_0,q_1,\ldots,q_n,æ_\mu,x)}{\theta_{\mu\nu}(q_0,q_1,\ldots,q_n)+\Delta_{\mu\nu}(q_0,q_1,\ldots,q_n)} \right\} \exp(-j\gamma_\alpha z), \tag{4.41}$$

$$\vec{E}_{\alpha+1}(q_0, q_1, \ldots, q_n, \gamma_{\alpha+1}, x, z) = \left\{ \frac{\vec{E}_\mu(q_0,q_1,\ldots,q_n,æ_\mu,x)\left[\theta_{\mu\nu}(q_0,q_1,\ldots,q_n)+\Delta_{\mu\nu}(q_0,q_1,\ldots,q_n)\right]+K_{\mu\nu}(q_0,q_1,\ldots,q_n)\vec{E}_\nu(q_0,q_1,\ldots,q_n,æ_\nu,x)}{\theta_{\mu\nu}(q_0,q_1,\ldots,q_n)+\Delta_{\mu\nu}(q_0,q_1,\ldots,q_n)} \right\} \exp(-j\gamma_{\alpha+1} z), \tag{4.42}$$

$$\gamma_\alpha = \frac{1}{2}\gamma_\nu + \frac{\Delta\gamma_\nu(q_0, q_1, \ldots, q_n)}{2} + \frac{1}{2}\gamma_\mu + \frac{\Delta\gamma_\mu(q_0, q_1, \ldots, q_n)}{2} - \theta_{\mu\nu}(q_0, q_1, \ldots, q_n), \tag{4.43}$$

$$\gamma_{\alpha+1} = \frac{\gamma_\nu + \gamma_\mu}{2} + \frac{\Delta\gamma_\nu(q_0, q_1, \ldots, q_n)}{2} + \theta_{\mu\nu}(q_0, q_1, \ldots, q_n). \tag{4.44}$$

Thus, the intrinsic hybrid surface waves of a haemoglobin have three transverse and longitudinal components of the electric and magnetic fields, which are more conveniently represented through electric and magnetic waves of the reference structure (cross-sectional functions):

$$E_{x\alpha}(q_0, q_1, \ldots, q_n, æ_\alpha, x) = -\frac{K_{\mu\nu}(q_0, q_1, \ldots, q_n)E_{x\mu}(q_0, q_1, \ldots, q_n, æ_\mu, x)}{\theta_{\mu\nu}(q_0, q_1, \ldots, q_n) + \Delta_{\mu\nu}(q_0, q_1, \ldots, q_n)}, \tag{4.45}$$

$$E_{y\alpha}(q_0, q_1, \ldots, q_n, æ_\alpha, x) = E_{y\nu}(q_0, q_1, \ldots, q_n, æ_\nu, x), \tag{4.46}$$

$$E_{z\alpha}(q_0, q_1, \ldots, q_n, æ_\alpha, x) = -\frac{K_{\mu\nu}(q_0, q_1, \ldots, q_n)E_{z\mu}(q_0, q_1, \ldots, q_n, æ_\mu, x)}{\theta_{\mu\nu}(q_0, q_1, \ldots, q_n) + \Delta_{\mu\nu}(q_0, q_1, \ldots, q_n)}, \tag{4.47}$$

$$E_{x(\alpha+1)}(q_0, q_1, \ldots, q_n, æ_{\alpha+1}, x) = E_{x\mu}(q_0, q_1, \ldots, q_n, æ_\mu, x), \tag{4.48}$$

$$E_{y(\alpha+1)}(q_0, q_1, \ldots, q_n, æ_{\alpha+1}, x) = -\frac{K_{\mu\nu}(q_0, q_1, \ldots, q_n)E_{y\nu}(q_0, q_1, \ldots, q_n, æ_\nu, x)}{\theta_{\mu\nu}(q_0, q_1, \ldots, q_n) + \Delta_{\mu\nu}(q_0, q_1, \ldots, q_n)}, \tag{4.49}$$

$$E_{z(\alpha+1)}(q_0, q_1, \ldots, q_n, æ_{\alpha+1}, x) = E_{z\mu}(q_0, q_1, \ldots, q_n, æ_\mu, x). \tag{4.50}$$

Then the magnetic vectors of asymmetrical waves can be represented as follows:

$$\vec{H}_\alpha(q_0, q_1, \ldots, q_n, \gamma_\alpha, x) = \left\{H_{x\alpha}(q_0, q_1, \ldots, q_n, æ_\alpha, x), H_{y\alpha}(q_0, q_1, \ldots, q_n, æ_\alpha, x), H_{z\alpha}(q_0, q_1, \ldots, q_n, æ_\alpha, x)\right\} \tag{4.51}$$

$$\vec{H}_{\alpha+1}(q_0, q_1, \ldots, q_n, \gamma_{\alpha+1}, x) = \left\{H_{x(\alpha+1)}(q_0, q_1, \ldots, q_n, æ_{\alpha+1}, x), H_{y(\alpha+1)}(q_0, q_1, \ldots, q_n, æ_{(\alpha+1)}, x), H_{z(\alpha+1)}(q_0, q_1, \ldots, q_n, æ_{(\alpha+1)}, x)\right\} \tag{4.52}$$

As an example, the dependence of the longitudinal wave numbers of the first hybrid modes on the angle φ between the optical axis and the wave propagation direction for haemoglobin was calculated. Elements of the permittivity tensor, distributed according to the biquadratic law, were represented as: $\varepsilon_{xx}(q_2, q_4, x) = \check{\varepsilon}_{xy}(q_2, q_4, x) = \check{\varepsilon}_{xz}(q_2, q_4, x) = \check{\varepsilon}_{yx}(q_2, q_4, x) = \check{\varepsilon}_{zx}(q_2, q_4, x) = 0$,

$$\check{\varepsilon}_{yy}(q_2, q_4, x) = [\varepsilon_H(q_2, q_4, x) - \varepsilon_0(q_2, q_4, x)]\sin^2\phi, \tag{4.53}$$

$$\check{\varepsilon}_{yz}(q_2, q_4, x) = \check{\varepsilon}_{zy}(q_2, q_4, x) = [\varepsilon_H(q_2, q_4, x) - \varepsilon_0(q_2, q_4, x)]\sin\phi\cos\phi, \tag{4.54}$$

$$\overset{\vee}{\varepsilon}_{zz}(q_2,q_4,x) = [\varepsilon_H(q_2,q_4,x) - \varepsilon_0(q_2,q_4,x)]\cos^2\phi, \tag{4.55}$$

$$\varepsilon_0(q_2,q_4,x) = \varepsilon_{xx}(q_2,q_4,x) = \varepsilon_{yy}(q_2,q_4,x) = \varepsilon_{m,0} + \varepsilon_{n,\text{н}}\left(1 - q_2x^2 + q_4x^4\right), \tag{4.56}$$

$$\varepsilon_H(q_2,q_4,x) = \varepsilon_{zz}(q_2,q_4,x) + \varepsilon_{m,\text{г}} + \varepsilon_{\text{н},\text{г}}\left(1 - q_2x^2 + q_4x^4\right). \tag{4.57}$$

Here we took into account the fact that the optical axis lies in the plane *yz* of the structure.

The gradient parts of the dielectric permittivity profiles of the electric and magnetic modes of the reference composition structure depend on the angle φ. At the investigated angles φ the spatial distributions were restored $\varepsilon_{\text{н}}(x)$ and $\varepsilon_0(x)$. As an example, Figure 4.1 shows the dependence of the longitudinal wave numbers of the first hybrid modes on the angle φ for various parameters of the gradient of the spatial profiles of the elements of the permittivity tensor in the compositional haemoglobin solution.

4.4 CONCLUSIONS

It is clear from them that the degree of dependence of the longitudinal wave numbers for the hybrid modes on the angle φ is determined by the comparative composition of the ordinary and extraordinary modes of the discrete spectrum in them for the waveguide structure of comparison. It can be shown from Equations (4.31)–(4.32) that γ of the hybrid mode, which is formed mainly by extraordinary waves, decreases monotonically with an increasing of an angle φ.

This is mainly due to the fact that the surface of the change in the elements of the permittivity tensor $\varepsilon_H(q_2,q_4,x)$ was a rotational ellipsoid with variable semiaxes. If the modes of the haemoglobin solid prevail in the composition, then the angular dependence is much weaker, since the surface of the variation of the corresponding elements of the tensor $\overleftrightarrow{\varepsilon}$ is a sphere with a varying radius and is determined only by the gradient of the anisotropy of the artificial internal environment of the structure. It is clear from Figure 4.1 that when the angle φ and the gradient parameters are varied, the curves of the variation of the longitudinal wave numbers of the hybrid modes $HE_{\mu\nu}$, $EH_{\mu\nu}$ both with the same and with different indices ν, μ can intersect, that is, in certain directions of mode propagation. So we noted the fact that an effective transformation of the intrinsic hybrid modes of the haemoglobin film is possible. We proved in our results that it is possible to increase the accuracy of determining the composition and concentration of haemoglobin in the blood.

We defined differential equation in partial derivatives of a special kind and found its solution in the layer using the integral transformation for Fourier-image of the field. Then we studied the asymptotic behaviour of the particular solutions at infinity. On the basis of this we determined Fourier transforms of the falling and the reflected wave beams. An integral equation for the electromagnetic field in the Fourier transform of the nonlinear media for the conditions of continuity of the tangential component of the electric and magnetic vectors was obtained. It gave us the possibility to take into account the effect of dependence between the complexity of the non-linear waveguide medium, and the parameters, and characteristics of the reflected optical beam.

However, the assessment of the limits of applicability of this approach involves obtaining higher approximations for the solution of the integral equation of the field. We used an approximate distribution of variables, which were based on the special characteristics and structure conditions of the falling laser beam. For example, we have taken into account an effective variation of the waves with infinite phase front entering into the wave vector. Then slowly varying amplitude was defined from the expression of the Fourier transform of the reflected beam. Then we simplified the integral operator using the partial integration of the transverse and longitudinal wavenumbers. And differentiating it for the longitudinal coordinate, we got the special differential equation for the amplitudes of modes of discrete wave spectrum in the constructed beam.

Considering the extreme solutions of the equation, we obtained an algebraic equation. It may have one or three real roots, depending on the structure of the equation.

$$\overset{\vee}{\varepsilon} = \frac{\varepsilon_{\text{н}}}{\varepsilon_{0,m}} = 0,931,\ \overset{\vee}{\varepsilon}_1 = \frac{\varepsilon_1}{\varepsilon_{0,m}} = 0,97,\ \overset{\vee}{\varepsilon}_3 = \frac{\varepsilon_3}{\varepsilon_{0,m}} = 0,9804;$$

$$1 - q_2 = q_4 = 0; \quad 2 - q_2 = 6\cdot 10^{-2}, q_4 = 36\cdot 10^{-4}; \quad 3 - q_2 = 10^{-2}; \quad q_4 = 10^{-4}.$$

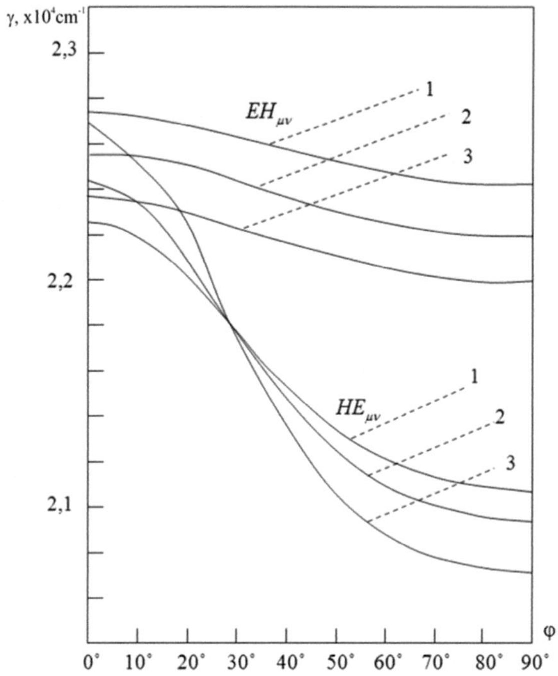

Figure 4.1. The dependence for the longitudinal wavenumber of the first hybrid modes in the haemoglobin film on the angle φ for various parameters of the gradient profiles of the elements of the permittivity tensor.

Taking into account the decisions of Cardano, we determined the conditions of existence of the three roots. Our choice of the solutions was based on Tikhonov's theorem. So we took into consideration those of the solutions, which were asymptotically stable. Choosing a solution was dependent on the proximity of the initial conditions to a specific branch of solutions. Modal solution of the equation for the incident beams of Gaussian and stepped profiles also were considered for verification.

A blood sample was placed on the substrate underneath the glass, and the process of propagation of optical radiation in it was examined. External glasses have constant relative magneto-dielectric permittivities. The sample clearly had the anisotropy of the optical properties. We observed, how far the light wave has deviated during its propagation in the investigated medium from the optical axis. We determined the level of the haemoglobin in solute basing the uniaxial anisotropy, which aroused under the optical radiation. We carried out an analysis of the longitudinal wave numbers of surface waves when the hybrid waves are the own waves of the mixed spectrum. We defined an angular dependence of the discrete spectrum of modes for a number of sample parameters based on the results, which were obtained.

REFERENCES

Arce-Diego, J. L., Pereda-Cubian, D. & Muriel, M. A., 2004. Polarization effects in short-and long-period fibre gratings: a generalized approach. *J. Opt. A.: Pure Appl. Opt.* 6(3): 45–51.

Chernozatonsky, L.A., Sorokin, P.B. & Artyukh, A.A. 2014. New nanostructures based on graphene: physical and chemical properties and applications. *Advances in Chemistry* 83(3): 251–279.

Fan, Z., et al. 2010. A three – dimensional corbon nanotube: grapheme sandwich and its application as electrode in supercapacitors. *Advanced Materials* 33: 3723–3728.

Gonzalez, J., Gtuinea, F. & Herrero, J. 2009. Propagating, evanescent, and localized states in carbon nanotube-graphene junctions. *Phys. Rev. B* 79(6): 165–434.

Hanson, G.W. 2008. Dyadic Green's functions and guided surface waves for a surface conductivity model of grapheme. *J. Appl. Phys.* 103:197–203.

Harris A., Kamien R.D. & Lubensky T. C. 1999. Molecular Chirality and Chiral Parameter. *Reviews of Modern Physics* 71(5): 1745–1757.

Ivanov, O.V. 2010. *The propagation of electromagnetic waves in anisotropic and bianisotropic layered structures.* Ulyanovsk: UlSTU publishing house.

Ivanov O.V. & Shuty A.M. 2007. Induced uniaxial optical activity of haemoglobin solutions in constant magnetic field. *Proc. SPIE* 6791: 679108.

Jagard, D.L. & Sun, X. 1992. Theory of chiral multilayers. *J. Opt. Soc. Am. A.* 9(5): 804–813.

Kalvach, A., & Szabó, Z. 2015. Isotropy analysis of metamaterials. *Informatyka, Automatyka, Pomiary w Gospodarce i Ochronie Srodowiska* 5(4): 52–54. https://doi.org/10.5604/20830157.1176576

Kireeva A.I. & Rudenok I.P. 2017. Some elements of investigation the transformation of surface and pseudosurface modes in an open asymmetric thin-film structure with a synthetic medium. *Proc. SPIE* 10466: 104662A.

Labunov, V.A. et al. 2010. Composite nanostructure of vertically aligned carbon nanotube array and planar graphite layer obtained by the injection CVD method. *Semiconductor Physics, Quantum Electronics and Opto-electronics* 13(2): 137–141.

Rao, Y. J., Zhu, T., Ran, Z. Ls., Wang, Y.P., Jiang, J. & Hu, A.Z. 2004. Novel long-period fiber gratings written by high freguency CO_2 laser pulses and applications in optical fiber. *Opt. Commun.* 229(1): 209–211.

Weiglhofer, W.S. 1998. A perspective of bianisotropy and bianisotropics. *Int. J. Appl. Electromagnetics and Mechanics* 9(2): 93–101.

CHAPTER 5

Metrological analysis of a neural network measuring system for medical purposes

O.A. Avdeyuk, Yu.P. Mukha & D.N. Avdeyuk
Volgograd State Technical University, Volgograd, Russian Federation
Volgograd State Medical University, Volgograd, Russian Federation

M.G. Skvortsov
Volgograd State Technical University, Volgograd, Russian Federation

Z. Omiotek, R. Dzierżak & M. Dzieńkowski
Lublin University of Technology, Lublin, Poland

A. Kozbakova
Institute of Information and Computational Technologies CS MES RK, Almaty, Kazakhstan
Almaty University of Power Engineering and Telecommunications, Almaty, Kazakhstan

ABSTRACT: The aim of our work was to make a metrological analysis of neural network measuring systems for diagnosing a person's condition. The approach methodology was based on the concept of the proposed class of measuring systems on neural networks for diagnosing of the state of complex objects. They are differ than the software (or software-hardware) implementation of the measuring system with the neural network environment, which is using at present time; considering a neural network as a super numerous channel measuring system; approach to the diagnosis of the state of the object as system measurements of the integral parameter; categorically-operational metrological description of neural network measuring functional converters. We proposed to consider neural networks as ordinary measuring instrument. The description of their operation can be form from the point of view of classical measurements with traditional metrological estimates. The procedure for bringing the neural network measurement methods to the classical ones is most constructed on the basis of formalisms of general algebra, graphs, theory of categories and functors, system and operational approaches. The metrological description of neural networks is based on a consistent description and analysis of measurement errors and their characteristics, which is formed from the accepted representation of the measurement procedure as a sequence of transformations of the input action. We presented some examples of the metrological analysis of neural network measuring systems for diagnosing a person's condition (acupuncture diagnostics of the bio-object condition, monitoring system of the main vital functions of a person). The categorical operational representation of the metrological description makes it possible to obtain traditional metrological estimates of the process of neural network measurements, to detail various types of errors in measuring transformations (for neurons, neuronal layers and measuring channels), to analyse the influence of the neural network structure on the measurement error, to perform the synthesis of neural network measuring systems with specified metrological characteristics. We can form a quantitative express diagnostics of internal organs, functional systems and the organism as a whole using neural network diagnostic system.

5.1 INTRODUCTION

A large number of modern objects (processes, phenomena) of research are complex systems (man, ecosystem and others), the determination of which is the primary task. Analysis of medical data and the formation of integrated assessments is the most actively developing area of modern medical diagnostics. The human body as an object of control is a complex system and differs in structural (hierarchical, multiply connected) and functional (nondeterminism and self-organisation of structure and connections) complexity. Correct control of a bio-object is possible only on the basis of a set of measured parameters that reflect its functional state. The condition of the body and the causes of its change are traditionally assessed by the totality of indicators (blood, urine, pressure, pulse, ECG). These indicators are formed under the influence of external and internal influences. Many authors did not take into account the contribution of biological objects of the body in the formation of the indicated set of different parameters.

A special feature of the task of assessing the functional state of bio-objects is a large amount of current data arriving in real time and requiring pre-processing. Existing difficulties in the implementation of many diagnostic methods arise due to the complex of the relationships between the measured values and the parameters for characterising of the condition of the bio-object (for example, the connection of Korotkov's measured tones with the parameters characterising blood pressure). Adequacy of the form of communication is established after the interpretation of the results of measurements on the formulated a priori mathematical model.

5.2 METHODOLOGY

The methodology of our approach was based on the description of the neural network as a measuring tool for the diagnosis of human condition, the category-operational metrological description of neural network measuring functional transformers, medical diagnostics by the integral parameter.

Currently, the actual task in medical diagnostics and scientific research is the applying of measuring systems on neural networks (MS/NN). The concept of the proposed MS/NN class (Mukha & Skvortsov 2007) for diagnosing of the condition of complex objects differs from the well-known neural network environment of software (or software-hardware) implementation of the measuring system. Because we considered a neural network as a supernumerous channel measuring system and approached to diagnosing of the condition of the object as system measurements of the integral parameter.

The methodology of developing of the neural network measuring systems includes a construction of a system function that is a function of the formation of a system state from the particular states of the elements of the system; a system functional converter for constructing of the scale of the integral parameter; a formation of the accepted standard of a norm for a condition of diagnosed object; a categorically-functorial description of the general synthesis of neural network measuring systems at the stages of their structural and parametric synthesis, functioning and training. We also carried out the stage of structural synthesis of neural network measuring transducers using the fractal neuron as the base one. We made quantitative estimation of the complexity of the synthesised structure and optimisation of the neuronal measuring converters (by functional realis-ability, inaccuracy, the number of interneuronal connections), channels and systems using the fractal dimension of the structure, which was represented in the form of a graph.

We concluded a metrological description (Tsvetkov 1992; Tsvetkov 2005) of neural network measuring systems by the definition and structuring of the total error of neural network converters (Mukha & Skvortsov 2007), the operationally-categorical description of errors at the stages of structural and parametric synthesis, the functioning and the training.

We used the following advantages of neural network technologies: the possibility of approximation using a limited set of data; work with incomplete and noisy data; flexible formation of the standard for training and autonomous selection of the standard for recognition; high parallelism, which ensures the work in real time mode; replacement of complex mathematical modeling with information modeling using the required amount of data, a nonlinear transformation function, and a given topology of the neural network; the ability of models to adapt. We provided a real-time mode by software and hardware implementation of the neural network measuring systems on the neural accelerator MC4.31 with neuro-chip NM 6403.

We proposed an approach (Mukha & Skvortsov 2007) for evaluation of the functional state of the body. This approach was based on the consideration of the functional state as a system reaction of the organism (interrelated hierarchical system) and the idea of systemic measurements of the integral

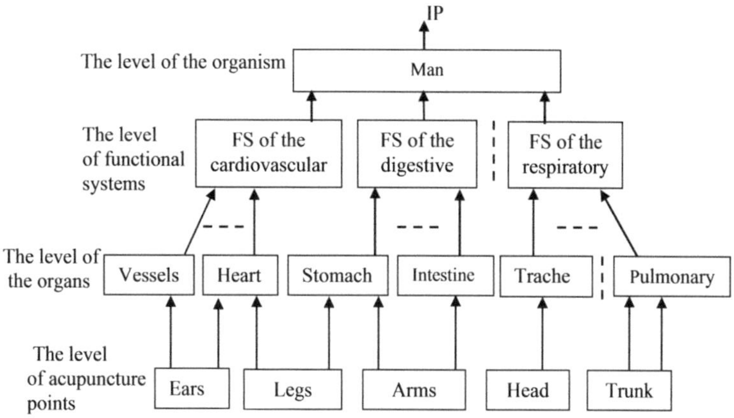

Figure 5.1. Hierarchical model of a bio-object.

parameter (with the formation of the hierarchical structure of the bio-object, the construction of the system function, integral parameters of each level of the hierarchy, joint registration and analysis of changes in diagnostic indicators at all levels of the hierarchy, taking into account the age, sex, weight of the patient).

We reduced the task of assessing of the state of an object to the construction of algorithms and functional mappings of a multidimensional space of parameters, which characterise a bio-object, into a one-dimensional space of estimates of its state. We defined the quantitative assessment of the general condition of the body (integral parameter) as the degree of deviation of the set of indicators of organs and functional systems of the body from normal indices. We needed to resolve the contradiction between the complexity of the problem of diagnosing an object in a modern setting and the limitations of the perception system of a physician, who makes decisions based on numerous results of medical measurements (no more than five to seven objects). That was our reason for constructing of an integral parameter (IP) for the functional state of an organism.

In solving the problems of information processing, the following requirements for measuring systems are advanced: information aggregation (transition from a large number of parameters to a small, in the limit to one, integral parameter); intellectualisation (the ability to select an expedient operation algorithm depending on the changing current tasks of measurement and control, input effects, an internal state); work with incomplete and contradictory information; transition to the receipt and use of not separate (point) values of the measured quantities, but of some set (fields) of the investigated quantities; the necessity to monitor all signals simultaneously and together.

Functions of neural network technology for assessing the state of a bio-object are: analysis of results (extraction of hidden dependencies between parameters); modelling of bio-objects, spatial-temporal characteristics of signals and investigated phenomena. So, we distinguished the following stages for the diagnostics of the bio-object condition: formalisation of the subject area (determination of the composition of the information base for constructing the NN model); building a system function and a hierarchical information model.

The hierarchical model of the bio-object, shown in Figure 5.1, is a four-level: the level of acupuncture points of the corresponding parts of the body; the level of internal organs; the level of functional systems (FS) by Anokhin P.K., with taking into account stasis regularities; the level of the organism as a whole.

To simulate the state of the corresponding bio-object, we used a neural network system functional converter (Mukha & Skvortsov 2007). The hierarchy of system functional transformations (SFC) that represent the hierarchical model of the bio-object was shown in Figure 5.2.

At the level of acupuncture points (the lower level of the hierarchy), the primary parameters for assessing the state of the object are formed as a result of acupuncture measurements. The state of the biologically active point reflects the functional state of the body organ. The system functional

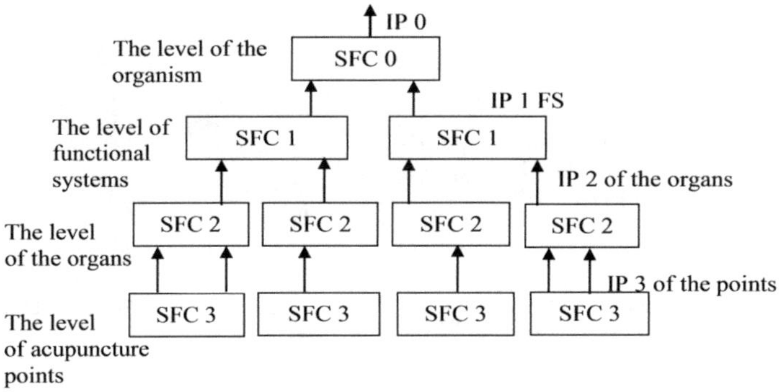

Figure 5.2. Hierarchy of the system functional transformations.

converter SFC 3 displays the formation of the state of the corresponding acupuncture point by the bio-converter of the organism with the formation of an integral parameter IP 3 at the output.

At the organ level, the status of the corresponding organ of IP 2 is determined in SFC 2. The system functional converter SFC 2 displays the formation of the state of the corresponding organ (according to the input signals of this organ coming from the acupuncture points located in different parts of the body: the auricle, arm, head) with the formation of an integral parameter IP 2 at the output.

At the FS level, their state is modeled in SFC 1 with the formation of an integral parameter IP 1. At the level of the body, the state of the bio-object as a whole is determined in SFC 0. The system functional converter SFC 0 simulates the formation of the organism state by input signals from all functional subsystems, output of integral parameter IP 0.

The scale for representing the state of bio-objects contains 100 conventional units. The norm for the state of the organs and systems in our test corresponds to 50–65 units of the scale. Values above the norm reflect the state of hyper-function (or inflammation) from toxic load (65–80 units), partial inflammation (80–90 units) to total (90–100 units). Values below the norm reflect the state of hypofunction from the initial stage (40–50 units), progressive degeneration (30–40 units), from significant degeneration (20–30 units) to complete atrophy (below 20 units).

Formation of the integral parameter of the state of the organism taking into account the scales used at all levels of the hierarchy was shown in Figure 5.3. At the levels of organs and functional systems, state graphs are depicted.

The configuration of the measuring system on neural networks MS/NN was represented by structural and parametric synthesis (Mukha & Skvortsov 2007). We developed the structure and set up the neural network SFCs based on the information area (training and test samples, formed from the a priori, a posteriori and current data base). We have been developed a program for engineering of the neural network system functional converters.

We showed the conditions for the organ and functional levels in Figure 5.3. We consider an organism as interconnected hierarchical system for estimation of its functional condition.

We formed an evaluation of the functional state of internal organs, systems and the organism as a whole on the basis of acupuncture measurements and hierarchy of integral parameters. Neural network diagnostic system allows us to form a quantitative express diagnostics of internal organs, functional systems and the organism as a whole.

In this part of our investigation, we proposed the solving of problems of processing, analysing measurement results, real-time information modeling with the help of neural networks that operate on the basis of information continuously coming from sensors.

In process of considering a neural network as a measuring tool for diagnosing the state of bio-objects, it is necessary to construct a metrological description for the measuring process in the neural network with known errors in the input signals. It is also necessary to consider the following components of metrology: the equations of measurement (interpreted either as a model of a procedure performed by a physically realised measuring circuit (Tsvetkov 1992; Tsvetkov 2005) or as a model

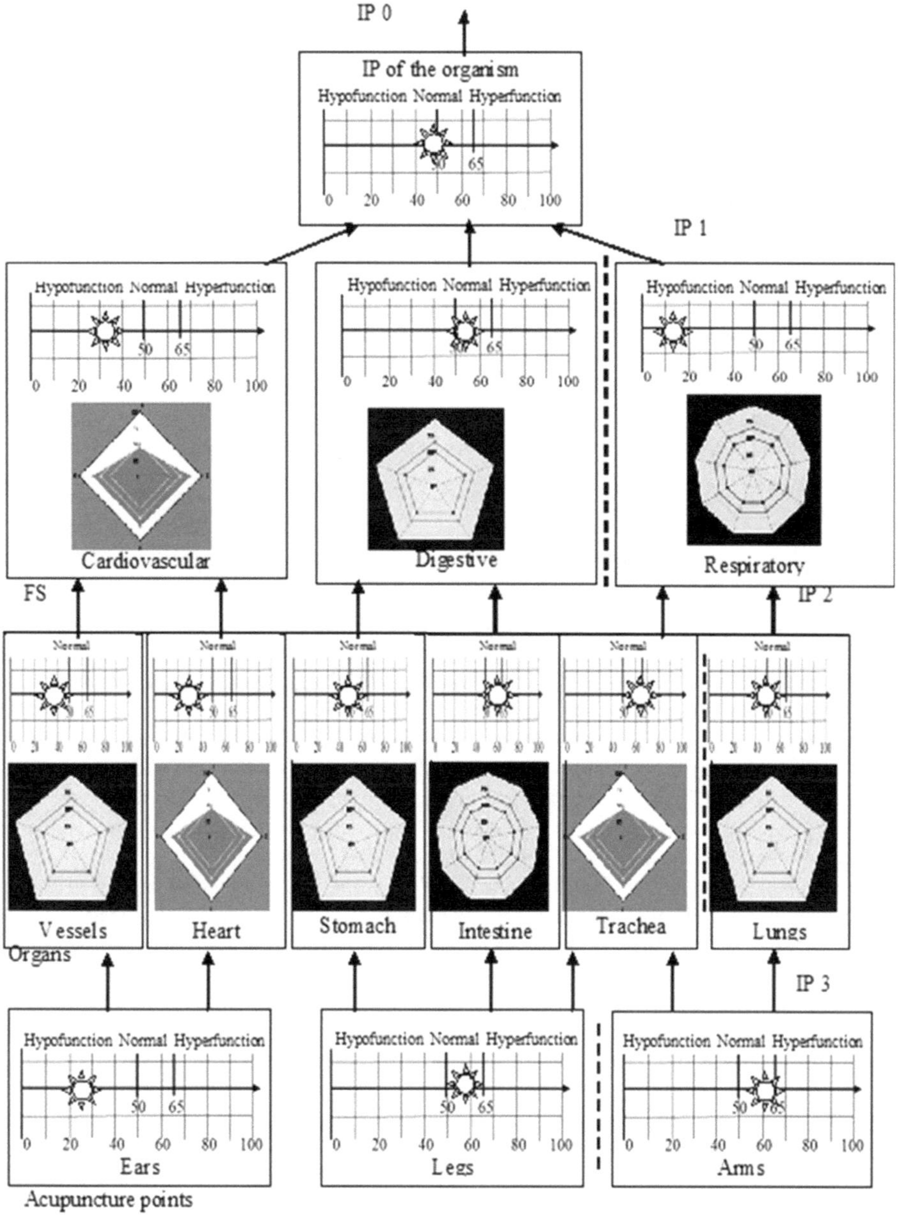

Figure 5.3. Hierarchical structure for the formation of the integral parameter of an organism.

of an ideal measuring procedure), structuring the total error (methodical and instrumental, systematic and random, additive and multiplicative, static and dynamic).

Formation of the integral parameter of the state of the organism taking into account the scales used at all levels of the hierarchy was shown in Figure 5.3. At the levels of organs and functional systems, state graphs are depicted. The configuration of the measuring system on neural networks MS/NN was represented by structural and parametric synthesis (Mukha & Skvortsov 2007). We developed the structure and set up the neural network SFCs based on the information area (training and test samples,

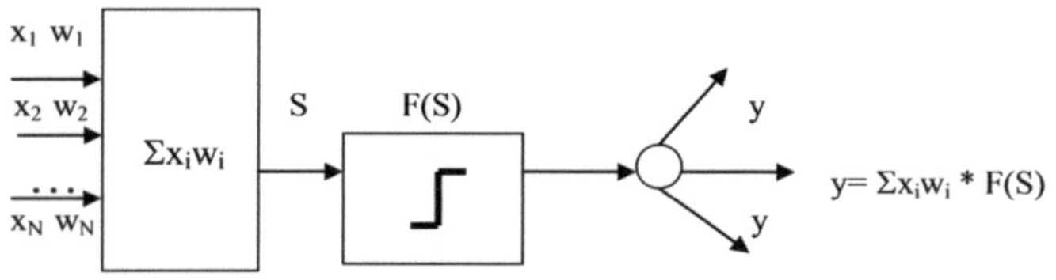

Figure 5.4. Measuring transformations in the neuron.

formed from the a priori, a posteriori and current data base). We have been developed a program for engineering of the neural network system functional converters.

We showed the conditions for the organ and functional levels in Figure 5.3. We consider an organism as interconnected hierarchical system for estimation of its functional condition.

We formed an evaluation of the functional state of internal organs, systems and the organism as a whole on the basis of acupuncture measurements and hierarchy of integral parameters. Neural network diagnostic system allows us to form a quantitative express diagnostics of internal organs, functional systems and the organism as a whole.

In this part of our investigation, we proposed the solving of problems of processing, analysing measurement results, real-time information modeling with the help of neural networks that operate on the basis of information continuously coming from sensors.

In process of considering a neural network as a measuring tool for diagnosing the state of bio-objects, it is necessary to construct a metrological description for the measuring process in the neural network with known errors in the input signals. It is also necessary to consider the following components of metrology: the equations of measurement (interpreted either as a model of a procedure performed by a physically realised measuring circuit (Tsvetkov 1992; Tsvetkov 2005) or as a model of an ideal measuring procedure), structuring the total error (methodical and instrumental, systematic and random, additive and multiplicative, static and dynamic).

We proposed to allocate in the neural network, as in any other measuring system, realisable, accepted and hypothetical measurement algorithms in accordance with the accepted in the theory of measurement postulates (Tsvetkov 2005). At the same time, the implemented algorithm is understood as the measurements made by a trained neural network created by software or hardware with all the errors that appeared both because of the features of the training and because of the imperfect implementation. Every investigator must take into account the adopted algorithm only learning errors. He understands the hypothetical algorithm as an ideal measurement algorithm, which allows him to obtain the true value for the measured value. However, it is difficult to formulate an ideal measurement algorithm in many problems (for a true value of the measured value, a priori known values of the output vector corresponding to the input vector can be adopted).

The separation of the total error into the methodological and instrumental is determined by the type of the applied measurement algorithm (due to the level and volume of a priori information used in describing the measurement procedure and measurement results). The degree of correspondence of the mathematical model of the accepted measuring procedure (accepted algorithm) to the procedure, which will be realised, increases, and then the degree of correspondence between the methodological and total errors increases.

We considered the functions of the neuron elements in the measurement aspect in more detail. The neuron consists of a linear connection, a multi-input adder, a nonlinear transducer, and a branch point (look at the Figure 5.4). The linear link has one tuneable parameter w_i (weighting coefficient), which receives a scalar signal x_i at the input, forms the product $x_i w_i$ at the output and can be realised using a resistor. A multi-input adder (without configurable parameters) has a vector input, generates an algebraic sum of the input signal components, it may be realised on the operational amplifier. An adaptive (having adjustable parameters w_i) multi-input adder is a composition of i-linear links and a multi-input adder.

A nonlinear threshold device (signal converter) with various activation functions F (S) (for example, threshold, sigmoidal) converts the input scalar signal in accordance with the selected nonlinear

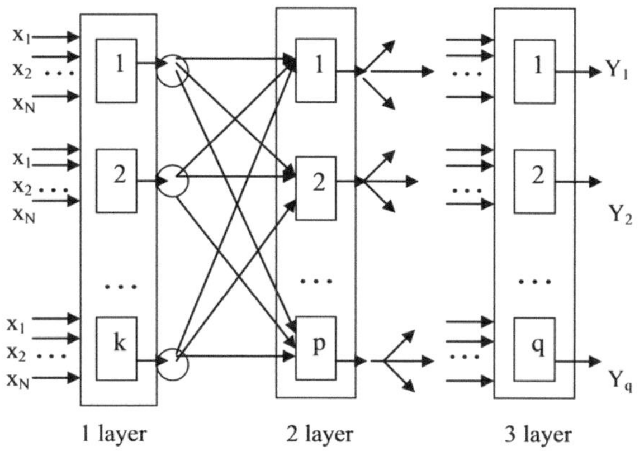

Figure 5.5. Three-layer neural network of direct propagation.

function. It is realised on the operational amplifier with the appropriate feedback, ensuring the local independence of the neuron operation in the neural network.

The branch point is the starting for the multiplication of the output signal of the neuron, it is implemented in hardware in the form of direct, cross and reverse (positive and negative) connections with increased load capacity at the output of the operational amplifier.

The adder implements the role of a functional switch, switching to the output a certain combination of the components of the input signal taken with different weight coefficients (weighted).

In the non-linear (threshold) device, the value of the signal passed through the commutator is measured by the method of comparison with the threshold value specified by the activation function. The result of the comparison of the measured quantity λ_j, passed through a switch with a standard (in this case with the accepted unit of measurement λ_1) depends on the size of the unit used $\lambda_0 = 1/\omega_I$ and the value of the activation function F in the working zone of the measured signal: $\lambda_1 = 1/(F\ \omega_i)$.

For a common three-layer structure of the neural network (look at the Figure 5.5)

We can obtain the following expressions for the output signals. We represented the output signal of the 1-st and the q-th measuring channels in the next equations respectively:

$$\left.\begin{aligned} Y_1^3 &= F_1^3\left(\sum_{k=1}^{L} F_j^2\left(\sum_{j=1}^{P} F_i^1\left(\sum_{i=1}^{N} w_i^1 x_i\right)\right)\right) \\ Y_q^3 &= F_q^3\left(\sum_{l=1}^{L} F_j^2\left(\sum_{j=1}^{P} F_i^1\left(\sum_{i=1}^{N} w_i^1 x_i\right)\right)\right) \end{aligned}\right\} \tag{5.1}$$

As a result, we got the integral value (parameter) at the output of the neural network with the integration frequency. This frequency is equal to the number of summing layers. In this case, the topology of the links between the layers makes it possible to obtain the necessary interrelation between the parameters due to the ability for self-organisation, the flexible formation of the standard at the stage of training or self-learning, and the autonomous selection of the standard in recognition.

We proposed to consider neural networks as ordinary measuring means, the description of their operation can be made from the point of view of classical measurements with traditional metrological estimates. Thus, if we consider a neural network as a multiply connected measuring system (with a heterogeneous measure across all channels), in which the basis is a single-channel measuring system, and the problem of pattern recognition is treated as a partial formulation of a more general problem of multi-parametric joint measurements on the basis of indirect ones, so we can bring new neural network measurement methods to classical ones with traditional metrological estimates.

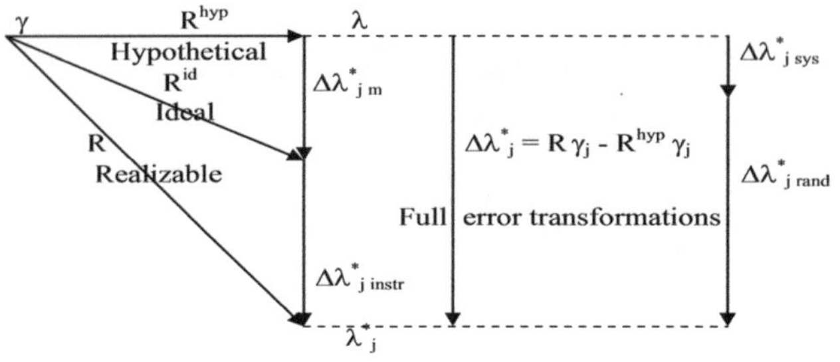

Figure 5.6. Expansion of the total error of the measurement transformation.

It is the most appropriate way to build the procedure of bringing neural network measurement methods to classical ones on the basis of formalisms of general algebra, graphs, theory of categories and functors, system and operational approaches. The analysis of the structural interrelation with the help of the indicated formalisms will allow us to construct linear equations of the interrelation of the required metrological estimates.

The metrological description of the neural network is based on a consistent description and analysis of measurement errors and their characteristics. Here we based on the accepted representation of the measurement procedure as a sequence of transformations of the input action (Tsvetkov 2005). From these positions, we formally defined widely used types and characteristics of errors included in the measurement procedure of neural network transformations (Skvortsov 2001).

We included auxiliary measurement transformations in the neural network measurement procedure to increase the metrological level (accuracy due to the introduction of adaptive and corrective transformations, expansion of the dynamic range), and also for the convenience of software implementation, and to make the system multifunctional. These transformations include: the transformation of the value (normalisation), the functional transformation (nonlinear, in general, the activation function), multiplexing (switching), filtering (smoothing), identical transformation (transfer), memorisation (fixation) of intermediate results.

The complexity of the problem, which we have solved for diagnosing the state of modern objects, requires the application of an adequate level of complexity of the formalisms of the representation of measurement transformations.

Categorical formalisms are used to describe the main types of measurements (direct, indirect, cumulative, joint, integral) based on which the categorical-operational representation (Mukha 2006) of measuring transformations in a neuron, in a multilayer neural network and neural network functional converters (ADC, normalisation, scaling device).

Consider the decomposition of the total error of the generalised measurement transformation R of the input quantity γ in the output value λ on the following components (Tsvetkov 2005): methodical ($\Delta\lambda^*_m$) and instrumental ($\Delta\lambda^*_{instr}$), systematic ($\Delta\lambda^*_{sys}$) and random ($\Delta\lambda^*_{rand}$). Figure 5.6 shows the R^{hyp} – hypothetical, R^{id} – ideal (taken as ideal for hardware implementation), R – realisable measurement transformations, as well as output quantity λ^*, weighed down by mistake.

The categorical representation of the measurement transformations in the neural network begins with the refinement of the measurement situation (description of the input signal model, the measurement procedure model, the model of the measuring instruments, and the model of the measurement conditions) (Tsvetkov 1992; Tsvetkov 2005). Specific metrological description of neural network measuring systems is (Mukha & Skvortsov 2007):

- The necessity to clarify the concept of input effects (input and output signals as an ordered set of elementary signals, which are specified by means of vectors);
- The necessity to describe the error of the basic measurement transformations of the neuron (multiplication by weight, weighted summation, non-linear transformation by means of the activation function);

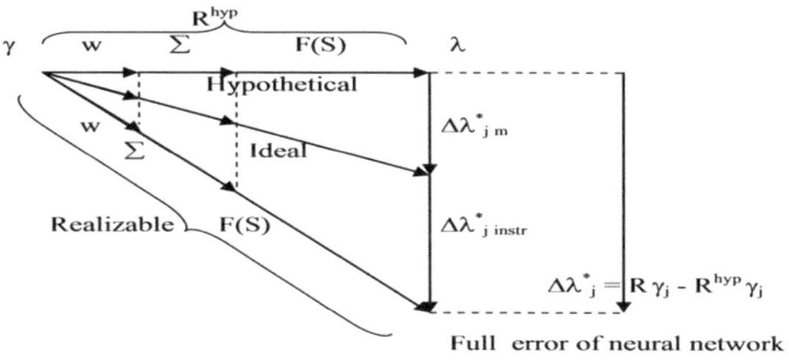

Figure 5.7. Decomposition of the total neuron error.

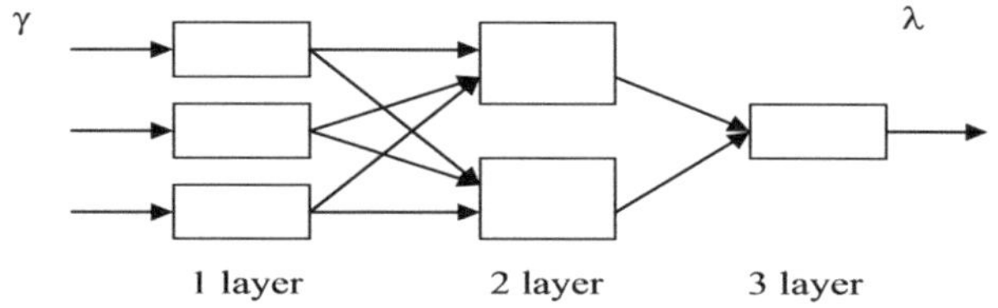

Figure 5.8. Three-layer neural network.

- The complexity of describing the contribution to the corresponding error of all components of the neural network structure (activation functions of neurons of each layer, all neurons in each layer, the number of measuring channels, the degree of interconnection of internal measuring channels, each neural layer);
- The necessity to describe the error of the learning stage (the training and test sample formed, the training method).

The total error of the generalised measurement transformation R is:

$$\Delta\lambda_i^* = R\gamma_i - R^{hyp}\gamma_i \tag{5.2}$$

Decomposition of the total error of the basic measurement transformations in the neuron (multiplication of the input signal γ by weight w, weighted summation $\sum \gamma_i w_i$, nonlinear transformation F (S)) of the input quantity γ in the output value λ on the following components: methodological ($\Delta\lambda_{\text{j m}}^*$) and instrumental ($\Delta\lambda_{\text{j instr}}^*$) is presented in Figure 5.7. In addition, hypothetical, ideal and realisable measuring neural network transformations are presented. Methodical component of the error $\Delta\lambda_{\text{j m}}^*$ includes the errors of the applied training method, the starting topology of the NS (the number of inputs and outputs of neurons, the number of neurons and the type of activation function in each layer, the number of layers, the starting matrix of weight coefficients), and the formation of training and test samples.

The error of the neural layer, which is formed by a parallel connection of unbound neurons, is determined by the error in the transformations of each neuron. The error of the measuring channel, which contains consecutively connected neurons, is determined by the sum of the errors of the transformations in each neuron (Mukha & Skvortsov 2007; Rymarczyk et al. 2018).

We considered a neural network of direct propagation and represented it in Figure 5.8. This neural network realise a normalising functional transformation and consists of three layers (input layer – 3 neurons, second layer – 2 neurons and output layer – 1 neuron) with cross links of internal measuring channels (when the output of each channel. The previous layer is connected to the inputs of all the channels of the next layer). Six measuring channels are formed in this network (3-2-1).

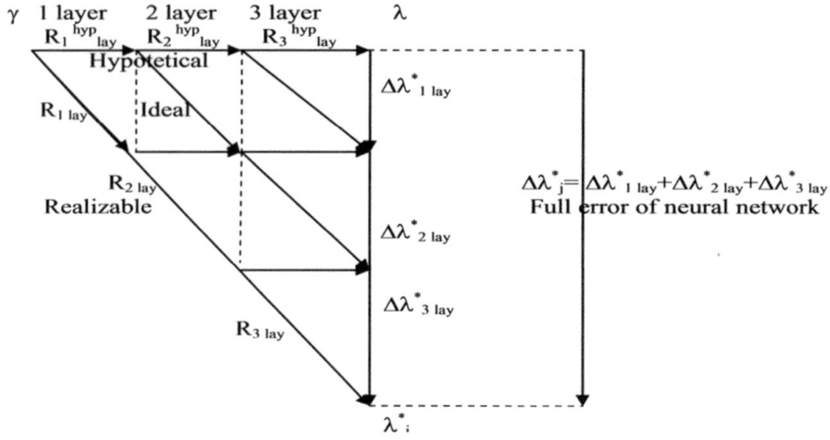

Figure 5.9. Decomposition of the total error along the layers of the neural network.

The categorical operational representation of the total error of the three-layer NN over the layers was shown in Figure 5.9. The expansion of the total error of the normalisation operation $\lambda_n = R_{3lay} R_{2lay} R_{1lay} \gamma$ by layers is:

$$\Delta\lambda^*_{1lay} = R_{3lay} R_{2lay} R_{1lay} \gamma - R_{3lay} R_{2lay} R_1^{hyp}{}_{lay} \gamma, \tag{5.3}$$

$$\Delta\lambda^*_{2lay} = R_{3lay} R_{2lay} R_1^{hyp}{}_{lay} \gamma - R_{3lay} R_{2lay}^{hyp} R_1^{hyp}{}_{lay} \gamma, \tag{5.4}$$

$$\Delta\lambda^*_{3lay} = R_{3lay} R_{2lay}^{hyp} R_1^{hyp}{}_{lay} \gamma - R_{3lay}^{hyp} R_{2lay}^{hyp} R_1^{hyp}{}_{lay} \gamma, \tag{5.5}$$

$$\Delta\lambda^*_i = \Delta\lambda^*_{1lay} + \Delta\lambda^*_{2lay} + \Delta\lambda^*_{3lay}, \tag{5.6}$$

$$\Delta\lambda^*_i = R_{3lay} R_{2lay} R_{1lay} \gamma - R_{3lay}^{hyp} R_{2lay}^{hyp} R_1^{hyp}{}_{lay} \gamma. \tag{5.7}$$

The categorical operational representation of the total error of a three-layer neural network (input layer – 3 neurons, second layer – 2 neurons and output layer – 1 neuron) for each layer, each neuron in the layer and for each measuring channel was shown in Figure 5.10. We accurately distinguished the contribution of each channel to the total error according to the indicated decomposition errors as well as change of the error of each channel, when the number of neurons in the channel changes.

The representation of the total error of a two-layer neural network (the first layer – 2 neurons, the second layer – 2 neurons) for each layer and two measuring channels in case of their interaction was shown in Figure 5.11. The contribution of the neurons of each layer to the total error of the corresponding channel, channel in the operations of switching and signal separation $\Delta\lambda^*_{cs1}$ (was shown in the area between the first and second layers), for the second channel is: $\Delta\lambda^*_{cs2}$. The error in the effect of the second channel on the first $\Delta\lambda^*_{21} = \Delta\lambda^*_{1full} - \Delta\lambda^*_1$ (where $\Delta\lambda^*_{1full}$ – total channel error, $\Delta\lambda^*_1$ – the error of the first channel without interaction). Similarly, the error of the effect of the first channel on the second $\Delta\lambda^*_{12} = \Delta\lambda^*_{2full} - \Delta\lambda^*_2$.

The analog-digital measurement transformation, formed by the operations of sampling, quantisation and rounding, was shown in Figure 5.12.

The measurement equation in the operator form for the ADC, containing the operations of sampling, quantisation and rounding, was represented as:

$$\lambda^*_j = \{R_r[R_q(R_{dis} \gamma_j)]\}. \tag{5.8}$$

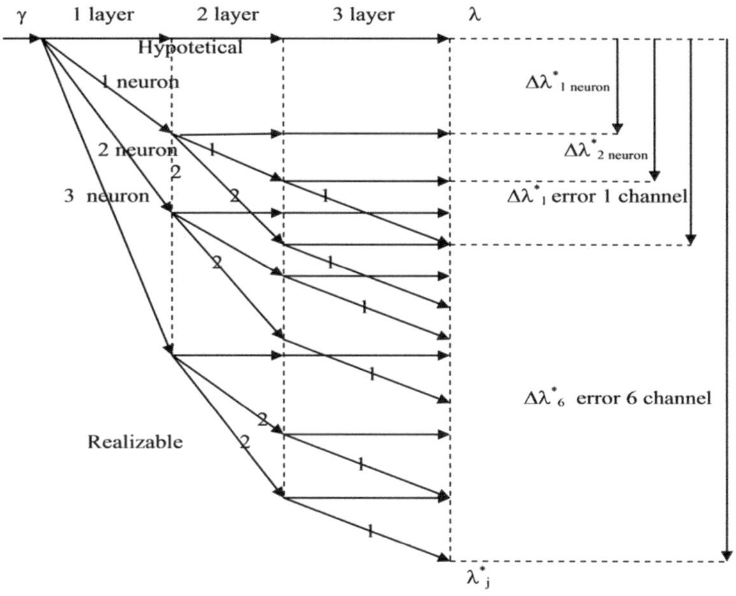

Figure 5.10. Decomposition of the total error in neurons, layers and channels of a neural network.

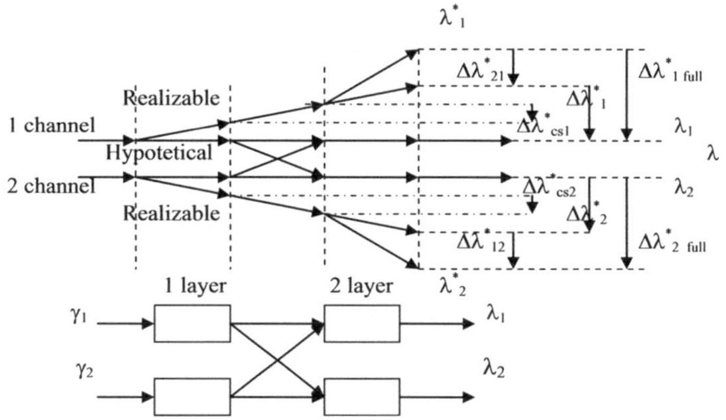

Figure 5.11. The expansion of the total error with allowance for interaction of neural network channels.

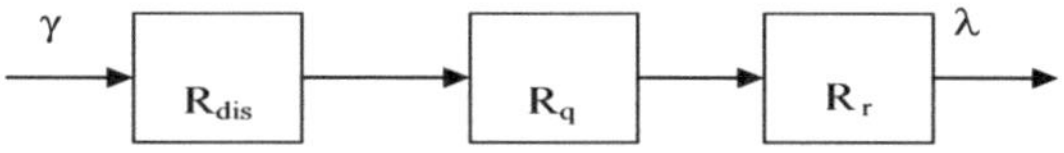

Figure 5.12. Analog-to-digital measurement conversion (ADC).

The total error of ADC (Mukha & Skvortsov 2007) is:

$$y_7 = R_{38} R_{37} R_{36} R_{35} R_{34} R_{33} R_{32} R_{31} X_7. \tag{5.9}$$

Categorical-operational representation of the total ADC error, in which the sampling operation was implemented by a three-layer neural network, was shown in Figure 5.13.

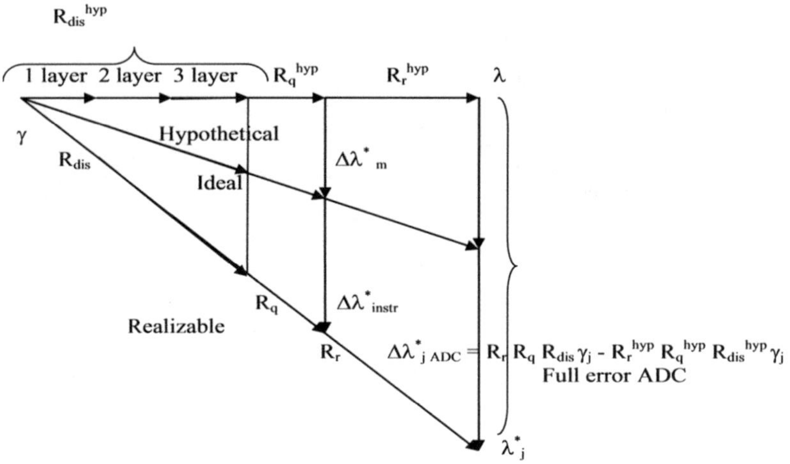

Figure 5.13. Decomposition of the total error of ADC.

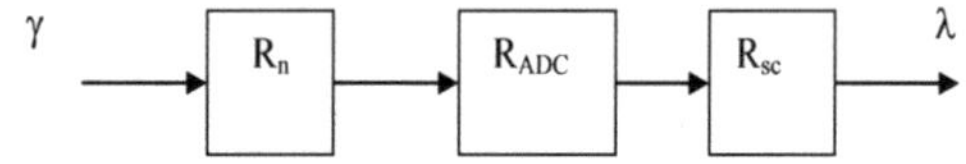

Figure 5.14. The minimum measuring channel.

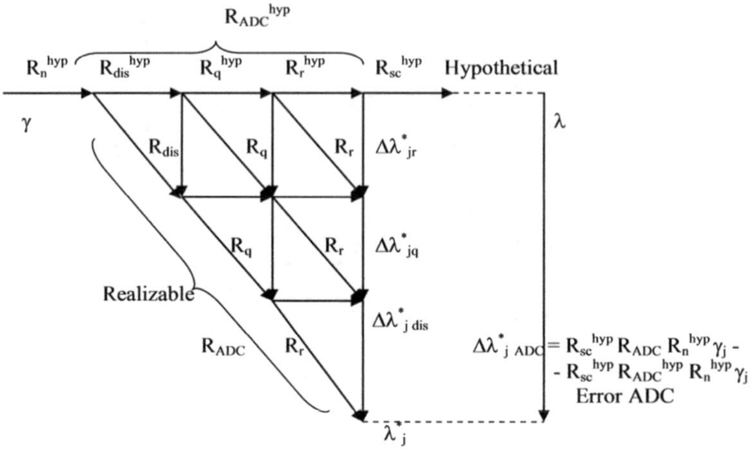

Figure 5.15. Representation of the ADC error in the minimum measuring channel.

The minimum measuring channel with neural network measurement transformations such as R_n, A/D conversion and R_{sc} was shown in Figure 5.14.

Figure 5.15 shows the categorically operational representation of the total analog-to-digital conversion (ADC) error in a neural network measuring channel.

Measurement equations for the minimum measuring channel (Mukha & Skvortsov 2007) are:

$$\lambda_j^* = \{R_{sc}[R_{ADC}(R_n \gamma_j)]\}. \tag{5.10}$$

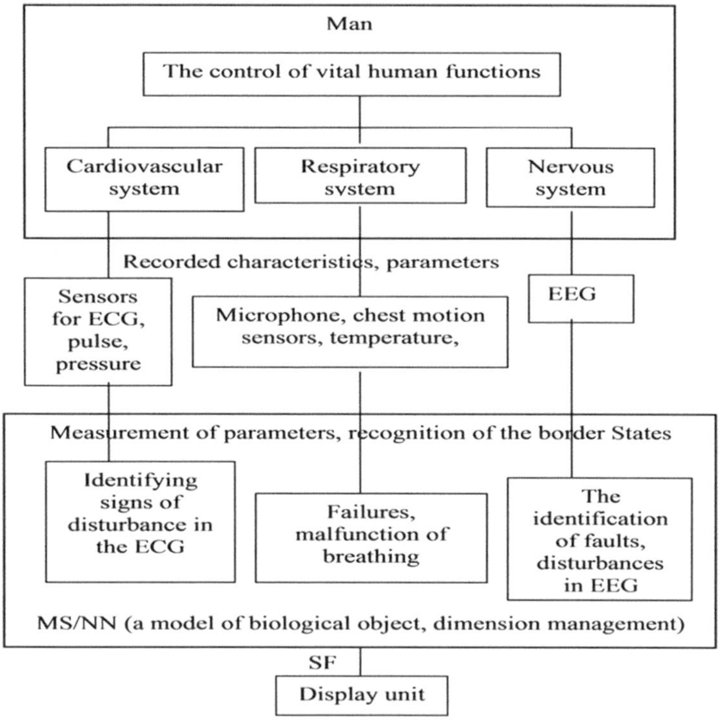

Figure 5.16. Diagnostic system.

Decomposition of ADC error in a neural network measuring channel for discretisation, quantisation and rounding operations:

$$\lambda^*_{1dis} = R^{hyp}_{sc} R_r R_q R_{dis} R^{hyp}_{id} \gamma_j - R^{hyp}_{sc} R_r R_q R^{hyp}_{dis} R^{hyp}_{id} \gamma_j, \tag{5.11}$$

$$\lambda^*_{jq} = R^{hyp}_{sc} R_r R_q R^{hyp}_{dis} R^{hyp}_{id} \gamma_j - R^{hyp}_{sc} R_r R^{hyp}_{q} R^{hyp}_{dis} R^{hyp}_{id} \gamma_j, \tag{5.12}$$

$$\Delta\lambda^*_{jr} = R^{hyp}_{sc} R_r R^{hyp}_{q} R^{hyp}_{dis} R^{hyp}_{id} \gamma_j - R^{hyp}_{sc} R^{hyp}_{r} R^{hyp}_{q} R^{hyp}_{dis} R^{hyp}_{id} \gamma_j, \tag{5.13}$$

$$\Delta\lambda^*_{jADC} = \Delta\lambda^*_{jdis} + \Delta\lambda^*_{jq} + \Delta\lambda^*_{jr}, \tag{5.14}$$

$$\Delta\lambda^*_{jADC} = R^{hyp}_{sc} R_r R_q R_{dis} R^{hyp}_{id} \gamma_j - R^{hyp}_{sc} R^{hyp}_{r} R^{hyp}_{q} R^{hyp}_{dis} R^{hyp}_{id} \gamma_j. \tag{5.15}$$

Similarly, a categorical-operational representation of the total error of other measuring functional converters was constructed.

There are representations of the instrumental and methodical, systematic and random components of the total error (sometimes the absence of components of any kind) for all measuring transformations.

Categorical representation allows us to obtain traditional metrological evaluations for the process of neural network measurements, to detail various types of errors in measuring transformations (for neurons, neural layers and measuring channels), to analyse the influence of the neural network structure on the measurement error, to perform synthesis of neural network measuring systems with the specified metrological characteristics.

We considered an application of the operational description of the metrological analysis of the proposed diagnostic system for monitoring the vital functions of a person (see Figure 5.16). This system was used for solving of important problems of prevention, diagnosis and treatment of cardiovascular diseases (ECG, pulse, arterial pressure, and temperature), brain damage (EEG), and sudden impairment of the respiratory system: asthmatic attacks, difficulty breathing (microphone, sensors of chest movement).

We can distinguish three types of structures (measuring channels) of the measurement procedures in this diagnostic system. These are the structures of the first type (temperatures, estimates of the magnitude of the movement of the chest), consisting of normalisation operations (R_{11}), ADC (R_{12}) and scaling (R_{13}).

Complex structures of the second kind (carrying out the signal transformations not only in analog but also in a digital form, for example, determination of oxygen content in blood, heart rate, blood pressure) are represented by analog filtering operations (R_{21}), normalisation (R_{22}), ADC (R_{23}), averaging (R_{24}), functional transformation (R_{25}) and scaling (R_{26}).

The third kind of structures are complex measurements with recognition (detection of malfunctions, disorders of the functioning of the nervous system according to EEG, malfunctions, cardiac dysfunction of ECG using electrocardiographic features.

They were not used in the usual evaluation of curves because of the complexity and difficulties of calculations, despite their high information content. Such type of structures also give a complete measurement procedure for malfunctions of the respiratory system. They consist of analogue filtering operations (R_{31}), normalisation (R_{32}), ADC (R_{33}), averaging (R_{34}), functional transformation (R_{35}), scaling (R_{36}), digital filtering (R_{37}) and recognition (R_{38}).

We wrote the measurement equations for connecting of the input (X_i) and exit (y_i) corresponding measuring channel to obtain the operator form of the measurement procedure model (taking into account the sequence and nature of the elementary measurement transformations).

Temperature measurement channel is:

$$y_1 = R_{13}R_{12}R_{11}X_1. \tag{5.16}$$

The channel for estimating the magnitude of the movement of the chest during breathing:

$$y_2 = R_{13}R_{12}R_{11}X_2 \tag{5.17}$$

Blood pressure measurement channel is:

$$y_3 = R_{26}R_{25}R_{24}R_{23}R_{22}R_{21}X_3. \tag{5.18}$$

Blood oxygen measurement channel is:

$$y_4 = R_{26}R_{25}R_{24}R_{23}R_{22}R_{21}X_4. \tag{5.19}$$

The channel for determining the malfunctions, disturbances in the functioning of respiratory organs (respiratory failure, hypoxia, fever) is:

$$y_5 = R_{38}R_{37}R_{36}R_{35}R_{34}R_{33}R_{32}R_{31}X_5. \tag{5.20}$$

The channel for detecting failures, disorders of the functioning of the nervous system according to EEG (violation of regulation of arterial pressure, cerebral blood flow, neuronal functions, detection of generators of pathologically intensified excitation, which are the cause of sensitive, motor, vegetative disorders, and also the cause of disorders of higher nervous activity):

$$y_6 = R_{38}R_{37}R_{36}R_{35}R_{34}R_{33}R_{32}R_{31}X_6. \tag{5.21}$$

The channel for determining the malfunction, cardiac dysfunction of ECG (arrhythmia, circulatory failure due to worsening of the heart or changes in vascular function, heart rate), it was shown on Figure 5.17:

$$y_7 = R_{38}R_{37}R_{36}R_{35}R_{34}R_{33}R_{32}R_{31}X_7. \tag{5.22}$$

We considered the main features of the neural network structure of the diagnostic system.

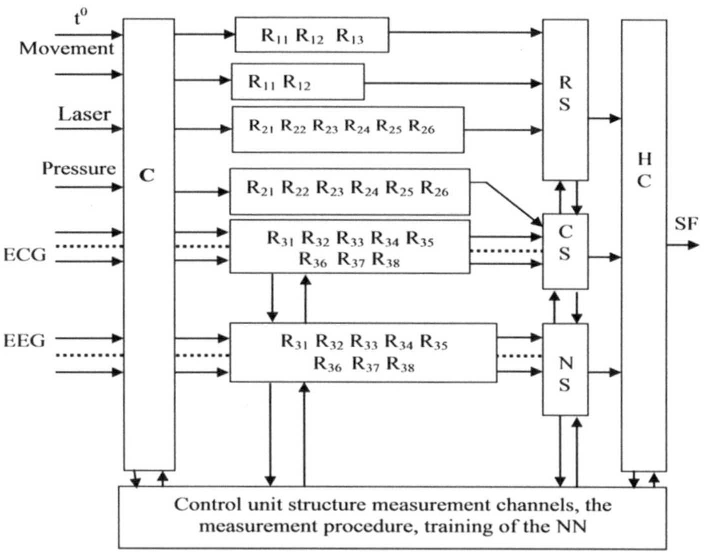

Figure 5.17. Neural network structure of the diagnostic system.

The input neuron layer (C) switches all input actions to the measuring channels of the medical diagnostic system. A system parameter SF is formed at the output of the investigated system. It makes it possible for us to determine the systemic state of a person. If the system parameter has a significant deviation from the nominal value (the norm, which is different for each person), then the system moves to a lower hierarchical level of representation (the level of subsystems – cardiovascular, respiratory, nervous) for identification of the expected causes. Further, at the sub-system level, the values of the subsystem parameters are analysed to determine the subsystems that make the maximum contribution to the deviation from the norm. Then the transition to the next level of detail is performed to search for the totality of the organs responsible for the pathological condition.

We used the control unit of the measurement channel structure and the measurement procedure to carry out the described measurement procedure (synchronisation of the work of all neurons, neural layers and networks, measurement order, comparison with the standard for a particular patient, on leaving out of the norm, transition to the lower subsystem levels, organs, primary measurements, set up the neural networks for the recognition of appropriate symptoms in norm and pathology).

5.3 RESULTS, CONCLUSIONS AND RECOMMENDATIONS

The metrological analysis of neural network measuring converters and measuring systems in the categorical operational representation differs from an existing ones by the definition and structuring of the total error of neural network converters, the description of the measurement situation, the categorical operational representation of errors at the stages of structural synthesis (neuron, neural network, neural measuring channel, functional measuring converter, a complete neural network measuring system), a parametrical synthesis (an applying of the priory data – training samples, test samples; instruction) at an operation step, at a step of additional training.

We can form the correct structure of the diagnostic systems on neural networks (MS/NN) for complete consideration of the system function of a complex bio-object (adequate to its behavior and level of condition for all its components), as well as for a measuring system based on neural networks as a tool for constructing of an object model.

Metrological analysis of measuring systems on neural networks (MS/NN) allows us to reveal additive, multiplicative and nonlinear components of error in links, and to derive formulas for these errors of the entire measuring device.

We can construct the measurement systems with a controlled error using the metrological description of different measuring systems on neural networks (MS/NN).

REFERENCES

Mukha Yu. P. 2006. The connection between metrological analysis and the theory of categories and functors. *Bulletin of SZF MA 17.*

Mukha Yu. P. & Skvortsov M. G. 2007. *Neural network measuring systems. Diagnosis of complex objects.* Moscow: Radio Engineering.

Rymarczyk, T., Stefaniak, B., & Adamkiewicz, P. 2018. Neural network and convolutional algorith to extract shapes by e-medicus application. Informatyka, Automatyka, Pomiary w Gospodarce i Ochronie Srodowiska, 8(3): 39–42.

Skvortsov M. G. 2001. Equations of measurement for neural networks. *Biomedical radioelectronics* 4: 48–52.

Tsvetkov E. I. 1992. *Algorithmic bases of measurements*. St. Petersburg: Energoatomizdat.

Tsvetkov E. I. 2005. *Fundamentals of mathematical metrology*. St. Petersburg: Politechnika.

CHAPTER 6

Neural network system for medical data approximation

A. Astafyev & S. Gerashchenko
Lipetsk State Technical University, Russia

N. Yurkov, N. Goryachev & I. Kochegarov
Penza State University, Russia

A. Smolarz & E. Łukasik
Lublin University of Technology, Lublin, Poland

M. Kalimoldayev
Institute of Information and Computational Technologies CS MES RK, Almaty, Kazakhstan

ABSTRACT: The chapter describes the Kaczmarz algorithm for the neural network. A distinctive feature of this algorithm is finding a solution by iterations that have proven to be effective in solving complex computational problems. It will be implemented in form of the cascade-correlation neural network. Its efficiency is shown on example in medicine tasks that contain many input factors.

6.1 INTRODUCTION

To solve the task of medical data approximation, it is proposed to use a cascade-correlation neural network representing neuron pooling in the form of a cascade, in addition to the algorithm (Anisimov et al. 1989; Bortnyk et al. 2018; Dmitriev et al. 2017). In the learning process, the algorithm considered both determine the weights and adjusts the structure of the network itself. The advantages of the algorithm are increased learning rate in comparison with similar algorithms and setting the architecture for a specific problem.

The architecture of cascade correlation was originally proposed by S. Fahlman (Fahlman & Lebiere 1997) in order to simplify the network topology, and contains the following main concepts: hidden layers are added once and remain unchanged, and the learning algorithm has the ability to add new hidden units. In the hidden units, the algorithm maximises the correlation value of the output node and the error (Anisimov et al. 1989; Lysenko et al. 2018). The general topology of a cascade network is shown in Figure 6.1.

The general structure for obtaining a decision is as follows:

1. There is a minimum neural network, shown in Figure 6.2, which consists of an input and output layer, and there are connections between all units in the network. The number of inputs and outputs is selected based on the task. Output neurons may contain arbitrary activation functions (Pashchenko & Pashchenko 2012; Andreev et al. 2016).
2. Training of the output layer connections is done until the error reduction stop.
3. The units are added one by one, and the weights of the input connections are added as well. Candidate units that are linked with all existing units are fixed.
4. There is a minimisation of the target function value and a maximisation of the correlation of new units and the residual network error. Learning can take place using both standard algorithms and more specific ones.
5. Learning is finished when the correlation indicators stop improving, and the error lies in an acceptable interval. Otherwise, the technique of unit connection to the network is repeated.

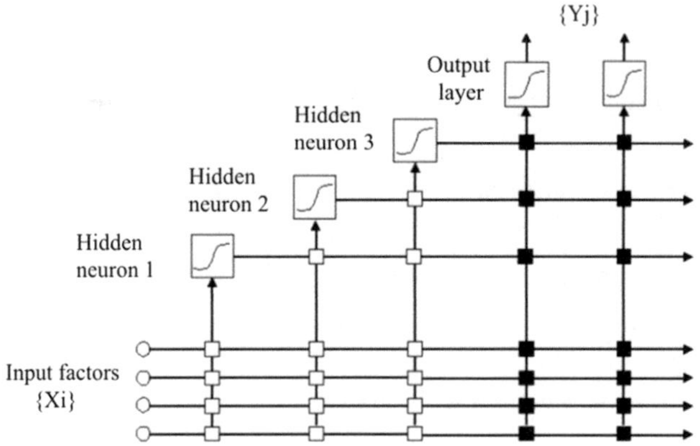

Figure 6.1. Topology of the cascade-correlation network with three hidden units (black intersections are trained).

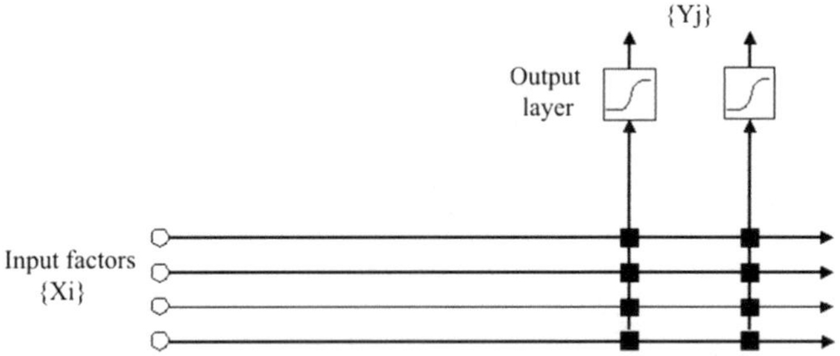

Figure 6.2. Topology of the cascade-correlation network at the initial stage of training.

The ultimate learning goal is to select such weights in which the correlation between the activity of the added neuron and the error value at the output of the network is maximised and determined by the correlation coefficient S.

$$S = \sum_{j=1}^{M} \left| \sum_{k=1}^{p} (v^{(k)} - \bar{v})(e_j^{(k)} - \bar{e_j}) \right|, \tag{6.1}$$

where p is the number of learning samples; M is the number of output neurons; $v(k)$ is the output signal of the candidate neuron for the k-th learning sample; $e_j^{(k)}$ is the error value of the j-th hidden neuron for the k-th learning sample; $\bar{v}$ and $\bar{e}$ are mean values.

After reaching the maximum S value, the candidate neuron is included in the network structure, the calculated weights of its connections are fixed, and the process of selecting the weights of output neurons to minimise the target function continues. Learning takes place simultaneously for several candidate neurons.

To train the network, a learning algorithm of direct propagation is used, in which localised excitation of neurons occurs. However, for more accurate adjustment of the weights, it is possible to use an iterative algorithm for adjusting several weights of candidate neurons. In general, a mathematical model for calculating weights can be represented as:

$$\begin{bmatrix} \bar{x}_{11} & \bar{x}_{12} & \dots & \bar{x}_{1n} \\ \bar{x}_{21} & \bar{x}_{22} & \dots & \bar{x}_{2n} \\ \dots & \dots & \dots & \dots \\ \bar{x}_{k1} & \bar{x}_{k2} & \dots & \bar{x}_{kn} \end{bmatrix} \cdot \begin{bmatrix} w_1 \\ w_2 \\ \dots \\ w_n \end{bmatrix} = \begin{bmatrix} \bar{y}_1 \\ \bar{y}_2 \\ \dots \\ \bar{y}_k \end{bmatrix}, \tag{6.2}$$

where $\bar{x}_{kn}$ is the network input; w_n is the weighting coefficient; $\bar{y}_k$ is the output signal (Kaczmarz 1937; Il'in 2006; Artamonov et al. 2018).

This equation cannot often have an exact solution; therefore, it can only be approached, minimizing the solution error w_n. The training error should not exceed the set value Δ.

$$\Delta > \Delta\bar{y}_i = \bar{y}_{pi} - \bar{y}_i, \quad i = \overline{1, k}, \tag{6.3}$$

where $\bar{y}_{pi}$ is the calculated response; $\bar{y}$ is the required response.

System training is to minimize the output signal error compared to the learning sample.

$$y_j = \sum_{i=1}^{N} w_{ji} x_i, \tag{6.4}$$

where y_{ji} is the output signal of the j-th neuron; w_{ji} is the weighting coefficient between the j-th neuron and the i-th component of the input vector; N is the dimension of the input vector. The input signal vector $X = [x_0, x_1, \ldots x_N]$ contains a component $x_0 = 1$, that generates a bias signal.

The weighting coefficients are calculated by taking into account the minimization of the output neuron error Δy_j:

$$\Delta y_j = y_j - d_j, \tag{6.5}$$

where d_j is the reference learning signal.

There is a comparison of the values obtained at the output neuron Δy_j with the reference signal: if the permissible threshold is exceeded, then the weights of connections of the j-th neuron are adjusted:

$$w_{ji}(t+1) = w_{ji}(t) + \Delta w_{ji}(t), \tag{6.6}$$

where t is the previous adjustment cycle; $(t + 1)$ is the current adjustment cycle; $\Delta w_{ji}(t)$ is the correction value of the weighting coefficient, calculated as:

$$\Delta w_{ji} = k \cdot x_i \cdot \Delta y_j, \tag{6.7}$$

where k is the accepted coefficient that determines the dynamics of learning to prevent getting into local minima.

The study is completed provided that the stop condition is met as a minimisation of the sum of squares of the error ΔY, calculated by the formula:

$$\Delta Y = \sum_{k=1}^{P} \frac{1}{2} \sum_{j=1}^{M} (\Delta y)^2, \tag{6.8}$$

where P is the dimension of the learning sample; M is the number of neurons of the output layer [10] (Farhat et al. 1994).

If ΔY excesses the acceptable threshold and the learning process loops, there is an addition of extra neurons. As a result of learning, the network architecture is dynamically formed with the optimal structure according to the presented set of the data sample. Connections between network elements are not formed randomly and in a predetermined order, but depending on the totality of the input vector, presented a set of solutions, and the previous network structure. As a result, the adequacy of the system also depends on the initial data and the specified parameters (Danilova et al. 2017). Under these conditions, it is of particular interest to evaluate the dependence of the system's adequacy on the post-processing functions of the final signal: linear, sigmoidal, hyperbolic tangent, as well as the criterion of learning accuracy, changes in the estimated error in the learning process, and learning data samples.

To study the characteristics of the neural network, the hepatitis patient assessment data were used (description of the system is given below). The final signal of each network element is post-processed by a specific activation function. In this research, three functions were used that are the most common

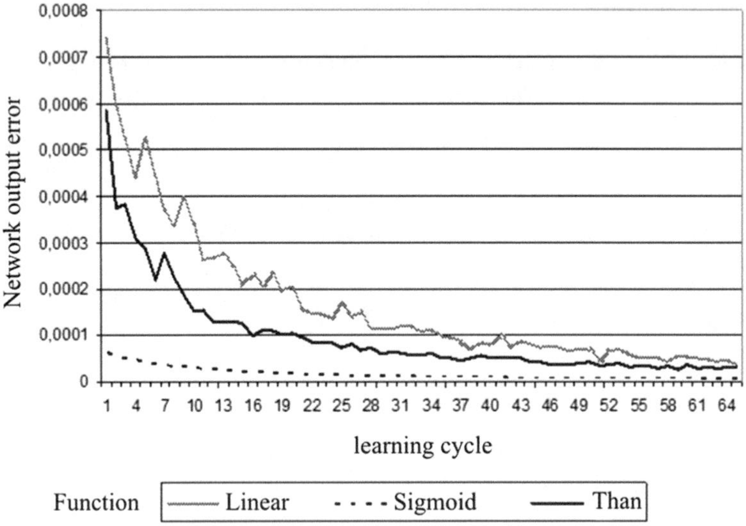

Figure 6.3. The dependence of the network response error on the type of neuron activation function and the number of learning cycles for the learning sample.

and, as a result, the most studied ones in the design of neural networks. Here are the characteristics of the functions:

1. Linear activation function $Y = X$, where X is the weighted sum of all synaptic inputs (induced field) of the neuron. This function is the simplest one used in the mathematical model of neural networks for the first time, and it is the least expensive for hardware resources.
2. Sigmoidal (logistic) activation function or the Fermi function $Y = (1 + \exp(-X \cdot a))^{-1}$. A characteristic feature of this function is asymmetry, which is expressed in the fact that the value of the output signal of any network element belongs to the interval [0, 1], which indirectly affects the shift of the weights of the overlying network elements. This function is everywhere differentiable (that is, smooth), and the presence of nonlinearity plays a key role in the functioning of the network, without which the input-output mapping can be reduced to an ordinary single-layer perceptron.
3. Hyperbolic tangent activation function $Y = a \cdot \tanh(b \cdot X)$ with the coefficients $a = 1.716$ and $b = 0.667$. For the given coefficients, in addition to the continuous derivative, the function has a useful property, namely, at the origin, the effective angle (that is, a slope) of the function is close to unity: $\varphi(0) = 1.716 \cdot 0.667 = 1.142$. This function is an even function of its argument, or asymmetric, that is, $\varphi(-v) = -\varphi(v)$. The final signal of any neuron will have a higher probability of zero mean since it belongs to the interval $[-1, 1]$.

The dynamics of training error changes in the formation process of the network structure, depending on the activation function (Fig. 6.3), shows that the smallest value of the training error is achieved with the sigmoidal activation function $\delta_{av.sigm.} = 0.000162$. The largest value is for the linear function $\delta_{av.lin.} = 0.000402$, and it is $\delta_{av.tg.} = 0.000326$ for the hyperbolic tangent function. The graph of changes in the network response error when using the sigmoidal activation function is smoother. The error reduction process is more stable and intensive.

However, based on the data presented in Figure 6.4, which reflect the dependence of the test error in the learning process, the results can be interpreted more objectively. These results show that good indicators achieved with the sigmoid function for training error were obtained due to the deterioration of the accuracy of the forecasting system $\delta_{av.sigm.} = 0.003056$. The hyperbolic tangent function shows the best results, which gives the smallest test error $\delta_{av.tg.} = 0.000609$ for a given number of learning cycles on data not presented for the formation of the network structure. The use of the sigmoid function can lead to excessive learning in the presented sample, which can lead to a deterioration of forecasting

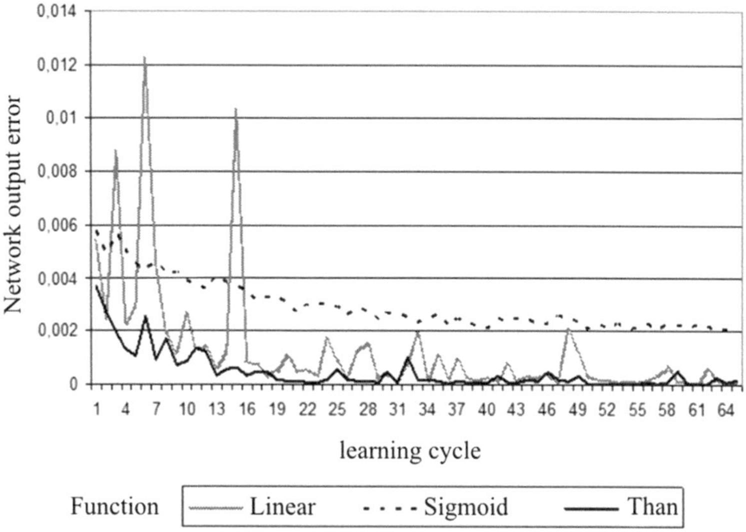

Figure 6.4. The dependence of the network response error on the type of neuron activation function and the number of learning cycles for the test sample.

indicators in real use. The linear function data show that, in comparison with other functions, its use is not justified, as it gives a test error $\delta_{av.lin.} = 0.001593$.

6.2 PRACTICAL IMPLEMENTATION OF THE SYSTEM

A hepatitis treatment assessment system can be proposed as an application of the approximation algorithm. A wide variety of techniques for treating hepatitis causes difficulties in their effective selection and assessment. Hepatitis itself has different variations of viruses, acute and chronic forms, and aetiology, causing difficulties to assess the treatment technique. However, it is worth noting that the cost of hepatitis treatment is not a guarantee of cure [12] (Fouad et al. 2012). The problem of effectiveness assessment can be solved by using intelligent systems that simulate the experience of a specialist.

The use of treatment effectiveness assessment by analysis of changes of the patient's state will allow determining the best treatment technique, assessing the effectiveness of treatment, and also carrying out accurate dosing of pharmaceutical medications, reducing the negative consequences for the body. Given these factors, it is possible to reduce the cost and duration of treatment, improving its quality. An intelligent system makes an assessment of a patient's state according to his data entered into the system. A response based thereon is equivalent to the patient's state. Comparison of the response over time allows a conclusion about the effectiveness of the applied pharmaceutical medications and treatment technique. The assessment of the state takes into account values of 20 factors of biological analysis, transferred into an intelligible scale by the system using the experience of specialists, presented in Table 6.1.

It is possible to use the generally accepted scales of APACHEII, APACHEIII, SAPS2, SAPS3, and SOFA for assessing the state as the response of the system. But for more effective evaluation, it is better to use a five-grade scale of assessment that combines the advantages of the above, in which 1 is a set of factor values characteristic for a healthy person; 2 is the patient's satisfactory state; 3 is the patient's state of moderate severity; 4 is the moderate state; 5 is the state characteristic for a seriously ill person. The operating window of the system is shown in Figure 6.5.

The approach under consideration was tested to analyse the severity of the patient with hepatitis, as well as to determine the nosological form of hepatitis. An intelligent system consists of the main

Table 6.1. Source factors.

Factor name	Group	Range of change
Sex	Physiological data	Male/Female
Age	Physiological data	1–70 years old
Leucocytes	Blood cells	$(1–15) \times 10^9$/l
Erythrocytes	Blood cells	$(2–10) \times 10^{12}$/l
Hemoglobin	Blood cells	80–270 g/l
Platelets	Blood cells	$(50–800) \times 10^9$/l
Autoantibody	Immune system	yes/no
NK cells	Immune system	40–750 $^{\mu}l^{-1}$
B cells	Immune system	80–700 $^{\mu}l^{-1}$
CD4+	Immune system	200–1500 $^{\mu}l^{-1}$
CD8+	Immune system	150–1050 $^{\mu}l^{-1}$
Polymerase chain reaction (PCR)	Polymerase chain reaction (PCR)	+/−
Number of copies	Polymerase chain reaction (PCR)	1–100,000 copies
Total bilirubin	Liver function indicators	0–100 $^{\mu}$mol/l
Conjugated bilirubin	Liver function indicators	0–30 $^{\mu}$mol/l
Thymol turbidity test	Liver function indicators	0–30 units
Alanine transaminase (ALT)	Liver function indicators	0–1000 unit/l
Collagen 4	Other	0–300 units
Thyroid-stimulating hormone (TSH)	Other	Yes/No
Circulating immune complex (CIC)	Other	0–220 mcg/ml

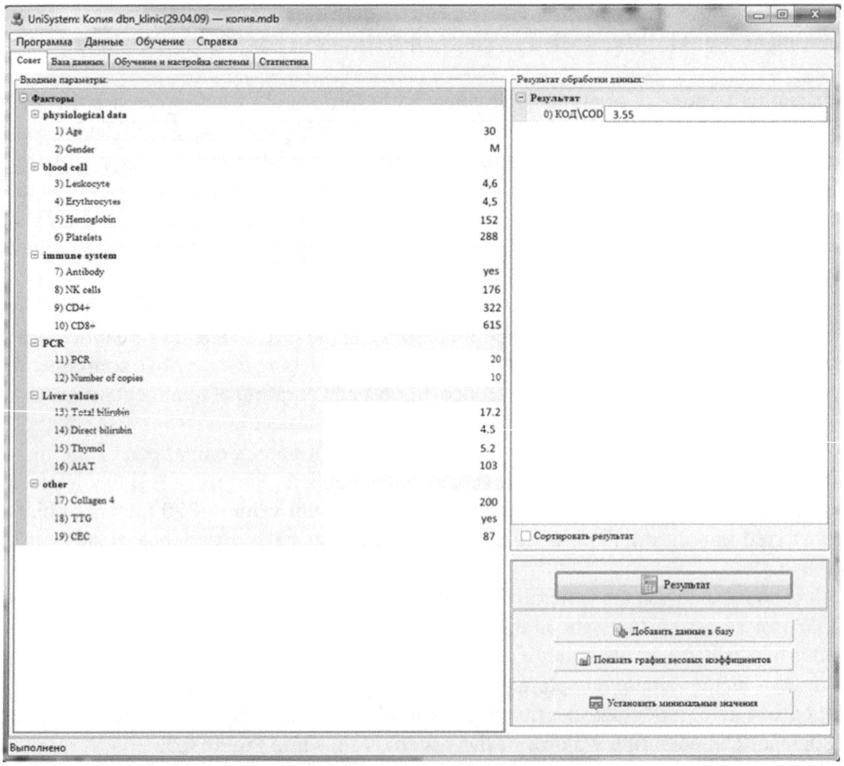

Figure 6.5. The operating window of the system.

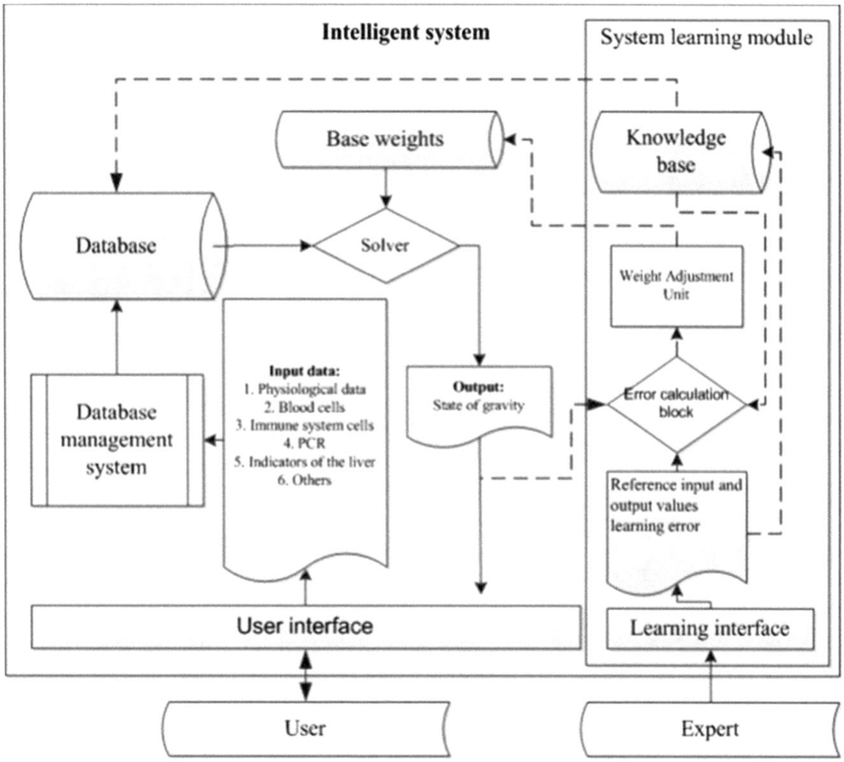

Figure 6.6. Structural diagram of the intelligent system.

module, which calculates the system response based on the input factors, as well as the system learning module that forms the weighting coefficients.

The general structural diagram of the system is given in Figure 6.6 (Fouad et al. 2012; Ostreikovsky et al. 2018; Elble et al. 2010).

It is necessary to consider the example of using the Kaczmarz algorithm in the system (Strohmer & Vershynin 2009). The formation of the weighting coefficients in the system was done through the presentation of the values of 280 images. The training error threshold was 0.25. It took the system 250 iterations to achieve the required training error (Fig. 6.7).

The main task when designing intelligent systems is the formation of a learning sample, which should take into account the experience of specialists and the influence of diverse factors on the situation in hand. There are two approaches to the formation of a learning sample of the system: a sample containing real patients' data, covering the maximum possible states, and a sample containing the basic rules of the states. A learning sample with real data is difficult to be implemented, it has a large volume of options, so it should be constantly checked to avoid the state of relearning.

To train the intelligent system, a sample was designed that takes into account the intervals of changes of biomedical factors for each state. The sample was additionally supplemented with factors with real estimates of patients' states having the greatest error (Strohmer & Vershynin 2009; Elble et al. 2010). The sample containing the basic rules for changing states includes 18 examples, and the sample containing real data of patients numbers 45 examples.

The approbation of the created intelligent system was carried out by comparing the assessments of the patient's states obtained by the system and set by an expert. Evaluation histograms are presented in Figure 6.8. Assessing the state changes over time, the effectiveness evaluation of a group of medications for treating hepatitis C was carried out.

The correlation coefficient of the intelligent system and the expert assessment is 0.9 for Medication 1, and 0.8 for Medication 2, which is acceptable for medical expert systems.

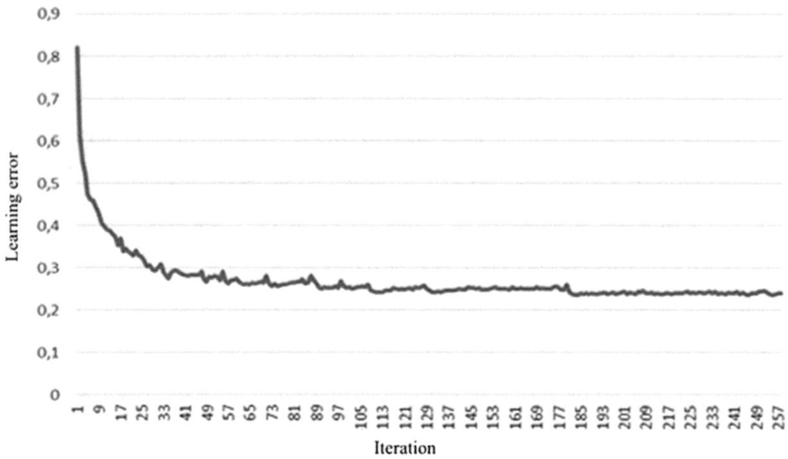

Figure 6.7. Graph of the training system.

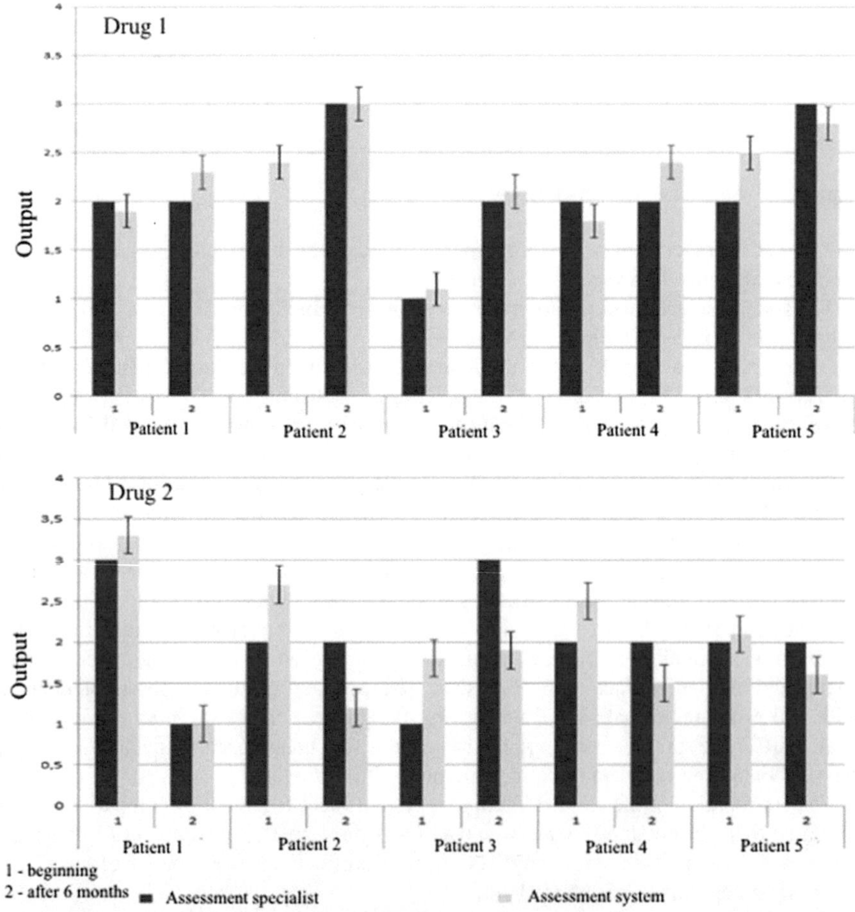

Figure 6.8. Histograms of a patient's state comparison (1 – at the beginning, 2 – six months later).

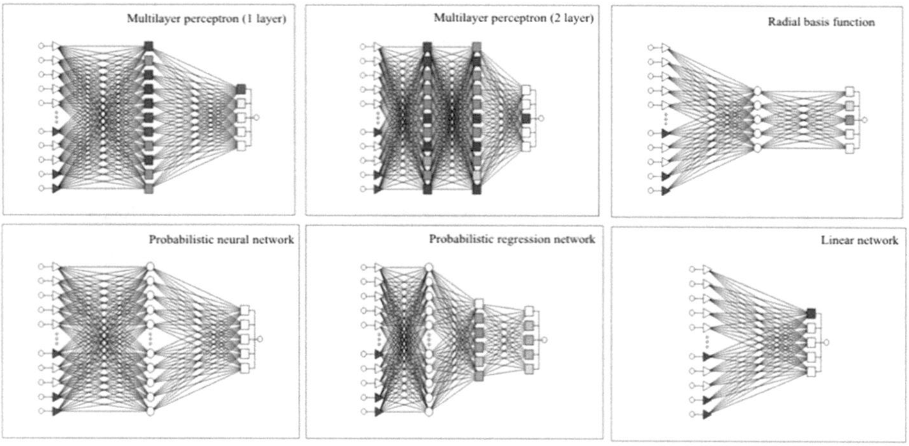

Figure 6.9. Architecture of neural networks participating in the comparison.

Table 6.2. The results of the calculations.

Neural network topology	Error
Perceptron with one layer	0.3
Perceptron with two layers	0.52
Radial basis function network	0.65
Probabilistic neural network	0.13
Probabilistic regression neural network	1.78
Linear multilayer neural network	0.65
Neural network with the Kaczmarz algorithm	0.02

The introduction of the developed system will allow improving the quality of treatment by constant monitoring its effectiveness to change the general state. Due to the general informatisation of medical institutions, the use of information systems for solving medical problems is a priority, since increasing volumes of information, improving diagnostic techniques, and expanding treatment techniques broadens the tasks of data processing and interpretation (Kaczmarz 1937).

6.3 EVALUATING THE ALGORITHM'S EFFECTIVENESS

Comparison of the proposed algorithm's effectiveness was carried out by assessing the average training errors calculated in analysing the learning sample and several examples of the test sample. The calculations are presented in Table 6.2, and the architectures of the neural networks participating in the comparison are found in Figure 6.9. Comparing the errors obtained during the calculation, we can conclude that the proposed algorithm is effective. The algorithms were compared in the Automated Neural Networks component of Statistica 10.3, based on learning and test samples. The Automated Neural Networks component has automatically carried out the selection of the most efficient neural networks for the samples presented.

6.4 CONCLUSIONS

The chapter describes the Kaczmarz algorithm for the neural network. A distinctive feature of this algorithm is finding a solution by iterations that have proven to be effective in solving complex computational problems. The application of the described approach in medicine for tasks that contain one or many input factors allows improving the quality of diagnosis.

REFERENCES

Andreev, P. G., Yakimov, A. N., Yurkov, N. K., Kochegarov, I. I. & Grishko, A. K. 2016. Methods of calculating the strength of electric component of electromagnetic field in difficult conditions. *Conference Proceedings 2016 International Conference on Actual Problems of Electron Devices Engineering, APEDE 2016.*

Anisimov, A. S., Kononov, V. T. & Chikildin, G. P. 1989. Comparison of Nonstationary Parameters Current Identification Methods. *IFAC Proceedings* 22(16): 35–40.

Artamonov, D. V., Litvinov, A. N., Yurkov, N. K., Kochegarov, I. I. & Lysenko, A. V. 2018. A technique for conducting experimental and theoretical dynamic research in design of instrument devices. *Proceedings of 2018 Moscow Workshop on Electronic and Networking Technologies, MWENT*: 1–5.

Bortnyk, G., Vasylkivskyi, M. & Kychak, V. 2018. Analog-digital path of radio-technical systems with digital processing of high-frequency signals. *Proc. 14th International Conference on Advanced Trends in Radioelecrtronics, Telecommunications and Computer Engineering (TCSET)*: 1162–1165.

Danilova, E., Kochegarov, I. & Yurkov, N. 2017. The construction of information measuring system of defects detection in conductive patterns of printed circuit boards. *Proceedings of 14th International Conference the Experience of Designing and Application of CAD Systems in Microelectronics, CADSM*: 183–187.

Dmitriev, G.A. & Astaf'ev, A.N. 2017. Sistema podderzhki prinyatiya reshenij pri opredelenii nozologicheskoj formy gepatita. *Programmnye produkty i sistemy* 4: 754–757.

Elble J. M., Sahinidis N.V. & Vouzis P. 2010. GPU computing with Kaczmarz's and other iterative algorithms for linear systems. *Parallel Comput.* 36 (5–6): 215–231.

Fahlman, S. & Lebiere, C. 1997. The Cascade-Correlation Learning Architecture. *Advances in Neural Information Processing Systems* 2.

Farhat C., Mandel J. & Roux, F. X. 1994. Optimal convergence properties of the FETI domain decomposition method. *Computer methods in applied mechanics and engineering* 115(3–4): 365–385.

Fouad, R.H., Ashhab, M.S., Mukattash, A. & Idwan, S. 2012. Simulation and energy management of an experimental solar system through adaptive neural networks. *IET Sci. Meas. Technol.*: 1–5.

Il'in, V.P. 2006. Ob iteratsionnom metode Kachmazha i ego obobshheniyakh. *Sibirskij zhurnal industrial'noj matematiki* 9(3): 39–49.

Kaczmarz, S. 1937. Angenäherte Auflösung von Systemen linearer Gleichungen. *Bulletin International de l'Académie Polonaise des Sciences et des Lettres. Classe des Sciences Mathématiques et Naturelles. Série A, Sciences Mathématiques* 35: 355–357.

Lysenko, A. V., Kochegarov, I. I., Yurkov, N. K. & Grishko, A. K. 2018. Optimizing structure of complex technical system by heterogeneous vector criterion in interval form. *Journal of Physics: Conference Series* 1015(4).

Ostreikovsky, V. A., Shevchenko, Y. N., Yurkov, N. K., Kochegarov, I. I. & Grishko, A. K. 2018. Time Factor in the Theory of Anthropogenic Risk Prediction in Complex Dynamic Systems. *Journal of Physics: Conference Series* 944:012085.

Pashchenko, F. F. & Pashchenko, A. F. 2012. Imitation models in decision-making systems. *Proc. 7th IEEE Conference on Industrial Electronics and Applications (ICIEA)*: 486–490.

Strohmer, T. & Vershynin R. 2009. Randomized Kaczmarz Algorithm with Exponential Convergence. *Journal of Fourier Analysis and Applications* 15(2): 157–165.

CHAPTER 7

Structural diagrams of algorithms for measuring of the probabilistic characteristics of a stationary segment of the EEG

Yu.P. Mukha
Volgograd State Medical University, Volgograd, Russian Federation
Volgograd State Technical University, Volgograd, Russian Federation

D.Yu. Ketov
Volgograd State Medical University, Volgograd, Russian Federation

A. Kotyra & M. Plechawska-Wójcik
Lublin University of Technology, Lublin, Poland

B. Amirgaliyev
Astana IT-University, Nur-Sultan, Kazakhstan

ABSTRACT: The authors examine the technique of model formation for the test signal of a special shape. This test signal is the base for monitoring the technical condition of electroencephalographic equipment during operation. They solve all tasks of synthesis of structural schemes and algorithms for forming a model of the test signal, and obtain structural diagrams of the algorithms for calculating the probabilistic characteristics. The authors perform a metrological analysis for the subsequent estimation of errors at each stage of data processing during the modelling of the test signal of a special shape.

7.1 INTRODUCTION

We establish the conformity of the quality indicators of electroencephalographic equipment to the requirements of normative documentation (ND) using technical tests. So, we can reveal the actual values of these indicators, check whether the medical product meets the requirements of standards, and compare the quality of products with the quality of analogues.

First of all, we mean that it is necessary to use the tests as the main form of assessing the technical level and quality. The effectiveness of all tests is determined primarily by avoiding damage from the use of poor-quality medical measuring products. We identified the most important component of the test: the system should be the range of issues ensuring the unity of tests, the achievement of the required accuracy and reproducibility of their results.

We also include here the whole complex of tasks of metrological support of measurements carried out during testing. We will use the following methods to evaluate the evaluation of the effectiveness of electroencephalographic equipment and to monitor its technical condition:

1. We make the test using the laboratory equipment, which is intended for special, control, acceptance testing of various objects. The objects are subjected to loads that are comparable or exceed to the loads in real conditions during these tests.
2. The purpose of such tests is to find out the response of an object to specific conditions and limiting load values.
3. The structural test stand is a set of working field (plate, or something else for fixing the device during a test), subsystems of sample load (vibrational, electrical or other depending on the type of the tests) and the instrumentations designed for measuring of a response of the sample to the load.

7.2 PROBLEM STATEMENT

Nowadays, many investigators use various functional generators, such as GF-05 and Diatest-04, for the testing equipment for evaluating the condition of electroencephalographic equipment (Plechawska-Wójcik 2015; Plechawska-Wójcik et al. 2017). As a rule, they have limited functionality that does not allow them to make full implement of the techniques described in the operational documentation in the absence of the ability to the modeling of the various waveforms. Even if it is possible to form a variety of test signals for testing equipment, the model of the test signal does not correspond to a real electroencephalogram (that is, it is possible to form a signal having nothing to do with the real electroencephalogram).

When we are monitoring the technical state, it is necessary to choose an adequate test procedure that takes into account the parameters reflected in the normative technical and operational documentation of the product. As a rule, these issues are solved on the basis of the techniques described in the operational documentation or using the "MI 2523-99" methodological recommendations (Gurevich 1988; Shilyaev 2008).

There is only one waveform that realises the possibility of an analysis of the amplitude-time dependencies in those recommendations. And we cannot say anything about the correctness of the reproduction of the waveform using in a test. Therefore, the creation of a model of a test signal should be considered in terms of the changes in the parameters and shape of the electroencephalogram of a healthy person and its changes in various diseases and pathologies.

Electroencephalography is an independent area of clinical diagnosis, which establishes a correspondence between the changes in electrical potentials observed on the EEG and the terms used to designate them.

EEG analysis consists of three interrelated components:

1. Evaluation of recording quality and differentiation of artefacts from the actual electroencephalographic phenomena;
2. The frequency and amplitude characteristics of the EEG, identification of characteristic graph elements on the EEG (phenomena such as "acute wave", "spike", "spike-wave", etc.), determination of the spatial and temporal distribution of these phenomena on the EEG, assessment of the presence and nature of transient phenomena on the EEG, such as "flashes", "discharges", "periods", etc., as well as determining of the localization of sources of various types of potentials in the brain;
3. A physiological and pathophysiological interpretation of the data and the formulation of the diagnostic conclusion.

We mean a certain type of electrical activity corresponding to a certain state of the brain and associated with certain cerebral mechanisms as the term "rhythm" in the EEG. Accordingly, when we are describing the rhythm, we know its frequency, which is typical for a certain state and region of the brain, the amplitude and some characteristic features (shapes) of its changes in time with accordance to changes in the functional activity of the brain.

There are usually four types of rhythms in the clinical studies: delta, theta, alpha and beta rhythms. An alpha-rhythm with a frequency of 8–13 Hz and an amplitude of up to 100 μV is the main one for preliminary detection of abnormalities. The amplitude of the alpha-rhythm, even in the same state, varies from a minimum to a maximum forming spindles – horizontally oriented amplitude modulations. Disorganization of the alpha-rhythm – frequency irregularity, change in the shape of waves, growth of amplitude and disruption of spatial distribution across the cerebral cortex, arises when the visual tuber is affected. Reduction (weakening) of alpha activity – a decrease in the index, the amplitude of the oscillations, slowing of the rhythm, usually accompanies to the local or diffuse lesions of the cortex of the cerebral hemispheres, as well as non-rough lesions of different levels of the brainstem.

Beta-rhythm with a frequency of 14–40 Hz and amplitude of up to 15 μV is the leading rhythm of active wakefulness. Usually, the beta-rhythm is expressed rather weakly (3-7 μV) and can be masked by noise and electromyogram (EMG). For healthy people, in a state of alertness, a diffuse, low-amplitude, unchanged Beta-rhythm, which does not change under any stimuli, is released. This form is intensified before the spontaneous development of convulsive seizures for patients with epilepsy. At the same time, the rhythm has a frequency of 24–22 per/sec first, then it slows down to 18–16 per/sec, often accompanied by the appearance of "peak-wave" complexes at that time.

Slow rhythms: theta rhythm with a frequency of 4–6 Hz and a delta rhythm with a frequency of 0.5–3 Hz have an amplitude of 40–300 μV and are normal in some states of sleep in the normal state. Diffusically pronounced theta-activity is observed for patients with clinical signs of lesion of the diencephalic region. Intermittent theta-activity in the posterior parts of the brain is noted for patients with mental disorders.

Delta activity is normally recorded during physiological sleep. In pathology, it is the most characteristic sign of impairment of the functional state of the brain. The hypoxia, a disorder of metabolism, discirculations and disorders in the lymph circulation and blood circulation are factors that cause changes in the activity of cortical neurons with the appearance of delta activity.

We use EEG to evaluate such properties of the brain as physiological maturity, functional state, the presence of focal lesions, cerebral disorders and their nature. As a result, EEG is the main method of diagnosing human diseases such as epilepsy, brain tumours and sleep disorders.

Epileptiform activity is a phenomenon typically observed in the EEG of epileptic patients. They arise as a result of highly synchronised paroxysmal depolarisation shifts in large populations of neurons, accompanied by the generation of action potentials. As a result of this, high-amplitude potentials of acute form arise, which have corresponding names:

1. Spike (spike is a peak) – negative potential of acute form, duration less than 70 ms, amplitude >50 μV (sometimes up to hundreds or even thousands of μV).
2. The sharp wave differs from the spike by stretching in time: its duration is 70–200 ms.
3. Sharp waves and spikes can be combined with slow waves, forming stereotyped complexes. A spike-slow wave is a complex of spike and slow-wave. The frequency of the spike-slow wave complexes is 2.5–6 Hz, and the period, respectively, is 160–250 ms. An acute-slow wave is a complex of an acute wave and the slow-wave, which follows after the acute wave. The period of the complex is 500–1300 ms (Fedoseyeva 1996; Khomskaya 2003; Kukes 2006).

An important characteristic of spikes and sharp waves is their sudden appearance and disappearance, and a clear difference from background activity, which they exceed in amplitude. Acute phenomena with corresponding parameters, vaguely different from background activity, are not designated as acute waves or spikes. Combinations of the phenomena described are indicated by some additional terms:

1. Flash is a term designating a group of waves with a sudden appearance and disappearance, clearly differing from the background activity by frequency, shape and/or amplitude.
2. Discharge is a burst of epileptiform activity.
3. The pattern of epileptic seizure is a discharge of epileptiform activity, typically coinciding with a clinical epileptic seizure. The detection of such phenomena is also characterised as a "pattern of epileptic seizure", even if it is not possible to clearly assess clinically the patient's state of consciousness.
4. Gypsarrhythmia (greek → "high-amplitude rhythm") is continuous generalised high-amplitude (>150 μV) slow hypersynchronous activity with acute waves, spikes, spike-slow wave complexes, polyspike-slow wave, synchronous and asynchronous. The gypsarrhythmia is an important diagnostic sign of West's syndrome and Lennox-Gastaut's syndrome.
5. Periodic complexes – the high-amplitude bursts of activity, characterised by a constant shape for the concrete patient. The most important criteria for their recognition are: close to a constant interval between complexes; continuous presence throughout the entire recording in case of the constant level of functional activity of the brain; intra-individual stability of the form (stereotype). Most often they are represented by a group of high-amplitude slow waves, sharp waves, combined with high-amplitude, the acuminate delta or theta-oscillations. Sometimes they have the form which is reminiscent to the epileptiform acute-slow wave complexes. The intervals between the complexes range are from 0.5–2 to tens of seconds. Generalised bilaterally synchronous periodic complexes always attest to the presence of deep disorders of consciousness and indicate severe brain damage. If they are not caused by the pharmacological or toxic factors (alcohol abstinence,

an overdose or sudden withdrawal of psychotropic and hypnosedate drugs, hepatopathy, carbon monoxide poisoning), then, as a rule, they are the consequence of severe metabolic, hypoxic, prion or viral encephalopathy. If intoxications or metabolic disturbances are excluded, then periodic complexes with high reliability indicate a diagnosis of panencephalitis or prion disease.

The EEG is substantially uniform and symmetrical. Functional and morphological heterogeneity of the cortex determines the features of electrical activity in different regions of the brain. Spatial change of types EEG of separate areas of a brain occurs gradually (Fedoseyeva 1996; Khomskaya 2003; Kukes 2006).

Many doctors considered all subtleties of the analysis of the electroencephalogram and diagnosed that it is very important for the simulation of the test signal to pay attention not only to the amplitude-time parameters of the signal, but also to the peculiarities of its shape change.

We examined a number of studies, in which authors showed that using a nonparametric segmentation made it possible to represent the EEG in the form of a set of stationary segments. So, the main goal of our scientific work was the creation of a correct EEG test signal model, which would make it possible to obtain an electroencephalographic signal model (Ketov & Mukha 2012; Ketov & Mukha 2014; Ketov & Mukha 2015; Tsvetkov 2008).

McEwen devoted his first paper to the analysis of the stationary properties of the EEG. He turned out that practically all EEG fragments were stationary with a duration of 2–4 s: with a larger EEG fragmentation, the statistical estimation of such short sections would become clearly untenable and the question of their stationarity would be lost meaning. We formulated the main conclusion of the study: the EEG signal may indeed be approximated by basic stochastic criteria of normality, ergodicity, Gaussianity, etc., but only on fairly short implementations, usually not exceeding 10–20 s.

It also became apparent for us that the use of the statistical characteristics, including, of course, the spectral-correlation is applicable to the EEG signal only after its preliminary segmentation into areas of relative stationarity. This work gave the base for our first steps to a completely new understanding of the organisation of the EEG as a piecewise stationary process.

Many authors devoted in their first papers to the analysis of the statistical properties of the EEG as a stochastic process. It was shown that the distribution of the amplitude values of the EEG corresponds to Gaussian parameters. Short segments of the EEG, up to 10 s, were usually well approximated by the Gaussian distribution. Long segments, up to 1 min, were not approximated by the normal law. Later, the specific data were obtained on the relationship between the correspondence of the Gaussian distribution and the length of the EEG estimation segments. It turned out that with an increase in the duration of the EEG from 4 to 64 seconds, the number of segments corresponding to the Gaussian distribution decreased from 90 to 20% with the discretisation of the EEG signal at the Nyquist frequency.

However, in practice, we usually control the constancy in time of the mathematical expectation, variance and parameters of the correlation function for a one-dimensional distribution of values for each sample of the dynamic process to monitor its stationary nature.

McEwen and Anderson estimated the EEG sections of different durations in that manner. They showed that Gaussianity and Stationarity are simultaneously observed only for 15–20% of the EEG sections of a record of 16 s for each of them. These conditions are met for 70–80% of the EEG record when the duration of those sections is reduced to 4 seconds.

It was found in numerous studies using EEG segmentation that the EEG actually consists of relatively stationary segments. The duration of the main mass of them varies according to the data of different authors in the range from 0.2 to 10–12 seconds. And their classification by spectral characteristics shows the existence of a fairly compact, within a few dozen, a set of typical segments.

7.3 RESEARCH

We obtained all the electroencephalographic signal models. As a result of consideration and analysis of the research data, we concluded that we need first apply nonparametric segmentation and perform subsequently a statistical estimation of the segments obtained.

We developed the technology of non-parametric EEG segmentation on the basis of the theory of the analysis of moments of abrupt changes or disruptions in time series having a clearly expressed piecewise-stationary structure. The discrepancies determined in this way are the marks of the boundaries between quasi-stationary fragments.

This technique is based on the use of a special statistical procedure for the detection of moments of "disagreements". We use a generalised version of the Kolmogorov-Smirnov statistics in that statistical procedure. We used these criteria in the technique of EEG segmentation taking into account their probability distributions. We estimated the confidence intervals of their positioning within the EEG fragment, which was being tested, and reliably detected of the boundaries of the segments.

Many authors have also shown that it is reasonable to use the normalised autocorrelation function of the EEG signal as the diagnostic sequence. The methodology of nonparametric analysis is based on two ideas. It was proved that the definition of changes in any distribution function or probabilistic characteristic can be reduced (with any degree of accuracy) to the determination of changes in the mathematical expectation of some other sequence formed from the original one. A new sequence will be called a diagnostic sequence. For example, we reduced the problem to the determination of changes in one of the sequences $V_t(\tau)$ considering autocorrelation functions.

$$V_t(\tau) = x_t x_{t+\tau},\ \tau = 0, 1, 2, \ldots$$

The changes in the autocorrelation values correspond to changes in the power spectra. The power spectrum is equal to the Fourier transform of the autocorrelation function. In particular, $V_t(0)$ is identical to the total power (by the Parseval theorem).

The second idea of the approach is in the using of the following set of statistics:

$$Y_N(n,\delta) = \left[\left(1 - \frac{n}{N}\right)\frac{n}{N}\right]^{\delta}\left[\frac{1}{n}\sum_{k=1}^{n} x_k - \frac{1}{N-n}\sum_{k=n+1}^{N} x_k\right] \quad (7.1)$$

where $0 \le \delta \le 1$, $1 \le n \le N-1$, $\{x_k\}_{k=1}^{N}$ is the implementation of the diagnostic sequence. N is the number of samples in this sequence (in our case in the entire EEG record). This set of statistics is a generalised version of Kolmogorov-Smirnov statistics, which is used to study of the coincidences or differences in the distribution functions of two sequences (of fixed size n). In other words, we calculated the difference between the average value of the first n samples and the last N-n samples multiplied by the coefficient as a function of δ. We performed this calculation is for all $n : 1 \le n \le N-1$. Then we compare the maximum of these n differences with a special threshold. The threshold is calculated on the basis of the limiting characteristics of statistics (*for* $N \to \infty$). We made a decision about the stationarity of the EEG implementation if this threshold is not reached, otherwise we consider this point to be the boundary of stationary segments (Brodsky 1998; Kaplan 1998; Kaplan 1999; Ketov & Mukha 2012).

The method can be characterised by such quantities as the probability of false alarm (the probability of making a decision about the existence of a boundary when it is not actually there), the probability of false peace (the probability that we will not notice the boundary where it really is) and time error of the segment boundary. For a given statistic, these quantities are functions depending on δ. We used an important property of the statistics: $\delta = 0$ ensures a minimum probability of false alarm, on the other hand, the case $\delta = 1$ ensures a minimum probability of false peace, and the case $\delta = 0.5$ ensures a minimum temporal error of the boundaries of segments.

We have done the nonparametric segmentation of the EEG taking into account the studies that were noted earlier. We considered a technique for calculating the statistical characteristics of the stationary EEG segments. They were in normal distribution law. We demonstrated the result of EEG on Figure 7.1.

In practice, it is not usually possible to use formulas for accurately determining the probabilistic characteristics of the real EEG signals. Therefore we performed their statistical estimation based on the realisations $X(t)$, which were obtained experimentally. We presented the obtained EEG segment data in the form of a table consisting of two rows. The first line contains the measurement numbers (time samples $t_1, t_2 \ldots t_n$), and in the second line, we set their results (voltage values $x_1, x_2 \ldots x_n$).

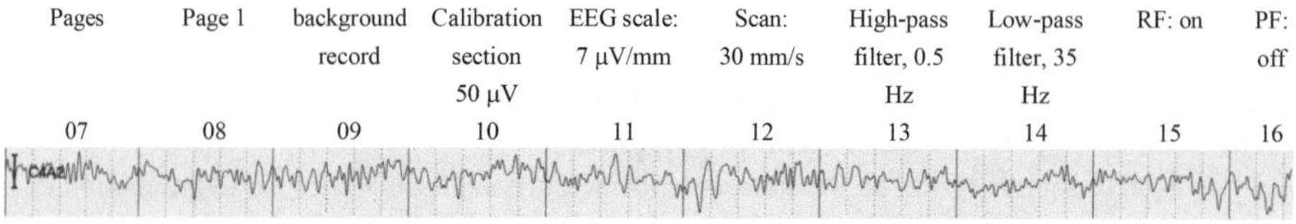

Figure 7.1. EEG-central lead C4A2.

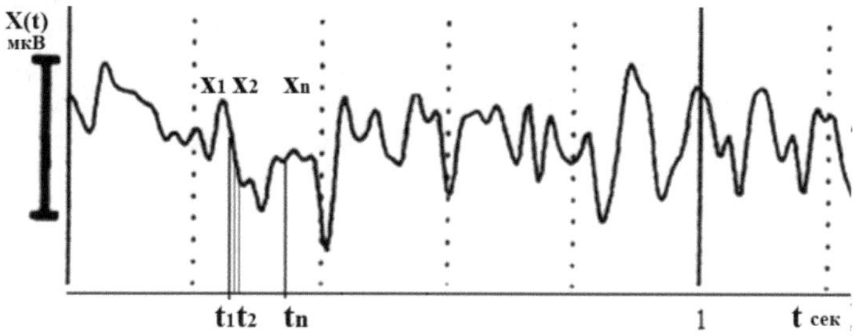

Figure 7.2. EEG segment.

Table 7.1. An interval table in the form of a statistical series.

Interval	Frequency f_i	Middle point of a class x_i	Relative frequencies	Accumulated frequencies	Accumulated relative frequency
x_i	f_i	$\bar{x}_i$	$\frac{f_i}{n}$	$\sum_{x_i<x} f_i$	$\sum_{x_i<x} \frac{f_i}{n}$
x_i, x_{i+h}	$\sum f_i = n$		$\sum \frac{f_i}{n} = 1$		

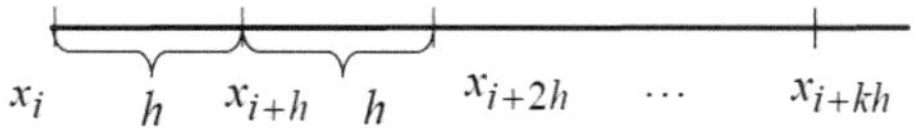

Figure 7.3. Bounds for the interval series.

$x_1(t_1)$, $x_2(t_2) \ldots x_n(t_n)$ are the observed values of the continuous random variable $X(t)$ of the EEG segment (Figure 7.2).

We transformed this series into a variational series, where all the observations are presented in ascending order, that is, in the form of:

$$x_1 \text{ min}, x_2, \ldots, x_n \text{ max},$$

where $x_1 \text{ min} \leq x_2 \leq x_n$ max.

On the next step, this variation series was represented by an interval table in the form of a statistical series (Table 7.1).

An interval of a series can be represented on a numerical axis (Figure 7.3).

The values $x_i, x_{i+h}, x_{i+2h}, \ldots, x_{i+kh}$ determine the boundaries of the intervals. Step h is equal to $h = (x_n \text{ max} - x_1 \text{ min})/k$, where k is the number of intervals. We took the point $(x_1 \text{ min} - h/2)$ for the beginning of the first interval. The middle point of the interval is defined as $x_{ik} = x_i$. The frequency f_i represents the number of the observations that fall within a given interval.

The law of large numbers in Bernoulli's form states that if the experiment is repeated n times under the same conditions, then the frequency f_i/n converges in probability to p_i (the values of f_i/n are approximated by probabilities p_i).

In the general case, the empirical distribution function is determined from the values of the accumulated frequencies from the following relation:

$$F_n(x) = \frac{1}{n}\sum\nolimits_{x_i<x} f_i \tag{7.2}$$

Since our random variable $X(t)$ obeys to the normal law of probability distribution, its distribution density is:

$$\varphi(x) = \frac{1}{\sigma\sqrt{2\pi}} e^{-(x-a)^2/(2\sigma^2)} \tag{7.3}$$

and the distribution function $F(x)$:

$$F(x) = \frac{1}{\sigma\sqrt{2\pi}} \int_{-\infty}^{x} e^{-(t-a)^2/(2\sigma^2)} dt \tag{7.4}$$

We applied the statistical methods of data processing to determine the distribution function of the EEG segment from experimental data in our case. We divided the range of the observed values $X(t)$ into intervals $[X_0, X_1], [X_1, X_2], \ldots, [X_{k-1}, X_k]$ of the same length ΔX. We accepted m_i as the number of observed values that fall in the i-th interval. We divided m_i by the total number of observations n and obtained the frequency P_i corresponding to the i-th interval: $P_i = m_i/n$, and $\sum_{i=1}^{k} p_i^* = \sum_{i=1}^{k} m_i/n = 1$

The empirical (or statistical) distribution function of a random variable is the frequency of the event, which means that the value of $X(t)$ takes a value less than x as a result of the experiment: $F^*(x) = P^*(\xi < x)$.

In practice, it is sufficient to find the values of the statistical distribution function $F^*(x)$ at the points $X_0, X_1, \ldots, X_k$, which are the boundaries of the intervals of the statistical series:

$$\begin{cases} F^*\left(X_0\right) = P^*\left(\xi < X_0\right) = 0 \\ F^*\left(X_1\right) = P^*\left(\xi < X_1\right) = \dfrac{m_1}{n} = p_1^* \\ F^*\left(X_2\right) = P^*\left(\xi < X_2\right) = \dfrac{m_1 + m_2}{n} = p_1^* + p_2^* \\ F^*\left(X_k\right) = P^*\left(\xi < X_k\right) = \dfrac{m_1 + m_2 + m_k}{n} = p_1^* + p_2^* + p_k^* = 1 \end{cases}$$

On the next step, we calculated the statistical parameters of the distribution of X(t). We defined the mathematical expectation $M(X(t)) = a$ and the dispersion $D(X(t)) = \sigma^2$ from the following equations:

$$M\left(x\left(t\right)\right) = lim\frac{1}{T}\int_0^T x\left(t\right) \tag{7.5}$$

$$a = \frac{x_1 + x_2 + \ldots + x_n}{n} \tag{7.6}$$

$$D[X] = M\left[(X - m_x)^2\right] \tag{7.7}$$

$$\sigma^2 = \frac{\sum_{i=1}^{n}\left(x_i - a\right)^2}{n} \tag{7.8}$$

If the estimate of the dispersion is deviated, then $\sigma^2 = \frac{\sum_{i=1}^{n}(x_i - a)^2}{n-1}$

If we have a large number of experiments, then a calculation of the quantities a and σ^2 is associated with too cumbersome calculations. Therefore, each of the observed values of the quantity $X(t)$, which falls in the i-th interval $[X_{i-1}, X_i]$ of the statistical series, is approximately equal to the middle c_i of this interval, i.e. $c_i = (X_{i-1} + X_i)/2$. We considered the first interval $[X_0, X_1]$. It contained m_1 from observed values of the random variable. We replaced each of them by the number c_1. Consequently, the sum of these values is approximately equal to m_1c_1. Similarly, the sum of the values of $X(t)$ in the second interval is approximately equal to m_2c_2, and so on. Therefore

$$a = \frac{x_1 + x_2 + \ldots + x_n}{n} \approx \frac{\sum_{i=1}^{n} m_i c_i}{n}$$

We obtained approximate equality for σ^2 in the same way:

$$\sigma^2 = \frac{\sum_{i=1}^{n} (x_i - a)^2}{n-1} \approx \frac{\sum_{i=1}^{n} m_i (c_i - a)^2}{n-1},$$

where $n = m_1 + m_2 + \ldots + m_k$, and k is the number of intervals of the statistical series.

We defined central moments of any order from an equation:

$$\mu_s = \int_{-\infty}^{\infty} (x-m)^s f(x)\,dx = \frac{1}{\sigma\sqrt{2\pi}} \int_{-\infty}^{\infty} (x-m)^s e^{-\frac{(x-m)^2}{2\sigma^2}} dx$$

Then we changed the variable $\frac{x-m}{\sigma\sqrt{2}} = t$, and obtained $\mu_s = \frac{(\sigma\sqrt{2})^s}{\sqrt{\pi}} \int_{-\infty}^{\infty} t^s e^{-t^2} dt$.

Then we applied the formula of "integration by parts" to the equation

$$\mu_s = \frac{\left(\sigma\sqrt{2}\right)^s}{\sqrt{\pi}} \int_{-\infty}^{\infty} t^{s-1} e^{-t^2} dt = \frac{\left(\sigma\sqrt{2}\right)^s}{\sqrt{\pi}} \left\{ -\frac{1}{2} e^{-t^2 t^{s-1}} \Big|_{-\infty}^{\infty} + \frac{s-1}{2} \int_{-\infty}^{\infty} t^{s-2} e^{-t^2} dt \right\},$$

and got $\mu_s = \frac{(s-1)(\sigma\sqrt{2})^s}{2\sqrt{\pi}} \int_{-\infty}^{\infty} t^s e^{-t^2} dt$, meaning that the first term inside the parentheses is zero. Then we obtained the following equation for μ_{s-2}:

$$\mu_{s-2} = \frac{\left(\sigma\sqrt{2}\right)^{s-2}}{\sqrt{\pi}} \int_{-\infty}^{\infty} t^{s-2} e^{-t^2} dt$$

We compared the right-hand sides of the last equations and saw that they differ only by the factor $(s-1)\sigma^2$. So, we obtained an equality $\mu_s = (s-1)\sigma^2 \mu_{s-2}$.

All the odd moments of the normal distribution are zero, as it follows from the formulas. The even moments are s: $\mu_2 = \sigma^2$, $\mu_4 = 3\sigma^4$, $\mu_6 = 15\sigma^6$

We found the moment of the s-th order for any even s in a form $\mu_s = (s-1)!!\sigma^2$, where the symbol $(s-1)!!$ means the product of all odd numbers from 1 to $(s-1)$.

The initial and central moments of any orders for statistical distributions are defined similarly:

$$a_s[X] = \frac{\sum_{i=1}^{n} x_i^s}{n} \tag{7.9}$$

$$\mu_s^*[X] = \frac{\sum_{i=1}^{n} \left(x_i - m_x^*\right)^s}{n} \tag{7.10}$$

In practice, we are interested in the correlation functions of the first two orders, since the significance of multiple correlations decreases with increasing order.

$$R_\tau(\tau) = \mathrm{M}[x(t)x(t+\tau)] = \lim_{T\to\infty} \frac{1}{T} \int_0^T x(t)x(t+\tau)\,dt \tag{7.11}$$

An estimation of the correlation function of a random process is

$$R^*(t_1, t_2) = \frac{1}{n} \sum_{i=1}^{n} \left[x_i(t_1) - m^*(t_1)\right]\left[x_i(t_2) - m^*(t_2)\right] \tag{7.12}$$

An estimation of the mutual correlation function of a random process is

$$R_x^*(t_1, t_2) = \frac{1}{n}\sum\nolimits_{i=1}^{n} \left[x_i(t_1) - m_\xi^*(t_1)\right]\left[x_i(t_2) - m_\eta^*(t_2)\right] \tag{7.13}$$

$$R_\tau(\tau) = \lim_{N\to\infty} \frac{1}{N}\sum\nolimits_{i=1}^{N} x(t)\, x(t+\tau) \tag{7.14}$$

We can find a complete description of Gaussian processes in the correlation theory. We considered a spectrum of power as spectral density of a process. By the Wiener-Khinchin theorem, spectral density of power for a stationary random process is the Fourier transform of the corresponding autocorrelation function. The spectrum of power characterizes the frequency distribution. We can define it from this equation:

$$\mathrm{S_x}(\omega) = \int_{-\infty}^{\infty} \mathrm{R_x}(\tau)\, \mathrm{e}^{-j\omega\tau} d\tau, \tag{7.15}$$

The mutual spectral density of the two realizations $X(t)$ and $Y(t)$ can be defined from an equation:

$$\mathrm{S_{xy}}(f) = \int_{-\infty}^{\infty} \mathrm{K_{xy}}(\tau)^* \,\mathrm{e}^{-j2\pi f\tau} d\tau,$$

We defined the spectral density for all frequencies, both positive and negative. The correlation functions are even functions. Their spectra are specified only by the real part of the Fourier transform:

$$S_x(f) = 4\int_0^{\infty} R_x(\tau) \cos 2\pi f\tau d\tau, \tag{7.16}$$

$$S_{xx}(f) = 4\int_0^{\infty} K_{xx}(\tau)^* \cos 2\pi f\tau d\tau,$$

$$S_{xy}(f) = 4\int_0^{\infty} K_{xy}(\tau)^* \cos 2\pi f\tau d\tau.$$

It is useful to determine the imaginary part of the Fourier transform for further finding of the phase shift function of processes, i.e.

$$Q_{xy}(f) = 4\int_0^{\infty} K_{xy}(\tau)^* \sin 2\pi f\tau d\tau$$

$$\theta_{xy}(f) = \mathrm{arctg}\left(\frac{Q_{xy}(f)}{S_{xy}(f)}\right).$$

For practical use, we can write the formula (7.16) in the form:

$$S_x(f) = 4\sum\nolimits_{\tau=0}^{T} R_x(\tau) \cos 2\pi f\tau,$$

$$S_{xy}(f) = 4\sum\nolimits_{\tau=0}^{T} K_{xy}(\tau)^* \cos 2\pi f\tau, \tag{7.17}$$

$$Q_{xy}(f) = 4\sum\nolimits_{\tau=0}^{T} K_{xy}(\tau)^* \sin 2\pi f\tau,$$

where T is the value of the time interval, which was taken for the analysis.

Then we explored the structural diagrams for measuring the parameters of the EEG segment (such as mathematical expectation, variance, correlation function, the spectral density of power) in accordance with the selected concept. We composed the corresponding measuring algorithms.

In a process of segmenting, we use the sets of statistics according to (7.1). The block diagram of this algorithm was shown in Figure 7.4, where SENS denotes the sensor, X_k is a measurement result, $X{:}Y$ – the operation of division, $x \cdot y$ denotes the operation of multiplication, SUB is a subtraction command, $[\ ]^2$ is the exponentiation operation, Σ denotes the operation of summation.

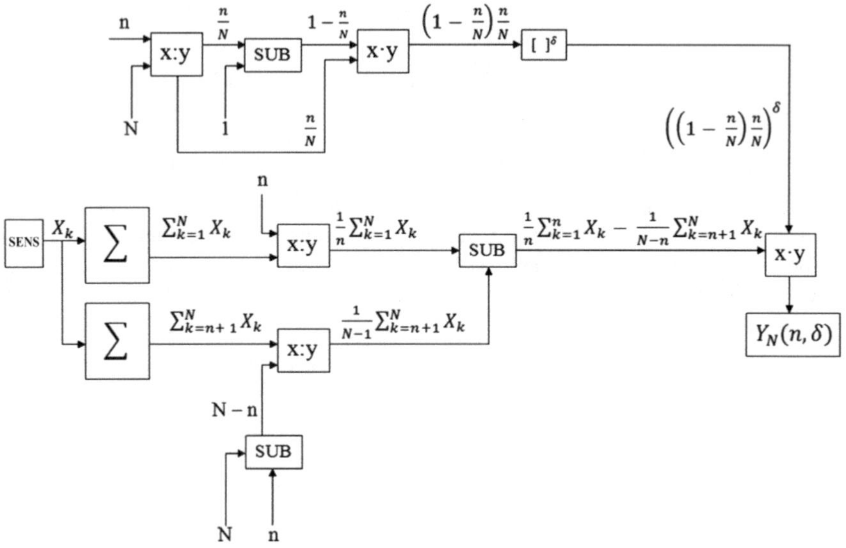

Figure 7.4. Structural diagram of the algorithm for calculating of the set of statistics.

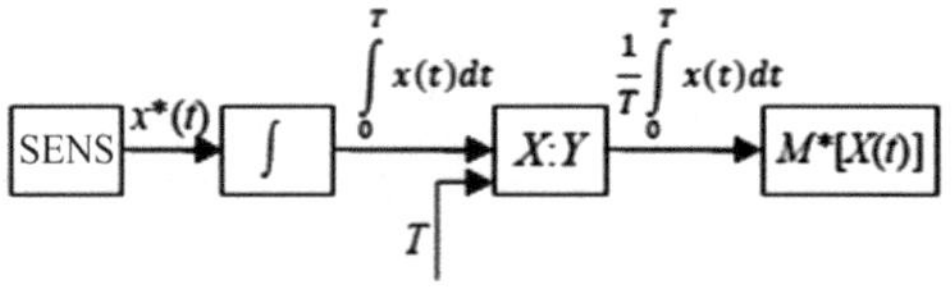

Figure 7.5. Structural diagram of the algorithm for measuring of the mathematical expectation.

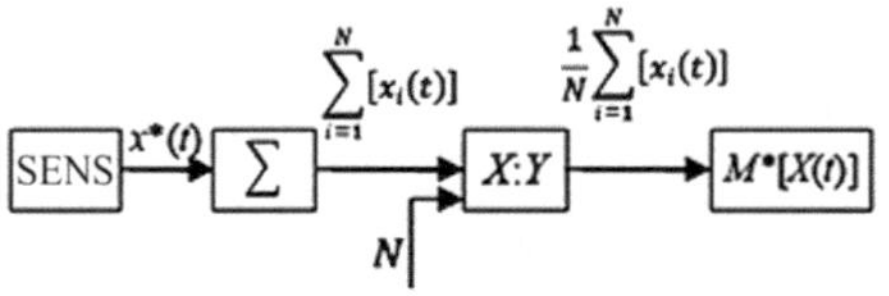

Figure 7.6. Structural diagram of the algorithm for measuring of the mathematical expectation from statistical data.

We use an Equation (7.5) to find the mathematical expectation from the realization of the random process $X(t)$. Then we constructed the block diagram of the algorithm for measuring the mathematical expectation takes in Figure 7.5, where SENS is a measuring sensor, $x^*(t)$ is a measurement result, $\int$ is the integration operation, $X{:}Y$ – the operation of division.

We found the mathematical expectation in the formula (7.6) with statistical estimation of the realization of the random process $X(t)$. The corresponding structural diagram of the algorithm for measuring of the mathematical expectation for statistical estimation is presented in Figure 7.6, where SENS is the measuring sensor, $x^*(t)$ – the measurement result, Σ denotes the operation of summation, $X{:}Y$ – the operation of division.

We use the Equations (7.3,7.4) to find the dispersion and write down the structural diagrams of the corresponding measurement algorithms – Figure 7.7 and Figure 7.8, where SENS is the measuring sensor, $x^*(t)$ – measurement result, $\int$ is the integration operation, $X{:}Y$ – the operation of division, SUB – subtraction command, $[\ ]^2$ is the exponentiation operation.

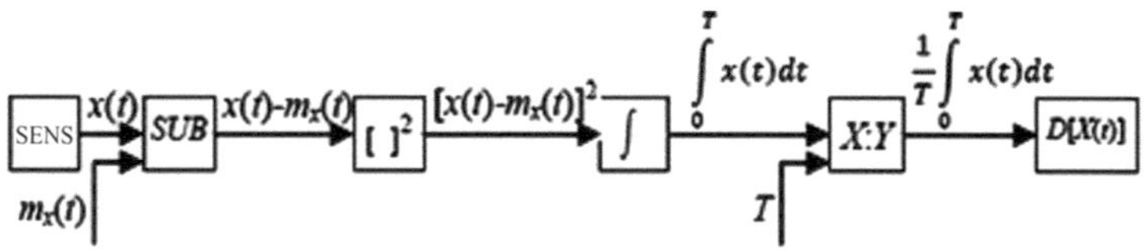

Figure 7.7. Structural diagram of the dispersion measurement algorithm.

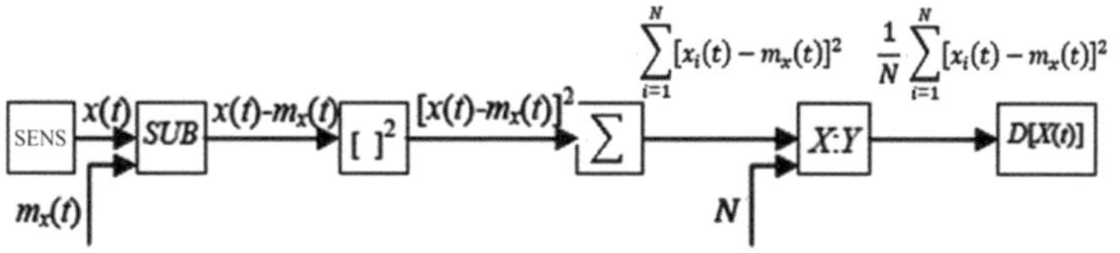

Figure 7.8. Structural diagram of the dispersion measurement algorithm according to statistical data.

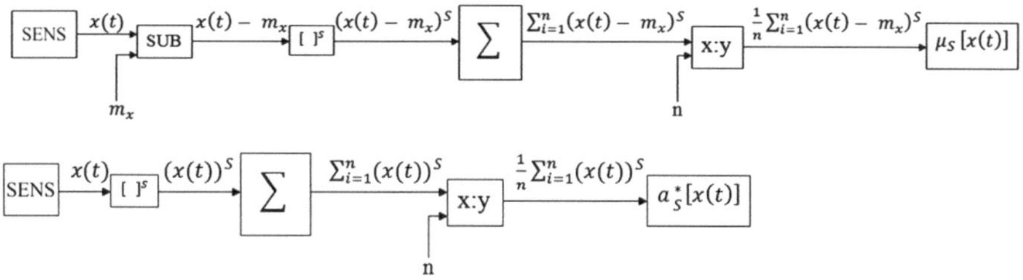

Figure 7.9. Structural diagram of the algorithm for measuring of the initial and central moments.

In statistical estimation, we took an Equation (7.8) to find the dispersion. According to the Equation (7.8), we have shown the block diagram of the dispersion measurement algorithm for statistical estimation in Figure 7.8, where SENS is the measuring sensor, Σ is the operation of summation, SUB is the subtraction command, $[\;]^2$ is the exponentiation operation, $X{:}Y$ – the operation of division.

We used the Equations (7.9,7.10) to find the initial and central moments of any orders for statistical distributions. We have shown a structural diagram of the algorithm for measuring of the initial and central moments in Figure 7.9, where SENS is the measuring sensor, Σ is the operation of summation, SUB – a subtraction command, $[\;]^2$ is the exponentiation operation, $X{:}Y$ – the operation of division.

Since our random variable $X(t)$ obeys to the normal law of probability distribution, the structural scheme of the algorithm for measuring of the distribution density and the distribution function from the Equations (7.3,7.4) was shown on Figure 7.10, where SENS is the measuring sensor, X – a measurement result, $X{:}Y$ – the operation of division, $x \cdot y$ denotes the operation of multiplication, SUB is the subtraction command, $[\;]^2$ is the exponentiation operation, $\int$ is the integration operation, e^x denotes exponential function.

We can define the correlation function for the stationary process $X(t)$ as the mathematical expectation of centred values at times t and $(t + \tau)$ and write it in the form of the Equations (7.11,7.12,7.13). The structural diagram of the algorithm for measuring the correlation function from expression (11) was shown in Figure 7.11.

We used an Equation (7.14) in the statistical estimation of the correlation function. The structural diagram of the algorithm for measuring of the correlation function for the statistical estimation was shown on Figure 7.12. Where SENS is the measuring sensor, $x(t)$ – the measurement result, $\int$ is the integration operation, $X{:}Y$ – the operation of division, $\frac{x}{y}\Big|^{xy}$ denotes the operation of multiplication.

The spectrum of power predetermined the distribution of frequency. We proved it in the Equation (7.15) (Figure 7.13).

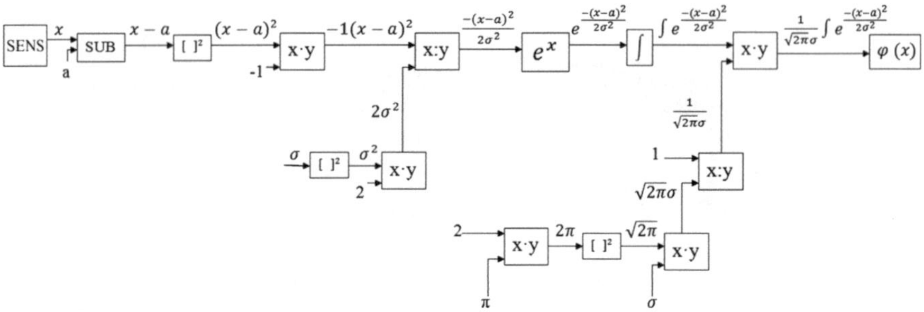

Figure 7.10. Structural diagram of the algorithm for measuring the distribution density and the distribution function.

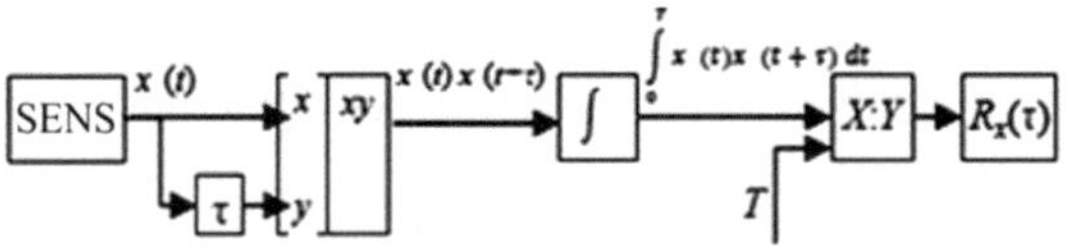

Figure 7.11. Structural diagram of the measurement algorithm of the correlation function.

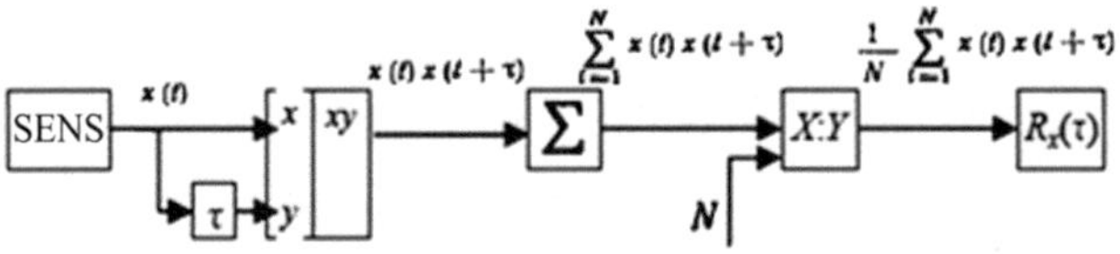

Figure 7.12. Structural diagram of the algorithm for measuring of the correlation function from statistical data.

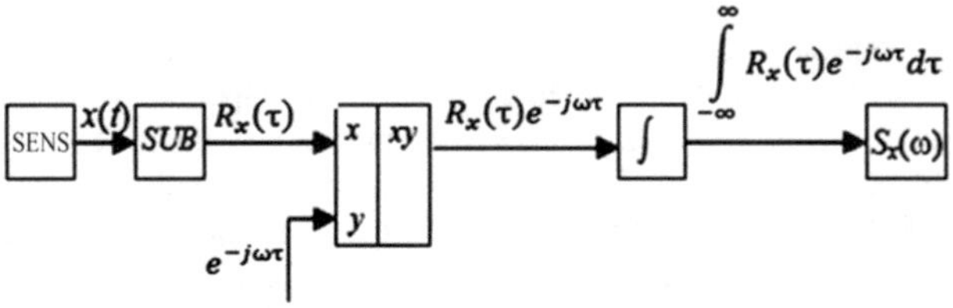

Figure 7.13. Structural diagram for an analyzer of power of a random process.

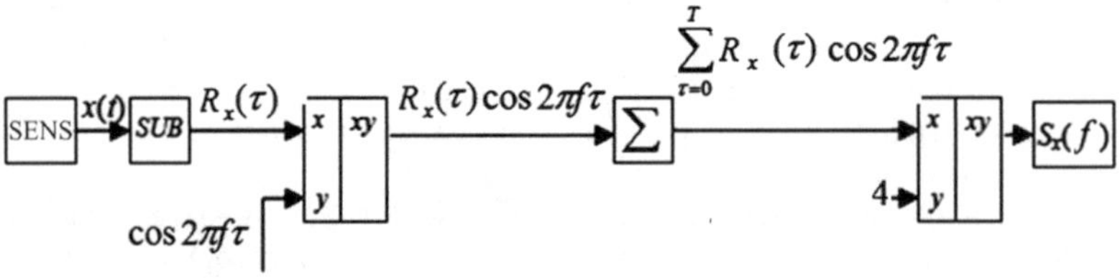

Figure 7.14. Structural diagram of the power analyzer of a random process.

Where SENS is the measuring sensor, $x(t)$- the measurement result, $\int$ is the integration operation, $X{:}Y$ – the operation of division, SUB – a subtraction command, $\left.{}^{x}_{y}\right|^{xy}$ denotes the operation of multiplication. The structural scheme of the algorithm for measuring the spectral density for statistical estimation was shown on Figure 7.14.

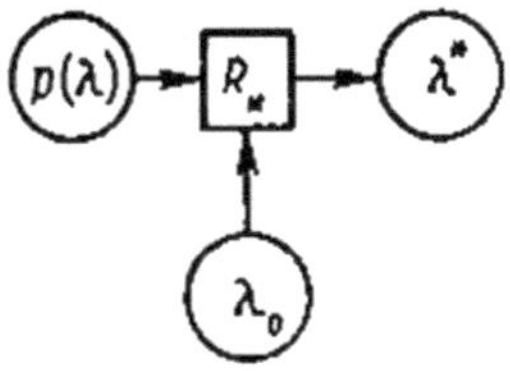

Figure 7.15. Structure of the measurement circuit for λ.

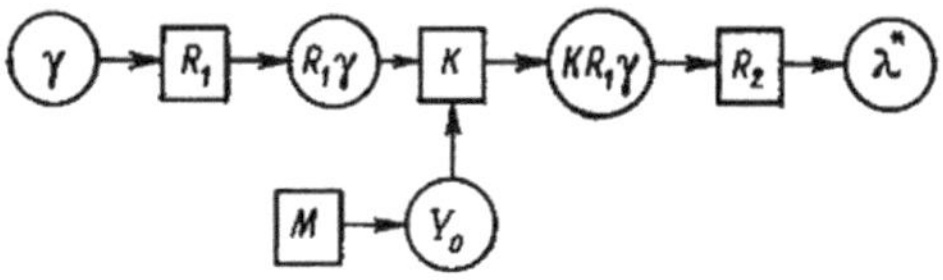

Figure 7.16. Structural diagram of the algorithm for measuring of probabilistic characteristics.

We onwards considered the structural scheme of the measuring element, M.s., in more detail. The evaluation of the value for the result, which was measured by the sensor λ^*, may be found by a formula:

$$\lambda^* = R_i[\mathrm{p}(\lambda), \lambda_0] \tag{7.18}$$

where R_i is an operator representing a measurement algorithm; $p(\lambda)$ – signal carrying information about the value of λ; λ_0 – the reference value underlying operation of comparison. We obtained an array of intermediate data during the implementation of the measurement algorithm – R_i. The structural scheme of finding λ according to the formula (7.18) was shown in Figure 7.15.

We made up the measurement equation for a formal description of the measurement procedures (algorithms, methods), measurement results and characteristics of the measurement results:

$$\lambda^* = \mathrm{R_2 K R_1}\gamma, \tag{7.19}$$

where R_1 – transformations performed during measurements in analogue form; K – comparison of the value of $R_{1\gamma}$ with the reference value (analogue-to-digital conversion); R_2 – transformations performed during measurements in numerical form; γ – an input effect (carrier of information on the value of the measured element). We showed the structural diagram compiled according to an Equation (7.19) on Figure 7.16. The symbols on the graph denote respectively: M – the reproduction operation of the sample value Y_0, the form of which corresponds to the form of the quantity $\mathrm{R_1}\gamma$, and K is a comparison operation.

We represented the operator K as follows:

$$\varphi^* = \mathrm{K} \cdot \varphi = (\varphi/\varphi_0) \cdot (\varphi_0/\varphi_1), \tag{7.20}$$

where φ_0 is a size of the reference value (measure value); φ_0/φ_1 – an established size of the reference value, expressed in units of measurement; φ_1 is accepted unit of the measurement φ. The ratio φ/φ_0 is determined in the measurement process and expressed in accepted units.

When we measure the probabilistic characteristics, it is always necessary to perform the following operations:

1. A transformation for determination of the probabilistic characteristic $g[\,]$;
2. Averaging over a sample S_d;
3. Comparisons with the standard value – K.

$$\theta_j^* [X(t)] = S_d g K \left[x_j(t)\right] \tag{7.21}$$

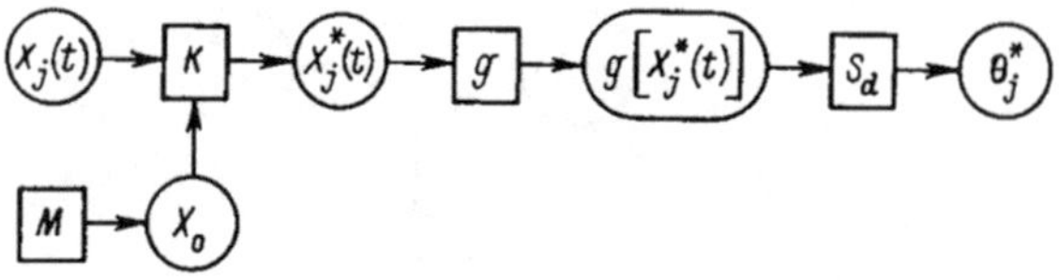

Figure 7.17. Structural diagram of the operation of comparison for measurements.

Substituting formula (7.20) in (7.21), we obtained the final expression for the operation of comparison for measurements and its structural diagram (Figure 7.17):

$$\theta_j^* [X(t)] = S_d g \left[\frac{x_j(t)}{x_0} \frac{x_0}{x_1} \right],$$

where X_0 is the sample value of the values of $X_j(t)$.

The comparison operation is built on the principle of analogue-to-digital conversion and always includes quantization and sampling operations. Considering it, we had clarified and rewritten the expression (7.20) as:

$$\varphi^* = K\varphi = \left(E\left[\frac{\varphi}{\Delta_k \varphi} \right] + s(\Delta_k \varphi) \right) \frac{\Delta_k \varphi}{\varphi_1} = [\varphi]^* \Delta_k \varphi,$$

where $E[\ ]$ is the integer part of the measured quantity; $\Delta_k \varphi$ – a quantization interval; $s(\Delta_k \varphi)$ – amendment, which is set on the basis of a priori information on the parameter φ.

We made several conclusions as a result of analyzing the obtained schemes for measuring probabilistic characteristics. Factors that reduce the accuracy of measuring the probabilistic characteristics of a random process include:

1. The finiteness of the amount of sample data;
2. The probability characteristics in the general case are expressed through the limits of the selective means:

$$\theta[X(t)] = \lim_{N \to \infty} \frac{1}{N} \sum_{i=1}^{N} g[x_i(t)]$$

where $g[x_i(t)]$ is the operator representing the transformations required to determine any of the probabilistic characteristics.

7.4 CONCLUSIONS

We obtained the structural diagrams of algorithms for calculating the probabilistic characteristics. Then we conducted the metrological analysis and the subsequent estimation of errors at each stage of data processing.

We can conduct accelerated tests of electroencephalographic equipment using our developed concept without detaching from the current operation. We also automate all measurement processes, which significantly simplifies the work of the service engineer and minimizes the risk of human factor influence on the technical testing process.

Further study of this issue is also relevant because electroencephalography as a method of research has found its application for development in the field of neurocomputer interfaces. If person perform any action, the electrical activity of the corresponding zones of the brain changes. These signals are reconed by an electroencephalograph and enter the computer in the form of digital data, where the calculation of signal characteristics of a particular mental process is performed. Then the feature set is divided into types, and the computer generates a command controlling the executive device. The user in real time observes the reaction of the system to his mental action. Such a system is called the neurocomputer interface (NCI). Such an interface will be useful both in a clinic for patients with impaired muscular control and in everyday life.

REFERENCES

Brodsky B.E. 1998. Nonparametric segmentation of brain electrical signals. *Automation and telemechanics* 2: 23.

Fedoseyeva, G. B. 1996. *Syndromic diagnosis of internal diseases*. St. Petersburg: Library of General Practitioner.

Gurevich, D. 1988. *Functional Generator GF-05*. Moscow: Ministry of Health.

Kaplan A.Ya. 1998. Nonstationary EEG: methodological and experimental analysis. *Successes fiziol. sciences* 29(3): 32.

Kaplan A.Ya. 1999. Problems of the segmental description of the human EEG. *The physiology of man* 25(1): 125.

Ketov D.Yu. & Mukha Yu.P. 2012. Metrological scheme of encephalograph tests. *Izvestiya VolgGTU*.

Ketov D.Yu. & Mukha Yu.P. 2014. Formation of test signal for verification of encephalograph *Izvestiya VolgGTU*.

Ketov D.Yu. & Mukha Yu.P. 2015. Automated network stand for operational tests of encephalograph *Izvestiya VolgGTU*.

Khomskaya, E. 2003. Neuropsychology. St. Petersburg.

Kukes, V.G. 2006. *Medical diagnostic methods: (examination, palpation, percussion, auscultation)*. Moscow: GEOTAR-Media.

Plechawska-Wójcik, M. 2015. Methods of EEG artifacts elimination. *Informatyka, Automatyka, Pomiary w Gospodarce i Ochronie Środowiska*, 5(2): 39–46. https://doi.org/10.5604/20830157.1159329

Plechawska-Wójcik, M., Wesołowska, K., Wawrzyk, M., Kaczorowska, M., & Tokovarov, M. 2017. Analysis of applied reference leads influence on an EEG spectrum. Informatyka, Automatyka, Pomiary w Gospodarce i Ochronie Środowiska, 7(2), 44–49. https://doi.org/10.5604/01.3001.0010.4837

Shilyaev, S.N. 2008. *Functional generator Diatest-4. The manual of VKFU.468789.109RE*. Moscow: Ministry of Health.

Tsvetkov, E.I. 2008. *Metrology (Lecture notes, Corrected and additions)*. St. Petersburg: KopiServis.

CHAPTER 8

Metrological aspects of a radio thermography in complex diagnostics of the inflammatory processes of an abdominal cavity

Yu.P. Mukha, S.V. Poroysky & M.V. Petrov
Volgograd State Medical University, Volgograd, Russian Federation
Volgograd State Technical University, Volgograd, Russian Federation

P. Kisała & J. Smołka
Lublin University of Technology, Lublin, Poland

A. Toigozhinova
Kazakh Academy of Transport and Communications named after M. Tynyshpayev, Almaty, Kazakhstan

ABSTRACT: Every physician needs an accurate and timely diagnosis of inflammatory processes in the abdominal cavity by a non-invasive method in a convenient form and without harmful effects on the body. At the same time, the polymorphism of clinical symptoms in combination with atypical manifestations of the disease imposes errors due to the method of conducting the study and subsequent hardware processing of the thermographic picture. Authors carried out a comparative metrological analysis of various methods of implementation of the thermographic studies in this chapter. They considered such factors as thermal imager resolution, thermal sensitivity, noise level (signal-to-noise ratio), affecting the quality of the resulting thermal image.

8.1 INTRODUCTION

A distinctive feature of non-invasive methods for studying the thermal radiation of bio-objects is their complete harmlessness with high information content. Radio thermometry (RTM-method) is a new method of medical diagnostics. The essence of the method is the non-invasive measurement of the deep temperatures of biological objects by registration of the radio emission power, which they radiate. The difference between the RTM-method and the well-known physical methods of investigation (palpation, x-ray studies, ultrasound methods, tomography) is in the fact that deviations are studied not in the anatomical structure of internal tissues but in deviation from normal metabolism processes. We investigate the effect of the metabolism processes on the distribution of temperatures in internal tissues in the case of inflammatory processes.

Experimentally, the RTM method has been successfully tested in various fields of medicine: neurology and neurosurgery; cardiology; gastroenterology; traumatology and orthopaedics; combobustology; diagnosis of ENT diseases; endocrinology; gynaecology. The RTM-method has special perspectives in oncology – it is used for early diagnosis of breast cancer.

Contact methods are actively being developed all around the world. They are realised by microwave receivers with different versions of antenna applicators. Such microwave receivers give the high information content of the absolute values of the deep temperature. However, when we are using the contact method for receiving thermal radiation from biological objects, a measurement error arises from the reflection of radiation at a border between an antenna and an object. The reflection coefficients can differ substantially due to the difference in the dielectric properties of the radiating tissues. We can avoid the influence of this coefficient with the relative method of measurements when we register the temperature difference at symmetrical points (Enander & Larson 1974).

We need to take into account the effect of the mismatch between the contact antenna and the human body at absolute measurements of the temperature. This effect influences the accuracy of measuring the radio brightness temperature of deep tissues or internal organs.

The temperature anomalies of internal tissues caused by inflammatory and other processes often precede the structural changes. This factor is very important for early diagnosis. In the early seventies for the first time, scientists researched the visualisation of infrared radiation in the epigastric region and established the dependencies of its magnitude and distribution on the functional states of the stomach. Then doctors recognised the fact, which was crucial for substantiating the clinical application of remote thermal methods of research. They confirmed that changes in the thermal radiation power of the skin surface in the epigastric region adequately reflect the temperature changes in the stomach. Subsequently, thermography was widely used in non-invasive diagnostics in abdominal surgery, angiology, neurology, neoplasms of the breast, skin, muscular and bone tissues, thyroid gland (Bogdanova et al. 2013, Mital & Scott 2007). Some authors noted an interesting fact in their numerous reports on the using of the thermal imaging method in diseases of the gastrointestinal tract: fatty tissue and underlying tissues absorb the basic amount of infrared rays, and this prevents the formation of heat-field zones on the skin surface (Lyutaya et al. 2010, Merla & Romani 2006). In the late 1970s, many authors positively evaluated the thermal imaging method for diagnostic of patients. They noted some changes in the temperature distribution on the surface of the anterior abdominal wall, which has various 16 features in peptic ulcer and stomach cancer. These changes were interpreted as a result of neuro reflex and vascular reactions of the organism in the corresponding zones (Zaretsky & Vykhovskaya 1976). There are always temperature changes on the surface of the human body, and even for perfectly healthy people, thermo-asymmetry is noted towards to the median line of the body, which in most cases does not exceed 1°C, while pathological thermo-asymmetry may reach 3–5°C. It was assumed that heat is transferred to the skin through thermal conduction through all layers of the skin and convective (vascular structures from the main vessels to the sites with a developed capillary network).

It is necessary to register and systematically analyse the structure of the thermographic image of the entire surface of the skin in order to obtain the most reliable thermographic data. It was found that in all people the navel and inguinal folds are the constant and brightest source of radiation in the abdomen. All folds of the abdominal skin area are more abundantly filled with blood in comparison with the surrounding areas. The cause of this is the excessive development of the intensity of infrared radiation.

However, asymmetric patches of "hot spots" are often observed in the mesogastric region. It makes an interpretation of thermograms more difficult. In healthy people, the radiation of these spots is slightly different from the surrounding areas, which allows them to differentiate from radiation sources caused by the development of pathological processes. It was shown that we cannot characterise the stage of disease by the magnitude of the temperature difference in the symmetrical regions of the abdomen. The maximum temperature zone does not always correspond to the projection of the pathological process and the temperature difference. In a series of studies, authors have been made some attempts to reproduce a thermal imaging picture for inflammatory diseases of the abdominal cavity (Vorobiev et al. 2005). Other studies emphasise the dependence of the distribution of thermal fields on the degree of development of subcutaneous adipose tissue of the anterior abdominal wall (Belokonev 2003). It was shown that the abdominal wall thermogram was monotonous of light grey colour without a clear drawing of borders of the structure of the thermal fields in all persons with reduced development of the subcutaneous fat layer. In this group, only the musculature of the abdominal wall demonstrated a noticeable effect on the character of the thermal image: the image was monophonic in the case of a weak development of the musculature; the image had regions of low infrared radiation (cold zones), coinciding in localisation and shape with the arrangement of straight lines muscles of the abdomen, in the case of a good development of the muscles of the abdominal press. A distinct increase in the contrast of the thermal image with age was noted in the group of patients with normal development of the subcutaneous fat layer. In persons over the age of 50, warm areas of any size had distinct boundaries; the cold intervals between them were of a rich dark shade, which together gave the thermos-image a contrasting appearance (Vorobiev et al. 2006). The cold regions appear on the thermograms, as the thickness of the subcutaneous fat layer in the lower sections of the abdominal wall, where fat is deposited, increases. The shape and dimensions of this cold area were determined by the thickness and location of the fat layer. At the same time, the upper abdominal wall, even with increasing of a structure of a fat layer, retained a distinct image structure. So, the authors had an opportunity to make an efficient analysis of the thermal processes taking place in the upper abdominal wall.

Characteristics of the physiological thermal symmetry, its degree and magnitude, first of all, depend on the individual features of thermoregulation and anatomical and physiological data of the patient. Thus, in healthy people, the physiological thermal symmetry locates towards the midline of the body. Physiological thermal asymmetry is characterised by an indefinite thermographic picture and a different magnitude of the temperature difference for each individual part of the body. The difference in temperature with vertical and horizontal thermal symmetry in most cases does not exceed 1°C for the anterior abdominal wall in healthy people. The researcher deals with the true projection of the affected organ on the front surface of the body in direct conductive heat transfer. We can give a concrete diagnosis of an affected body organ.

A conductive way of the increasing the temperature magnitude in the skin means depends on three factors – the magnitude of the change in temperature in the internal organs, the thickness of the abdominal wall and blood circulation in the tissues of the latter. Skin projections do not always correspond to the localisation of the pathological process in internal organs, although topographically located near them. Skin temperature depends on accompanying circulatory changes in pathological and adjacent tissue and, to a lesser extent, on metabolic processes and heat conduction (Agostini et al. 2009, Frize et al. 2003).

There is an opinion according to which an increase or decrease in the temperature of internal tissue structures does not lead to a change in the distribution of temperatures on the surface of the body due to heat dissipation and absorption to the surrounding tissues (Zayats & Koval 2010). The structure of the thermal image of the anterior abdominal wall, even in healthy individuals, is characterised by considerable polymorphism, which makes it difficult to classify and interpret the thermograms. Nevertheless, the distribution of temperatures on the surface of the body is characteristic of a concrete person and is reproduced from observation to observation under the standard conditions of the study. However, this distribution for all healthy people will demonstrate a lot of similarities.

Unfortunately, nowadays there are no generally accepted methods for thermal imaging diagnosis for various types of diseases. Most clinicians perform thermal imaging studies as follows. Preparation of patients consists in preliminary adaptation at a temperature of 21–23°C in a special room for 20–25 minutes through 2.5–3.5 hours after a meal. An examination of the patient is carried out in the supine position and with the turn of the corpus observed by 30–45 degrees right and left sideways forward. So, we increase the area of the study. Some authors consider that the comfort temperature for a naked and motionless person is 28°C, and lower temperatures act as a cooling one and can lead to a distortion of the results of the study (Vorobiev et al. 2006). Others are sure that thermography should be performed in 3 to 3.5 hours after meals, always at the same hours of the day, in the patient's standing or sitting position, and the study is preceded by a 15-minute adaptation of the patient's skin to laboratory air temperature (Ivanitsky et al. 2007). There is an opinion according to which the thermal imaging study should be carried out in the position of the patient lying down. The supine position on the right side is also possible. It was noted that the lying position is more convenient, since it minimises the possibility of any side movements of the patient, affecting the quality of the study (Vorobiev et al. 2005).

We noted some general rules for preparing a patient for thermography require:

- the using of mustard plasters, cans, hyperemia ointments should be stopped 2 days before the study;
- it is necessary to stop any physiotherapeutic procedures, massage one day before the study;
- stop taking any medicines (except for vital), alcohol and smoking;
- the patient should wear a loose, not embarrassing body clothing in the course of 1 day before the test;
- it is necessary to carry out a woman's test 10 days after the end of menstruation;
- finally, we must make the study in the morning on an empty stomach.

Unfortunately, it should be noted that most of the above recommendations in conditions of emergency abdominal surgery are most often not feasible.

We often use such terms and expressions in analysing of the thermograms, like "hot" zone with clarifications and "cold" zone. We look at such important parameters: their localisation, size, shape, severity, etc. It is possible to perform targeted thermography with unconvincing thermal imaging. For this purpose, we use a special screen, which was made of a material with low thermal conductivity. The screen is superimposed on the anterior abdominal wall so that the area of interest is located in the centre of the "window". Then thermography is performed in the "compensation" mode, which was selected individually. Many researchers have attempted to classify the thermal imaging patterns that are detected in practically healthy people.

For example, we discussed here one of the proposed classifications for the thermograms of the anterolateral wall of the abdomen in practically healthy individuals:

- a uniform type of radiation, when the temperature of the body surface differences less than 0.5°C;
- epigastric, mesogastric, hypogastric types, when the temperature exceeds not more than 0.5°C over the corresponding area;
- polysemantic, characterised by a particular case of a uniform but the irregular shape of the thermal field.

A uniform type of thermogram is more common in males (56.6%), the epigastric type is more common in women (42.6%), mesogastric type of radiation occurs in 12.5% of cases. Hypogastric type is observed only in 5% of men, and polysemantic occurs in 4.4% of all examined (Ring & Ammer 2012). In all thermograms, we pay the attention to the warm zone in the umbilical region, which is associated with the absence of a subcutaneous fat layer at this site. The mandatory presence of a warm zone in the navel area is a reliable guide for the subsequent comparison of the thermogram with the real object, i.e. with the surface of the abdominal wall. A quantitative criterion for evaluation of thermograms is the most promising for thermal imaging diagnosis, which could later be used for diagnostic studies in abdominal surgery. Also, we proposed a "relative temperature index" for the analysis of the thermograms, while the isothermal zones are isolated and their area is measured. So, it possible for us to determine the quantitative temperature characteristics of individual organs. We fix the thermographic images of the concrete person for the first time and call it the "basic" thermogram. We can use it as a standard, the changes of which signalled the development of a pathological condition. In this case, there was a significant change in the absolute temperature of the same areas of the body during the repeated studies. It indicates that the very concepts of "cold" and "hot" zones are relative. Since the advent of deep microwave radio-thermography, it has become possible for the early diagnosis of internal disease. The main difference between microwave radio thermometry and well-known infrared thermography is that infrared thermography allows to measure and visualise the temperature of the skin, and microwave radio-thermometry provides information on the temperature at a depth of up to 7 cm.

8.2 RADIOTHERMOGRAPHIC PICTURE OF THE ABDOMINAL CAVITY WITH APPENDICITIS

We indicated above that the diagnosis of acute appendicitis is often made on the basis of clinical-anamnestic and laboratory data. This is due to the fact that in the early stages of acute appendicitis does not have a characteristic clinic.

An alternative method to infrared thermography is the ultrasound instrumental research. This method is not overall common for the functional diagnosis of acute appendicitis as we can see in practice. We often obtain a sufficiently distinct picture of the destructively altered appendix in ultrasound investigation. It is possible in a number of cases (Golestani et al. 2014). However, the significant difficulties of ultrasonic imaging of the appendix are well known in most cases. Therefore, this technique is used very limitedly in the diagnosis of acute appendicitis. The laparoscopic examination (Zhukova & Naledko 2016) is used for the diagnosis of acute appendicitis in very rare cases. It is an operation, and we noted that the diagnosis of acute appendicitis serves as an indication for conducting the emergency surgical intervention, according to existing provisions in surgery. Therefore, timely and accurate diagnosis of acute appendicitis is important for determining surgical tactics. From this point of view, the study of the diagnostic capabilities of the thermal imaging studies in acute appendicitis is very actual and modern.

The appendix is closely located to the anterior abdominal wall. So, the possibility of repeated thermal imaging studies during the dynamic observation of the patient formed the basis for repeated studies of the diagnostic capabilities of thermal imaging in the early diagnosis of acute appendicitis and its complications. There is abundant evidence that the thermal imaging method is informative in the diagnosis of acute appendicitis (Kirillova & Brovka 2012). For example, according to the literature, doctors examined 71 patients with acute appendicitis, and they have found such zones in 68 patients, in which temperature increases more often with localisation in the right side of the abdomen according to thermal imaging studies. The temperature difference depended on the peculiarities of the flow, and for catarrhal appendicitis, it was 0.8°C, and for destructive appendicitis, it was 1.1°C or more. Thermal imaging of the posterior surface of the trunk with acute appendicitis revealed zones of thermal asymmetry in almost half of the patients. These zones were determined in the scapula and subscapular regions equally often to the right and left of the spine and had a relatively small isothermal gradient, which indicated a reflex-vascular pathway of their origin. The reflex-vascular character of the appearance of these zones was confirmed by low figures of the isotherm gradient.

The investigators obtained interesting results when comparing the thermogram of the right iliac region with the stage of inflammatory changes of the appendix. When the acute form of appendicitis was catarrhal on thermograms in the right ileal region, they determined temperature increase with moderate intensity. They ascertained it mainly in the form of an elongated spot that coincides with the projection of the cecum and the appendix. The hyperthermia on the thermograms of the right ileal region was in the same form as in catarrhal for the phlegmonous stage of acute appendicitis. It appeared in separate bright foci and had a low intensity. In the presence of effusion in the abdominal cavity, hyperthermia in the right iliac region was often combined with hyperthermia above the pubis. Two types of thermograms were determined in case of the gangrenous form of acute appendicitis. The first group was characterised by the presence of moderate hyperthermia in the form of spots of rounded shape, which tended to merge and occupying almost in the entire lower half of the abdomen. The second group of the thermograms was characterised by a perifocal reaction around the supposed location of the appendix, depending on the degree of inflammation spreading to the surrounding tissues. A comparative analysis of the thermograms revealed several types of thermographic patterns characteristic of various forms of acute appendicitis in the process of examining patients with various forms of acute appendicitis. Then we summed up all types:

1st type. Investigators defined temperature asymmetry relative to the midline and symmetrical regions, local hyperthermia was in the right iliac region with a corresponding positive drop in the radiation temperature.

2nd type. They defined the distribution of the hyperthermia zone along the ascending part of the large intestine.

3rd type. They found the presence of hyperthermia in the epigastric region, which had a fairly large area and was characterised by the luminescence brightness.

4th type. A combination of 1 and 3 types of thermograms was obtained. Most patients had a positive Kocher symptom in this case.

5th type. This type occurred with the complete gangrene of the cecum and swelling in the abdominal cavity, associated with the destruction of the appendix. This process was characterised by the presence of a perifocal reaction around the alleged location of the appendix, depending on the extent to which the surrounding organs and tissues are involved in the inflammatory process.

6th type. This is not so very common type. Reflex hyperthermia was noted in the left ileal region, i.e. in the side opposite to the vermiform appendage. The dimly expressed hyperthermia in the right ileal region was noted in the initial stage of effusion formation homogeneous. There was a decreasing of infrared radiation in the process of its accumulation. Such a thermographic picture can be explained by the possible screening of heat radiation from the inflamed process, as a result of accumulating effusion. Thus, we can note that the diagnostic capabilities of thermal imaging in acute appendicitis are quite wide, but the thermal imaging criteria for the different stages of acute appendicitis and the dynamics of healing of the postoperative wound, as well as appendicle infiltration, remain open.

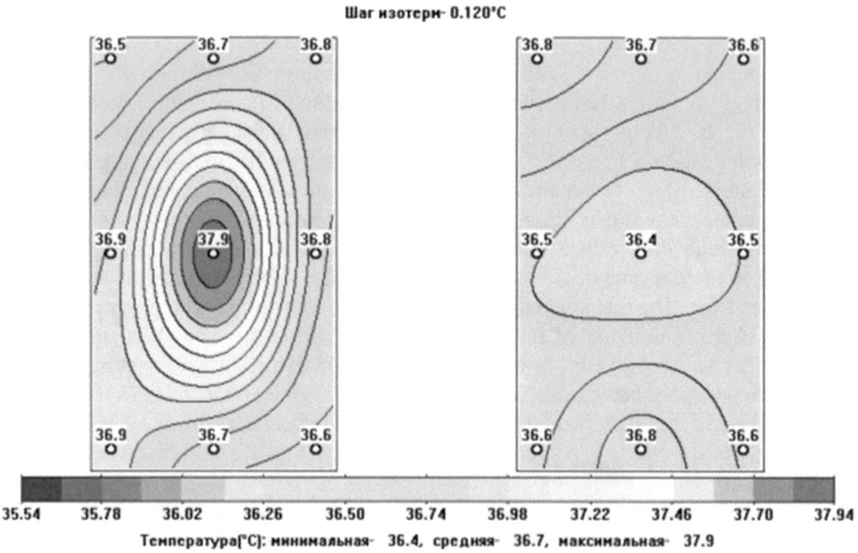

Figure 8.1. Thermogram of inflamed appendicitis.

Recently, the laparoscopic method has been successfully used in the diagnosis of acute appendicitis (Sazhin et al. 2009). However, domestic and foreign literature has accumulated sufficient material about the advantages and disadvantages of this diagnostic method. The advantages of diagnostic laparoscopy: the possibility of differential diagnosis from a comprehensive assessment of the obtained data during an examination of the appendix, and its instrumental palpation makes it possible to reliably distinguish destructive appendicitis from the secondary changes in the appendix. Along with this, the old age is an indication for diagnostic laparoscopy in connection with the atypical clinical picture of this age group. However, the high cost of equipment, the lack of qualified specialists, invasiveness, the possibility of damage to the internal organs and bleeding, the likelihood of relaparoscopy and relaparotomy, always nullify the advantages of this diagnostic method.

8.3 INVESTIGATION PART

Let us consider the thermal imaging patterns of the abdominal cavity at different positions of the appendix. The "hot zone" is often localised in the right iliac region with a typical location of the appendix. Figure 8.1 shows a thermogram of the abdominal region with typical appendicitis. It can define from Figure 8.1 that the focus of hyperthermia is of a rounded shape, it is clearly limited with a small degree of temperature asymmetry. Every physician characterises such an inflammatory process as an acute simple inflammation of the appendix according to this thermogram.

The "hot zone" was localised in the right lateral wall of the abdominal cavity and above the spinous crest of the right ilium in the retro-intestinal location of the appendix. The "hot zone" is biased towards the right in the pelvic location of the appendix than in the correct location of the appendage. According to Table 8.1, the patients with the diagnosis of "acute appendicitis" has a temperature asymmetry in the area of the projections of the appendix, with temperatures ranging from 0.6°C to 3.0°C. So, we proved the presence of an inflammatory process in the projection of the appendix.

The thermogram will change depending on the nature of the inflammation. We demonstrate the earliest stage of inflammation in Figure 8.2 when only the mucosa changes – catarrhal appendicitis. This stage lasts up to 12 hours. The next character of inflammation is the appearance of purulent changes – phlegmonous appendicitis (Figure 8.3). Pathological changes in the appendix develop for a short time (2–4 hours). Acute gangrenous appendicitis is a kind of purulent inflammation in which the irreversible destruction of its wall is based.

Table 8.1. Parameters of the radio-thermogram in patients with acute appendicitis, depending on the nature of the inflammatory process.

The nature of the inflammatory process in appendix	Mean temperature in the right iliac region, (°C)	Mean temperature in the left iliac region, (°C)
1. Catarrhal appendicitis	36.80 ± 0.04	36.21 ± 0.03
2. Phlegmonous appendicitis	37.58 ± 0.36	36.02 ± 0.02
3. Gangrenous appendicitis	38.01 ± 0.31	36.17 ± 0.04

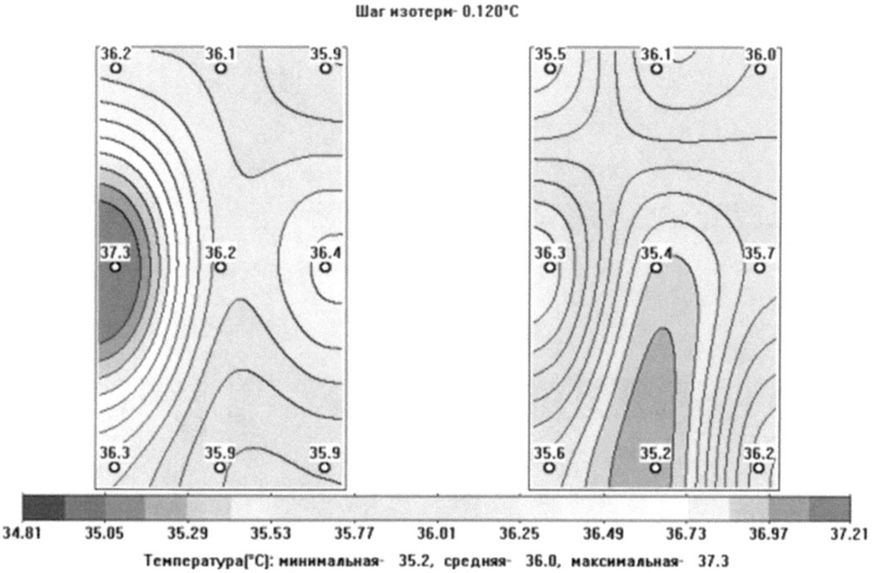

Figure 8.2. Thermogram of catarrhal appendicitis.

Factors, which determine the image quality of the thermal imager:

- Resolution of IR camera,
- Heat sensitivity,
- Noise level (signal-to-noise ratio).

The first parameter is the resolution of the resulting temperature-sensitive image (Figure 8.4). There are three accepted image resolution standards (may vary from manufacturer to manufacturer):

1. Low resolution – up to 19600 pixels (160 × 120 pixels).
2. Average resolution – up to 76800 pixels (320 × 240 pixels).
3. High resolution – up to 307200 pixels (640 × 480 pixels).

You need to determine the resolution by the applications for processing of making the image and by the quality level that you manually set in the settings first of all. Most users will not notice any difference when evaluating the image quality of cameras with 5 megapixels and 10 megapixels. Printing of an image with this resolution is quite problematic. If you are always going to print and demonstrate the full resolution images received by the thermal imager in the event, then it is enough for you to use the device with more modest parameters. The resulting thermal image will occupy only a part of the display of a modern computer even with a resolution of 640 × 480 pixels. You will print it out with the full required quality. Therefore, the number of pixels of the matrix is an important parameter for

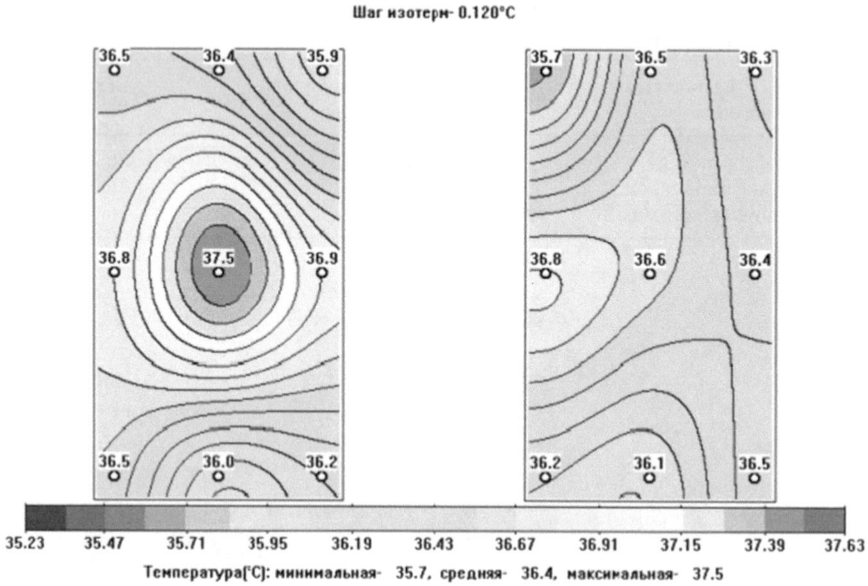

Figure 8.3. The thermogram of phlegmonous appendicitis.

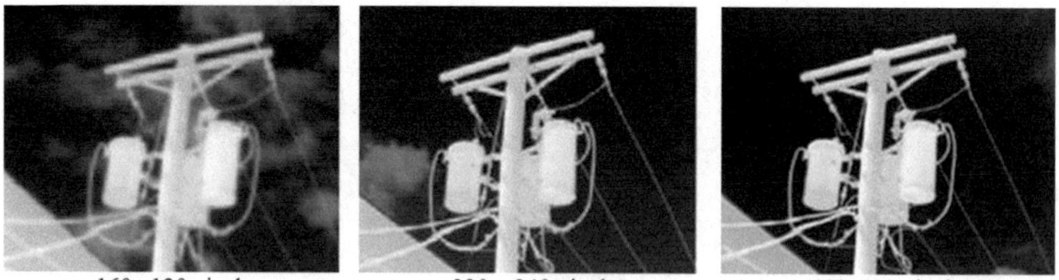

160 x120 pixels | 320 x 240 pixels | 640x480 pixels

Figure 8.4. Low-, average- and high-resolution thermal images.

assessing the quality of images, which were obtained with infrared cameras. But the most significant parameter is the image resolution level.

Another advantage of high resolution is the ability to scale shooting without losing image quality. The main part of thermal imagers is equipped with a standard optical system with a horizontal viewing angle of about 25°. The image quality of the device with a resolution of 640 × 480 pixels with the doubled magnification is equivalent to the quality of the IR camera with a resolution of 320 × 240 pixels (Figure 8.5). There is an expensive additional lens with a viewing angle of 12° in this IR camera. If you need to test objects at a distance of more than 20 feet, then you need to make a price choice between buying an IR camera with a resolution of 320 × 240 pixels with additional optics and a camera with a resolution of 640 × 480 pixels to obtain images of the same quality.

8.4 THERMAL SENSITIVITY

The thermal sensitivity of a pixel is the second most important parameter affecting the picture quality. The most significant test that determines the quantitative characteristics of this parameter is the evaluation of image quality with increasing contrast. The thermal sensitivity range of the thermal imager varies increases with the increasing temperature, depending on the temperature of the object

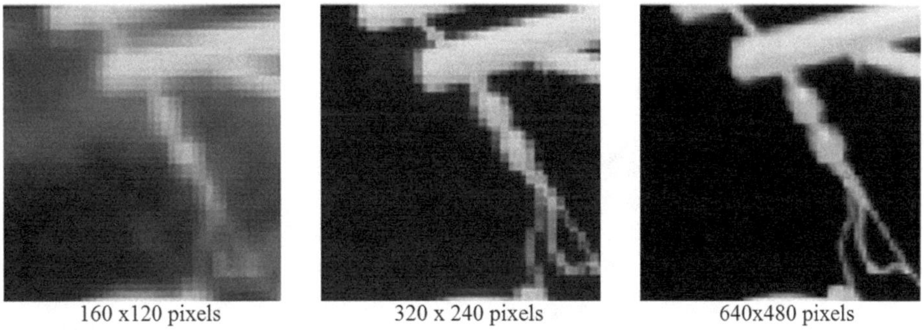

Figure 8.5. 4-fold magnification at various resolutions of a thermal image.

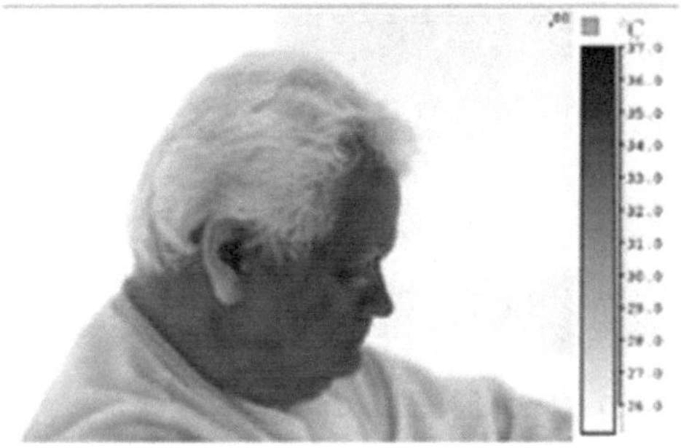

Figure 8.6. A snapshot at default settings.

as the signal level at the output of the detector. in other words, we improved the signal-to-noise ratio in the testing of the hot objects. But this is not always a positive quality, since there are situations in which the temperature of the object is low, and the temperature difference of the various sections of the object is small. A typical example of a low object temperature differential is the examination of walls inside a building. Small differences in temperature are recorded only by increasing the contrast between the test point (in which the temperature is determined) and the control point (in which the temperature is known). The thermal sensitivity of infrared sensors lies in the range of 0.05–0.25 K. Although the sensitivity in a quarter of a degree is high, noise is noticeable in a low-contrast image (the temperature difference of the object points is low). Thermal imagers reflect the thermal picture of the object, using a 256-colour palette or 256 gradations of grey. We determine that the temperature difference of the object is 0–256°C and each hue displays a difference of 1°C. We apply the same method to objects with a temperature range of 25–35°C. Now, each shade displays a difference of 0.03°C, which is less than the actual sensitivity of uncooled cameras. As a result, noise and errors appear on the image. In some situations, you need to set the smallest sensitivity range as possible to see the slightest temperature difference. If a device with a sensitivity of 0.25°C is used to create a thermal imaging picture and it is required to maintain the same noise level, then a temperature range of 65°C is required, at which a low-contrast picture is obtained. The difference between infrared cameras with a sensitivity of 50 mK and 100 mK is 100% rather than 0.05°C (Figure 8.6).

The sensitivity of 100 mK (Figure 8.7) is suitable for cases with a temperature range of more than 10°C. When the range is narrowed, the image quality drops significantly. The sensitivity of 70 mK (Figure 8.8) narrows the range of 5°C while maintaining the quality of the picture. The highest quality image is obtained with a sensitivity of 50 mK (Figure 8.9) competing with the quality of the images obtained on the cooled chambers.

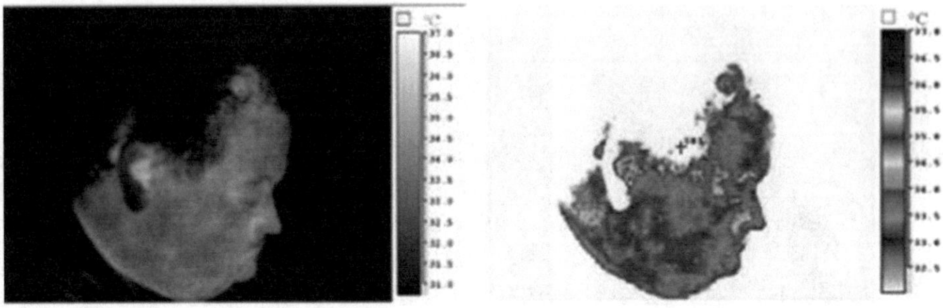

Figure 8.7. Resolution of 160 × 120, sensitivity of 100 mK.

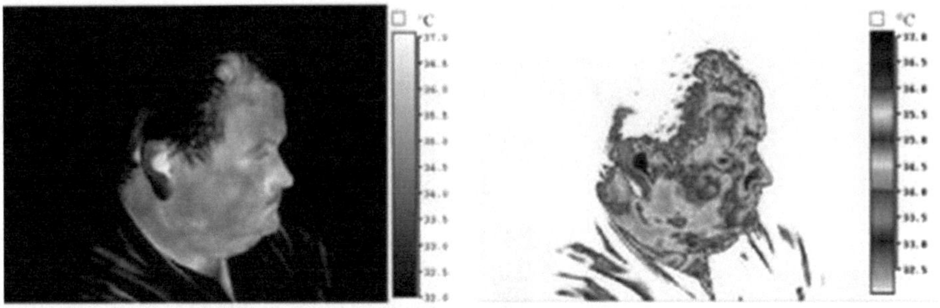

Figure 8.8. Resolution 320 × 240, sensitivity of 70 mK.

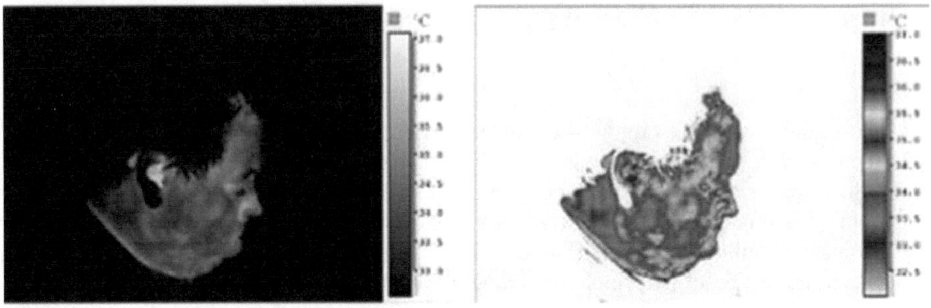

Figure 8.9. Resolution of 640 × 480, sensitivity of 50 mK.

8.5 NOISE LEVEL (SIGNAL TO NOISE RATIO)

The basis of the pixel structure of an uncooled infrared camera is a microscopic transition between a thin film of resistive material and an infrared-detecting layer located on the substrate. The outputs coming from the transition surfaces are connected to the silicon integrated circuit and transmit electric read signals to it. Reading takes place sequentially from each pixel by the multiplexing method and uses the IC protocol.

Infrared radiation, with a wavelength of 8–14 microns, falling on each pixel, is converted into heat, which changes the resistance of a thin resistive film. We sequentially read the voltage of the reading circuit, proportional to the amount of heat from each "microbolometer", and create a video image in real time.

The electrical scheme of the infrared sensor is shown in Figure 8.10. Each pixel is supplied with a bias voltage, and the change in resistance of the resistive film, based on the pixel temperature, is

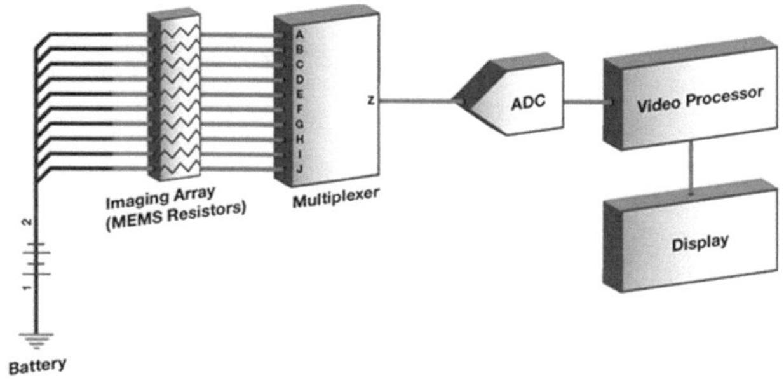

Figure 8.10. Electrical scheme of the infrared sensor.

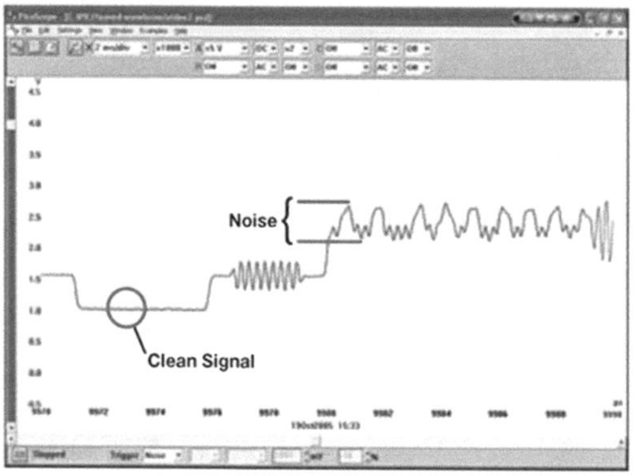

Figure 8.11. Image signal from the sensor.

translated into a digital value. Each analogue signal contains a certain noise level in a mixture with the signal detected by the sensor. The signal-to-noise ratio has a strong influence on the quality of the image since the amplification circuit increases both the useful signal and the noise component. As a result, we can see "snow" on the image (Figure 8.11).

We usually defined the ratio of the signal level to the noise level as the equivalent temperature difference. The noise occurs in almost all components as in any other electrical circuit. We determine the highest measurement of the signal-to-noise value from the noise level coming from the temperature-sensitive sensors. Then the noise increases in proportion to the amplification of the useful signal. Therefore, the temperature sensitivity to a large extent affects the quality of the resulting thermal image. The focal length of the camera lens is also very important. Lenses with a focal length of 1.0 (equal to the diameter of the lens) are considered as "fast". Increasing the focal length affects the quality of the device. For example, an optical system with $F = 1.4$ reduces the thermal sensitivity by a factor of 2, the system with $F = 2.0$ reduces the thermal sensitivity for 4 times. Therefore, the sensitivity of the 50 mK system will be 100 mK using optics with $F = 1.4$, which is acceptable. However, with the use of "slow" optics ($F > 1$), the thermal sensitivity of the 100 mK systems drops to unacceptable 200 mK. Temperature sensitivity has a very complex dependence on many factors. However, we can estimate the quality of the image using the most perfect device in the world of optics. We will distinguish the slightest nuances in the visual picture. As it was shown above, the heat-sensitive matrix consists of a set of microbolometers. They are tiny resistors with many connections between them. Each thermistor reacts to infrared radiation with a certain error. An increase in the range of errors is associated with an increase in the density of pixels and their thermal sensitivity. We used to correct this error by a process, which was called "uneven calibration" (NUC). The thermal imager must be normalised during manufacture. In other words, in the absence of a signal, the voltage level from each matrix sensor must be zero (Figures 8.12–8.14).

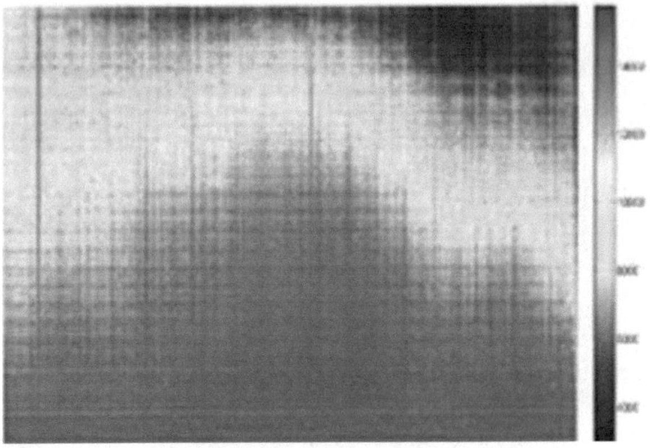

Figure 8.12. Failed image.

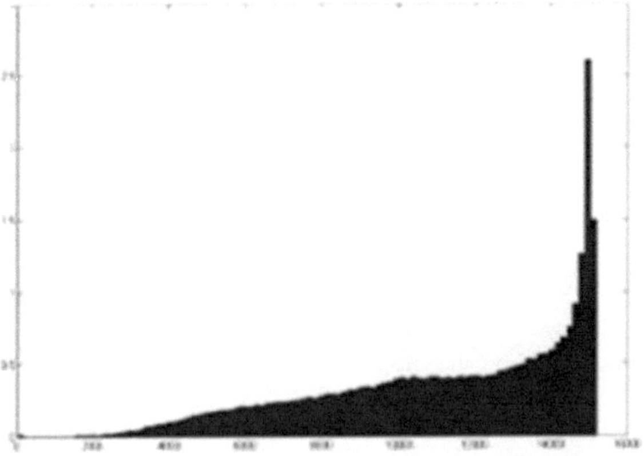

Figure 8.13. Uncorrected image histogram.

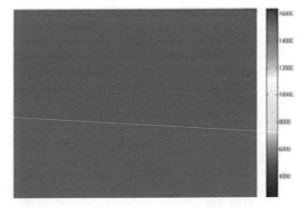

Figure 8.14. Corrected image.

We presented examples of uncorrected and corrected images above, as well as their histograms. A special screen was used for correction. We installed it before the temperature-sensitive sensor. This screen periodically obscured the sensor and occurred a programmable correction of the pixel readings to zero. We considered 2 tests and made a conclusion about the value of the ratio of the useful signal/noise. The first test determined the smallest temperature difference of the object, equivalent to

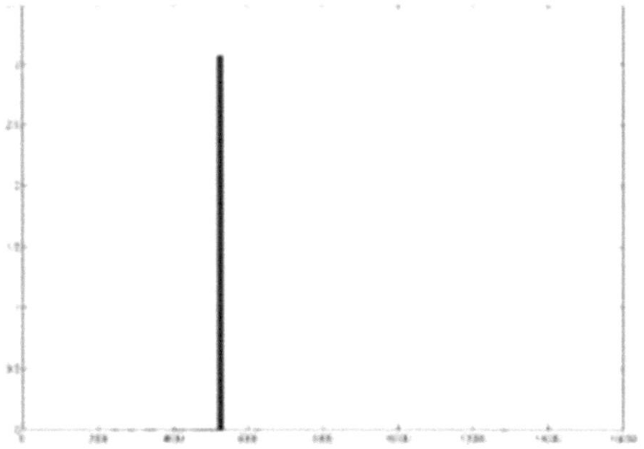

Figure 8.15. Corrected image histogram.

the internal noise characteristic of the detector or to the overall noise level of the device. Everybody as a potential thermal imager buyer needs to know the results of this test. We presented examples of uncorrected and corrected images above, as well as their histograms (Figure 8.15).

We presented examples of uncorrected and corrected images above, as well as their histograms. A special screen was used for correction. We installed it before the temperature-sensitive sensor. This screen periodically obscured the sensor and occurred a programmable correction of the pixel readings to zero. We considered 2 tests and made a conclusion about the value of the ratio of the useful signal/noise. The first test determined the smallest temperature difference of the object, equivalent to the internal noise characteristic of the detector or to the overall noise level of the device. Everybody as a potential thermal imager buyer needs to know the results of this test. The test setup consisted of a black body with a controlled temperature and several objects located next to the control body for simultaneous observation on the infrared camera screen. We set the temperature of the blackbody as close as possible to the temperature of the objects. An oscilloscope was connected to the output of the detector or the video output of the thermal imager, and the ratio of the recorded temperature difference to the noise level was clearly visible on the screen. It was defined as the ratio of the useful signal height to the noise height on the oscilloscope screen. The following test determined the minimum recorded temperature difference. This was a test system, not a sensor. The check was carried out by sequential observation of the picture of each of the three reference objects on the IR-camera screen. The reference object was a white plate, with four strips applied to it. Objects differed only in the colour of the strips. On the first object the strips were black (temperature difference 0.25°C), on the second – grey (temperature difference 0.05°C), on the third there were no strips (temperature difference 0°C). In both tests, the reference temperature was 30°C.

8.6 CONCLUSIONS

We can successfully use the RTM method for detection of the inflammatory processes in the abdominal cavity. The method was based on the identification of differences in the gradient of the deep temperature distribution in normal and abnormal metabolic process, which is expressed in the presence of a sharp transition and a strong asymmetry of the thermal field. In this case, it is necessary to take into account the presence of reflection on the antenna-object boundary. We got a more accurate picture of the pathological process in comparison with the surface thermometry. We used so deep thermometry and obtained data up to 7 cm in depth. We have shown that with age the contrast of the thermographic pattern increases due to an increase in the subcutaneous fat layer. We successfully applied the RTM method to identify the localization of the atypical location of appendicitis. The accuracy of this technique is comparable to ultrasound and shows a clear television image of the inflammatory process. According to the type of images, it is possible to distinguish the form of appendicitis: catarrhal, flegmona, gangrenous. We identified the type of appendicitis, so we got an opportunity to make more accurate planning of future surgical treatment. We have calculated all the parameters that characterize the thermal image and attained splendid accuracy of the image. These parameters are IR camera resolution, thermal sensitivity, noise level (signal-to-noise ratio). We explored a lot of examples of thermal images in dependence on those parameters. We proved the strong influence of the sensitivity of the infrared sensor on the analysis of the thermographic picture and saw the slightest difference in temperature with narrowing the sensitivity range. So the information content of the RTM method increased. The third parameter that has been discussed in detail is the signal-to-noise ratio of the infrared sensor. We proposed the recommendations for making of the conduct tests with correction of the image.

REFERENCES

Agostini V., Knaflitz M., Molinari F. 2009. Motion Artifact Reduction in Breast Dynamic Infrared Imaging. *IEEE Trans. Biomed. Eng.* 56(3): 903–906.

Belokonev V. I. 2003. Plastic surgery of the abdominal wall with ventral hernia in a combined way. *Surgery* 8: 24–26.

Bogdanova TM, Bakutkin VV, Lobanov V. V., Bolshakov A. A., Nalivaeva A. V. & Sinkeev M. S. 2013. Contact thermometry in clinical practice. *The Urals Medical Journal* 1 (106): 112–118.

Enander, B. & Larson, G., 1974. Microwave radiometric measurements of the temperature inside a body, *Electron. Lett.* 10:317.

Frize M., Herry C., Scales N. 2003. Processing thermal images to detect breast cancer and assess pain. *Proc. of the 4th Annual IEEE Conf. on Information Technology Applications in Biomedicine, UK*: 234–237.

Golestani N., M. Etehad Tavakol., Ng E. Y. K. 2014. Level set method for the segmentation of infrared breast thermograms. *EXCLI Journal* 13: 241–251.

Ivanitsky G. R., Deev A. A., Khizhnyak E. P., Khizhnyak L. N. 2007. Analysis of the thermal relief on the human body. *Technologies of living systems* 4(5–6): 43–50.

Kirillova E. S., Brovka N. V. 2012. Precision medical thermography in preventive examination of children. *10th Int. Confer. "Applied Optics-2012": Sat. Works of the Conference, SPb*: 99–100.

Lyutaya E. D., Podchaynov V. S., Poroysky S. V., Vorobiev A. A. & Beloborodova E. V. 2010. Thermal imaging method in the diagnosis of painful forms of adhesion of the abdominal cavity. *Bulletin of the Volgograd Scientific Center of the Russian Academy of Medical Sciences* 3:53–58.

Merla A., Romani G. L. 2006. Functional infrared imaging in medicine: a quantitative diagnostic approach. *IEEE Engineering in Medicine and Biology Society. IEEE Engineering in Medicine and Biology Society* 1: 224–227.

Mital M. & Scott E. P. 2007. Thermal detection of embedded tumors using infrared imaging. *J. Biomech. Eng.* 129(1): 33–39.

Ring E.F.J. & Ammer K. 2012. Infrared thermal imaging in medicine, *Physiol. Meas.* 33(3): R33–R46.

Sazhin A. V., Mosin S. V., Mirzoyan A. 2009. Laparoscopy in the diagnosis and treatment of periodic pain syndrome in the right iliac region. Endoscopic Surgery 1: 163.

Vorobiev A. A., Poroysky S. V., Lyutaya E. D., Podchainov V. S. 2005. Thermal imaging in the diagnosis of post-operative adhesion of the abdominal cavity. *Proceedings of the All-Russian Conference "Anatomical and Physiological Aspects of Modern Surgical Technologies", St. Petersburg*: 81–83.

Vorobiev A. A., Poroysky S. V., Lyutaya E. D., Podchaynov V. S., Legeza M. K. 2006. Development of the technique for thermal imaging study of patients with adhesive disease. *Proceedings of the All-Russian Conference dedicated to the 85th anniversary of the Astrakhan Society of Surgeons "Actual issues of modern surgery", Astrakhan*: 52–53.

Zaretsky V. V., Vykhovskaya A. G. 1976. *Clinical thermography*. Moscow: Medicina.

Zayats G. A., Koval V. T. 2010. Medical thermovision – a modern method of functional diagnosis. *Health. Medical ecology. The science.* 43(3): 27–33.

Zhukova E. M., Naledko V. A. 2016. Laparoscopy as a method of diagnosis of acute appendicitis in pregnant women. *Materials of the 62nd All-Russian Inter-College Student Scientific Conference with international participation with an open competition for the best student scientific work*: 154.

CHAPTER 9

Analysis of the information space used for the study of knee joints

S.A. Bezborodov
Volgograd State Medical University, Volgograd, Russian Federation

Yu.P. Mukha
Volgograd State Medical University, Volgograd, Russian Federation
Volgograd State Technical University, Volgograd, Russian Federation

A. Kotyra & M. Skublewska-Paszkowska
Lublin University of Technology, Lublin, Poland

M. Kalimoldayev
Institute of Information and Computational Technologies CS MES RK, Almaty, Kazakhstan

ABSTRACT: In this work we analyzed the information space of the knee joint for the purpose of effective implementation. For example, the concept of anatomical plasty of the anterior cruciate ligament (ACL) includes several principles: one of which is the anatomical location of the graft with the formation of the tibial and femoral tunnels in the areas of native attachment of ACL.

9.1 INTRODUCTION

The first step in the determining of the medical system is its structuring. That means isolation of certain functional elements and a definition of all links between them. This is the basis for determining the functions of the whole system and assigning a system formal parameter. This formal parameter will be an exit of an output element: the output element assigns an output parameter. Then we choose the system function which can be formed by sequentially transferring of the input action, that is, the action of the environment from the entrance to the selected output. That was obviously for us that the entrance would be the place of contacting with the outside medium.

9.2 PROBLEM STATEMENT

The proposed scheme of sequential formalization makes it possible to make the transition from a meaningful description to a formal description at levels of considerably greater complication and simplify stepwise the introduction of analytic-algorithmic descriptions preceding metrological analysis by regular formal transformations of category-functorial and graph schemes. The structuring process includes the following steps:

1. The set-theoretic formalism of the phase space (state space) is defined: a set of elements that determine the state of the object is established; the set of operations on the set of state elements is determined (set-theoretic mappings of any kinds, including various algebras); a set of rules for realizing mappings in the state space is established.
2. The phase space is analyzed in order to establish possible set-theoretic structures of mapping-operations defined earlier.
3. Information flows are formed, admissible essential set-theoretic mapping structures are established.

So structuring from a formal point of view is the establishment of successive transformations in the phase space in the form of specialized categories. All the suggested considerations regarding the structuring are well illustrated by the definition of systemic physiological functions within the technology of multidimensional measurements.

An analysis of the information space of the knee joint for the effective implementation, for example, of the concept of anatomical plastics of the anterior cruciate ligament (ACL) includes several principles: one of them is the anatomical location of the graft with the formation of the tibial and femoral tunnels in the areas of native attachment of ACL. The results of this approach should ensure the most complete restoration of the function of ACL and kinematics of the knee joint.

9.3 DEFINITION OF THE ELEMENTS FOR THE INFORMATION SPACE

Both axes of the knee joints (articulatio genus) are located on the same line in a relaxed state and in the frontal plane they can be considered in parallel. This position can be established at least due to a rotation in the hip joint. In this case, different individuals have a different rotation of the foot outside and torsion of the axis of the ankle joint with respect to the transverse axis of the hip and the axis of the knee joint. In the knee joint the shin moves relative to the hip and vice versa. The supporting skeleton of a shin is made up of two bones – the tibia and the fibula. But only the tibia forms an articular connection between the knee joint and the femur. The distal end of the femur extends and thickens, forming two, inner and outer, articular condyle, condylus medialis and lateralis. The deep intercondylar fossa (fossa intercondylaris) separate both condyles behind. The condyles are covered with a large articular surface in front. It consists of the patellar surface, fades patellaris, and two lateral convex for the tibia and its middle part is slightly concave for the patellar slip. Patella is a sesamoid bone located in the tendon of the quadriceps femoris. The front surface of the patella is roughened, the posterior surface is a joint surface covered with cartilage. The tibia is located on the inner side of the tibia and is much larger than the fibula. The proximal end of the bone has two articular condyles: medial and lateral, condylus medialis and lateralis. They are covered with two articular surfaces. The articular surface for articulation with the fibula (fades articularis fibularis) locates on the projection of the lateral condyle. There is a large rough outgrowth of the bone, tuberositas tibiae, in front of the junction to the body of the bone, corpus tibia. A strong tendon of the quadriceps muscle of the thigh is here (Figures 9.1 to 9.3).

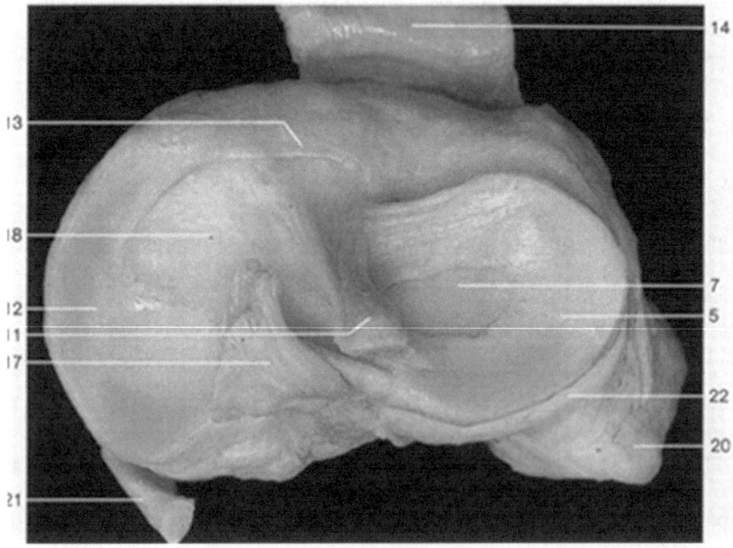

Figure 9.1. The joint surface of the tibia, meniscus and cruciate ligament.
Here 5 – lateral meniscus of the knee joint (the one that is outside the knee); 12 – the medial meniscus of the knee joint (the one that is adjacent to the inner part of the knee), 11 – the anterior cruciate ligament (it was cut here or disrupted off), 17 – the posterior cruciate ligament (and it was also cut here), 13 – the transverse ligament knee joint ; 14 – ligament of patella (= "knee cap"); 20 – head of fibula; 22 – posterior part of articular capsule of knee joint.

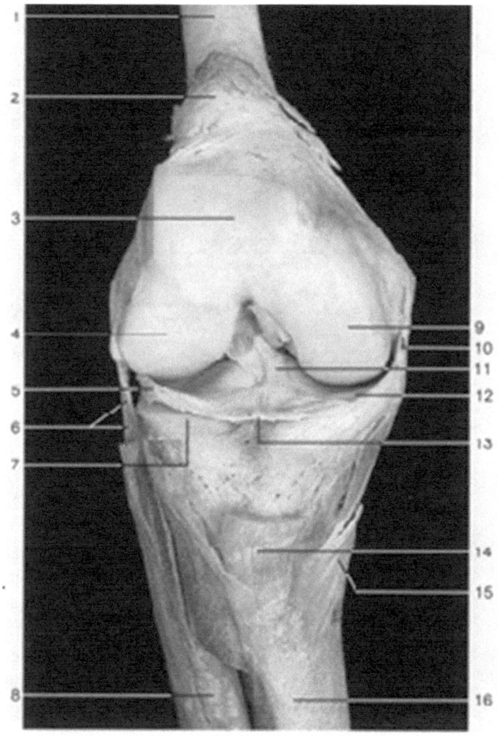

Figure 9.2. The right knee joint (opened) with ligaments (front view).
Here: upper bone – femoral, lower two – tibial with a fibula. This is the front view. The cuticle was cut off for clarity, cut off from ligament 14 (it was slightly higher). 5 – lateral meniscus; 11 – anterior cruciate ligament; 12 – medial meniscus; 13 – transverse ligament of the knee joint – connects the front of both meniscus.

9.4 DEFINITION OF BASIC FUNCTIONS IN THE INFORMATION SPACE

In the knee joint, two types of movements are performed: 1. Flexion and extension around the transverse axis of the condyles of the femur (axis of rotation or flexion) (Figure 9.4). The location of the intersection point of the compromise knee axis (according to Nietert) (Figure 9.5).

Average load distribution at the point of contact of the foot with support while supporting both limbs. Rotation inside and out around the longitudinal axis is possible only in the bent position (20–30°). The proximal articular end (epiphysis) is represented by the femoral condyles, which have a slight transverse curvature and much greater, not uniform curvature in the sagittal plane but with a gradually decreasing radius to the back. The distal articular end (epiphysis) is formed by both condyles of tibia bearing articular surfaces, fades articularis superiores. Both parts of the joint touch each other point-wise or linearly, since they, unlike other joints, do not fit well together. In order to make the contact between the two bony joints involved superficial and to compensate for their inconsistency, two interarticular cartilages are formed between them – menisci, which have the form of trihedral plates. The knee joint is characterized by strong tendon ligaments. The most important parts for the mechanics of this joint are the lateral collateral ligaments, the ligamenta colliteralia, and the cruciform ligaments of the ligamenta cruciata. Inner lateral ligament is anisotropic collateral ligament, ligamentum colliterale tibiale. It strengthens the capsule of the joint. It starts on the lateral epicondyle of the femur and attaches under the medial condyle of the tibia on its medial surface. The outer lateral ligament is the peroneal collateral ligament, ligamentum colliterale fibulare, a round, pencil-thick, independent ligament that extends from the lateral overcondyle of the femur to the fibular head. Lateral ligaments strain during extension and strengthen the knee in the support phase.

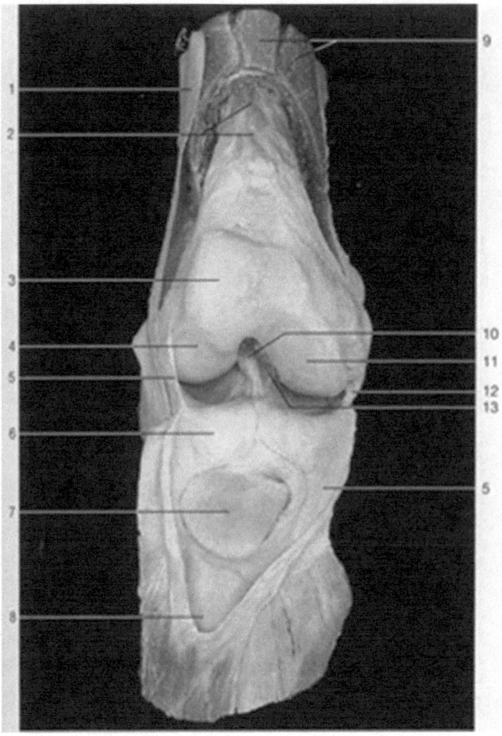

Figure 9.3. The right knee joint (opened). The patella with the knee ligament was bent.
Here: 2 – muscle; 5 – joint capsule; 9 – quadriceps femoris muscle; 10 – anterior cruciate ligament; 13 – posterior cruciate ligament.

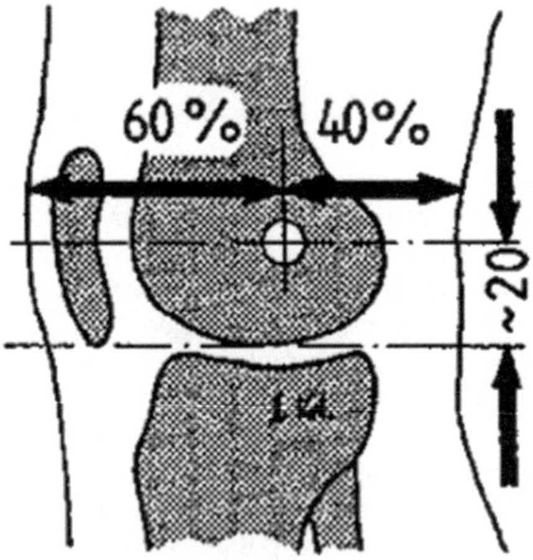

Figure 9.4. The axis of rotation of the knee.

It means that they prevent the "hogging" of the hip forward under the weight of the body. They relax in bending and allow rotational movements in this state. Cross-shaped ligaments, ligamenta cruciata, are two strong interbreeding ligaments located inside the cavity of the knee joint. There are anterior and posterior cruciate ligaments. Anterior, ligamentum cruciatum anterius, stretches between the anterior intercondylar field of the anterolateral bone, anterior area of the intercondilaris, and the medial surface of the lateral condyle of the thigh, condylus lateralis femoris. Posterior, ligamentum

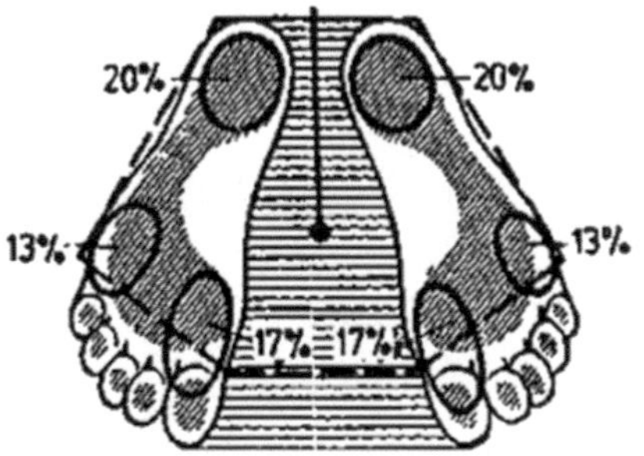

Figure 9.5. Load distribution at the contact point of the foot.

cruciatum posterius, begins on the lateral surface of the medial condyle, the condylus medialis femoris, and goes posteriorly downwards and attaches to the posterior intercondylar field above the tibia, area intercondilaris posterior.

The knee joint sets in motion the following muscles:

- Flexion: a group of muscles, a sciatic bone, a shin, ischiacrurale;
- Extension: the quadriceps femoris;
- Inside rotation: semitendinous muscle (semitendinosus), semimembranous muscle (semimembranosus);
- Rotation outward: biceps femoris.

The knee joint is polycentric, it performs not only rotational but also forward motion. Consequently, the femur not only rotates relative to the tibia but also moves anteriorly when flexing the knee. In addition, the femur rotates around the vertical axis. It turns outside approx. by 10° in bent and, on the contrary, by 10° inwards in extension. The final rotation occurs in the last phase of extension. The tibia rotates outward approximately about 5° at that moment. The effect can be compared with a bayonet shutter or with "screwing" parts of the joint. It stabilizes the extension of the joint.

9.5 DEFORMITIES OF THE KNEE JOINT

The hip and the shin are positioned in relation to each other not in a straight line in normal case (Gagala et al. 2014). The axes of the bones form an angle between them in the knee, which is 170° in the sense of the valgus. We always conclude about pathological genu valgum in the case when the angle is expressed more strongly than a normal valgus angle (Figure 9.6).

Deformations in the opposite direction, genu varum, occur less often than valgus deformities of the knee.In addition, deviations can also occur in the sagittal plane: we define the recurvation of the knee, genu recurvatum, if the knee is very out extended (see Figure 9.7). We can distinguish congenital and acquired irregular forms and positions in the region of the knee.

9.6 BIOMECHANICAL EVALUATION OF THE ORGANS OF HUMAN MOVEMENT

A specific feature of biomechanics is the biomechanical characteristics of movements. These are indicators of quantitative assessment, description and analysis of the mechanical state as a result of motor activity. We will draw up a block diagram of the structure of interactions between its elements using the anatomical scheme of the knee joint (Figures 9.1, 9.2, 9.3) (Figure 9.8):

A formal image of the structure of interelement interactions is a graph of the form (9.1). Here the following designations are accepted: CSL1,2 – cruciform ligament 1 and 2, respectively; TL – transverse ligament; TND – tendon; Fr is the friction; FB – femoral bone; CD – condyle;

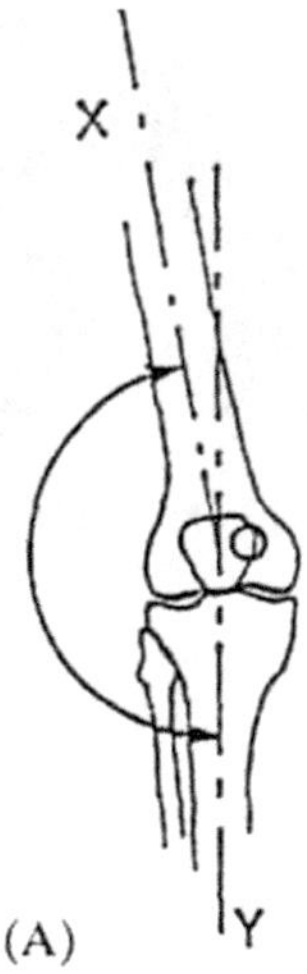

Figure 9.6. Normal position of the knee (angle Y – 0 – X = 170°).

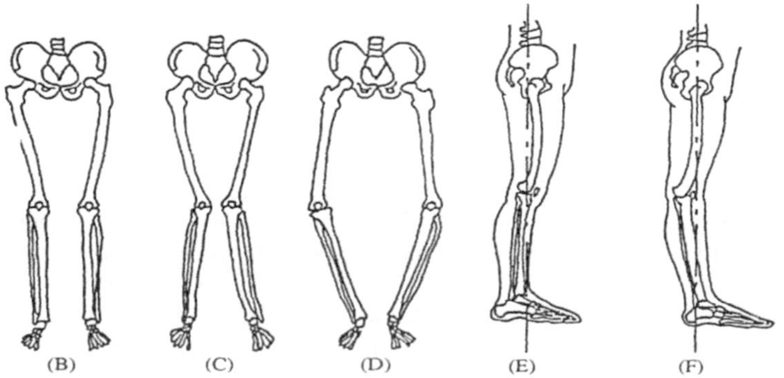

Figure 9.7. Incorrect position of the knees. B – Normal knee, C – Genu valgum (X-shaped legs); D – Genu varum (O-shaped legs), E – Normal knee F – Genu recurvatum (recurvation of the knee).

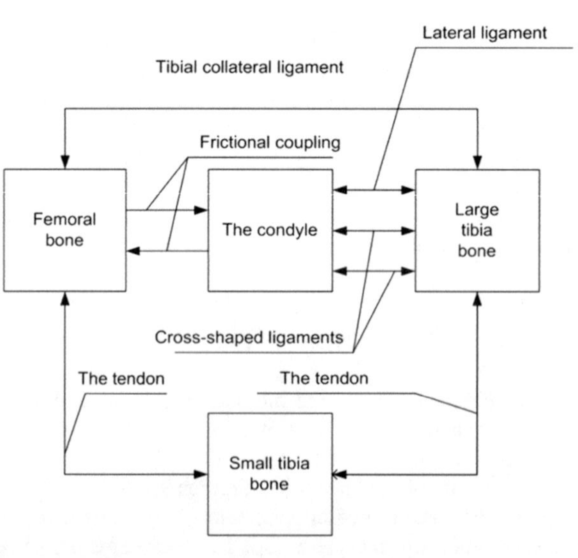

Figure 9.8. Structure of interelement interactions.

LTB – large tibia bone; STB – small tibia bone; MN is a meniscus; TCL – tibial collateral ligament; PT – patella; PTL– a patellar ligament; FBL – femoral ligament.

It is possible to form a categorical system (Malanin 2015) for power of interelement interactions (9.2) with the help of the graph (9.1). In this case, the indices 1,2,3 for categories.

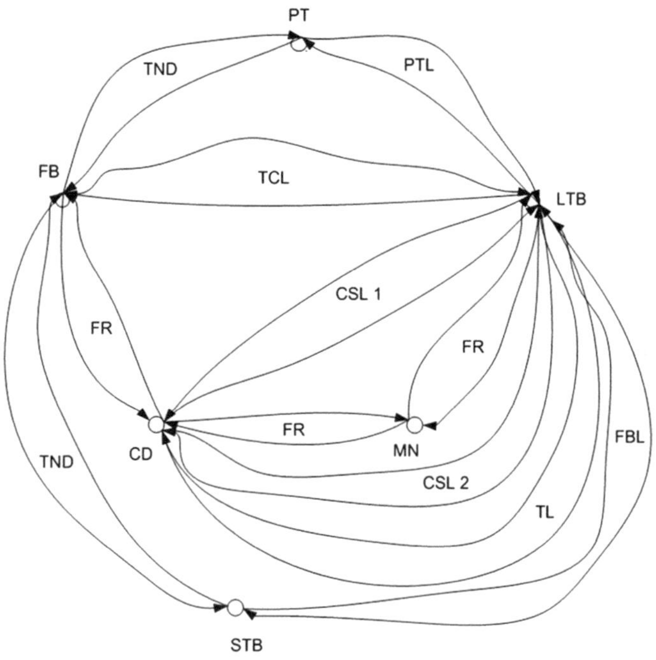

(9.1)

Correspond to the first and second cruciate ligaments (indices 1 and 2) and the transverse ligament (index 3). Since the elements of the BC, BBK, MN, MN, NK and MBK are included in this or that combination into all categories of the system (9.3), this system is correctly adequate to the model of the functional system.

$$
\left.\begin{array}{l}
\mathrm{M}_{fbpt} \subset (FB, PT) \cup (PT, FB) \\
\mathrm{M}_{ltbpt} \subset (LTB, PT) \cup (PT, LTB) \\
\mathrm{M}_{fbltb} \subset (FB, LTB) \cup (CB, LTB) \\
\mathrm{M}_{fbcd} \subset (FB, CD) \cup (CD, FB) \\
\mathrm{M}_{cdmn} \subset (CD, MN) \cup (MN, CD) \\
\mathrm{M}_{cdltb\,1} \subset (CD, LTB) \cup (LTB, CD)_1 \\
\mathrm{M}_{ltbmn} \subset (LTB, MN) \cup (MN, LTB) \\
\mathrm{M}_{fbstb} \subset (FB, STB) \cup (STB, FB) \\
\mathrm{M}_{ltbstb} \subset (LTB, STB) \cup (STB, LTB) \\
\mathrm{M}_{cdltb\,2} \subset (CD, LTB) \cup (LTB, CD)_2 \\
\mathrm{M}_{cdltb\,3} \subset (CD, LTB) \cup (LTB, CD)_3
\end{array}\right\} \quad (9.2)
$$

Category (9.2) can be supplemented with information on the types of connection of structural elements and the types of loading of connecting elements. To this end, matrix coupling types (Table 9.1) and loading types are constructed (Table 9.2).

Every model assumes the use of numerical characteristics of its individual elements, their character and pattern of distribution on the model. In this case, the assignment of numerical values is based on the fact that the ligaments are dense connective-woven cords and plates that connect the bones of the skeleton or separate organs. They are located mainly in the field of joints and strengthen them, limit or direct movement in them. All ligaments have physical characteristics in accordance with their individual purpose in this case.

Table 9.1. Matrix of communication types.

	FB	CD	LTB	STB
FB		Couple by friction	Collateral ligament	Tendon
CD	Couple by friction		Cross-shaped and transverse ligaments	
LTB	Collateral ligament	Cross-shaped and transverse ligaments		Tendon
STB	Tendon		Tendon	

Table 9.2. Matrix of types of loading.

	FB	CD	LTB	STB
FB		Sliding friction; compression	Deformation of stretching	Deformation of stretching
CD	Compression		Reaction to shear, reaction to compression	
LTB	Reaction to tension	Friction shear, compression reaction		Stretching, torsion
STB	Reaction to stretching/torsion		Reaction to stretching/torsion	

The correct choice of therapeutic and rehabilitation technologies due to the management of the force interactions of the joint elements is expedient to objectify by introducing the model of the diagnosed state:

$$\mathrm{M}_{DPS} = \{\mathrm{M}_{\mathrm{FUS}}, \mathrm{M}_{\mathrm{DDEF}}, \mathrm{M}_{PC}, \mathrm{M}_{CF}, \mathrm{M}_{\mathrm{SP}}, \}$$

Here MDPS is the model of the diagnosed physiological state; MFUS-model of the physiological functional system (FUS); MDDEF is the model of the domain of definition of the FUS; MPC-model of physical constants; MCF-model of conditions of functioning; MSP-model of the system parameter.

The contents of the model of the domain of definition are intervals of values of each component of the system (9.3), which we denote as follows:

$$\begin{aligned} M_{\mathrm{DDEF}} = & \left\{\langle \overline{FB}_{min}, \overline{FB}_{max}\rangle\right\}; \left\{\langle \overline{PT}_{min}, \overline{PT}_{max}\rangle\right\}; \left\{\langle \overline{LTB}_{min}, \overline{LTB}_{max}\rangle\right\} \\ & \left\{\langle \overline{CD}_{min}, \overline{CD}_{max}\rangle\right\}; \left\{\langle \overline{MN}_{min}, \overline{MN}_{max}\rangle\right\}; \left\{\langle \overline{STB}_{min}, \overline{STB}_{max}\rangle\right\} \end{aligned} \tag{9.3}$$

Here $\{\langle \overline{FB}_{min}, \overline{FB}_{max}\rangle\}$ means a set of concrete values, which corresponds to the use of the designation $\langle . \rangle$, the assemblages of parameters, which are indicated by a dashed line above the element name, the angle brackets have their own ordinal index i. The assemblage factor is denoted by curly braces. Among such parameters, it is necessary to note, first of all, the modulus of elasticity of the material of the element: FB, for example.

The M_PC model is a set of standing constants characterizing the elements of the object, that is, the knee joint, in a geometric or physical sense:

$$M_{PC} = \left\{ \langle \overline{FB}\rangle_{const}, \langle \overline{PT}\rangle_{const}, \langle \overline{LTB}\rangle_{const}, \langle \overline{CD}\rangle_{const}, \langle \overline{MN}\rangle_{const}, \langle \overline{STB}\rangle_{const} \right\}. \tag{9.4}$$

The model M_{CF} contains a list of various conditions under which the stability of the functioning of the knee joint is observed, and the permissible limits of these conditions are listed.

The model M_{SP} of the system parameter contains the name of a parameter or parameters which measurements allow to objectively evaluate the physiological functional system (FUS) and the equation of the measurement procedure. When detailing the behaviour of the joint in the phase force space, it is necessary to place the centre of the coordinate system for each of its elements and to consider the movement of each element under the influence of forces external with respect to the elements.

Graph (9.2) serves as the basis for determining the position of coordinate systems in the process of loading by interacting pairs. All interacting pairs realize the general equilibrium of the body in space and the interaction vector has an arbitrary operating direction, however, the coordinate axes of all coordinate systems are collinear with each other and with the resultant system. Therefore, in this case, it is expedient to organize coordinate systems with respect to all pairs of interactions. The resulting vector of force interactions of pairs taking into account the foregoing can be represented as follows:

$$\overline{F}_{\mathrm{SP}} = \overline{F}_{\mathrm{FB/CD}} + \overline{F}_{\mathrm{FB/LTB}} + \overline{F}_{\mathrm{FB/STB}} + \overline{F}_{\mathrm{CD/LTB}} + \overline{F}_{\mathrm{LTB/STB}} \quad (9.5)$$

The functional of each vector component is determined in accordance with the tables of the matrix types of the connection between the elements (Table 9.1) and the loading types (Table 9.2) of the connecting elements. The domains of definition and existence of functionals, as well as the coefficients and parameters, are taken in accordance with models (9.3) and (9.4). The initial and boundary conditions for the functionals in (9.5) are assigned by the model $\mathrm{M}_{\mathrm{FUS}}$. With allowance for (9.5), we got

$$M_{\mathrm{SP}} = \overline{F}_{\mathrm{SP}}. \quad (9.6)$$

As an example of the application of the analysis of the information space, we considered the loading model of the anterior cruciate ligament implant. This investigation used in the search for the optimal layout of implant placement in the knee space with the aim of its most effective anchoring (Mukha et al. 2013; Mukha et al. 2016).

9.7 STRUCTURAL MODEL OF LOADING

In accordance with the anatomy of the knee joint (Kapandji 2009) and the plastics of PKJ (Malanin 2015) (Figure 9.1), the structural model contains a representation in space of the elements of the knee, lower limb and implant PKJ. This model includes their interaction in the form of loads F_i, reactions R_j and angular momenta $M_{\mathrm{ROT...K}}$ under the assumption that the femur is considered rigidly fixed in the form of an "embedding" in the place of the hip joint, and the tibia is rigidly supported on the elements of the foot in the place of the ankle joint. It is possible in this case to present the following structural scheme of loading of PKS implant taking into account the conditions of the biomechanics of the knee joint: (Figure 9.9).

Here we use the following notation:

O_1 – the fixation point of the implant element on the surface of the lower knee condyle;
F_1 – the force of loading, acting on the LTB in the direction of its anatomical axis, caused by weight and external influence on the knee joint;
R_1 – the reaction force of the LTB applied to the implant equal to the projection of the total reaction force of the LTB along the direction along the anatomical axis of the LTB to the direction of the implant axis;
F_{OUT} – the force of external influence on the elements of the knee joint;
M_{ROT1OUT} – the torque applied to the implant element, from an external force F_{OUT} around the centre O_1;
$M_{ROT...r1}$ – reactive torque of rotation around the centre;
F_2 – the loading force acting on the femur from the body weight and external influence along the anatomical axis of the femur;
R_2 – the implant reaction force along the anatomical axis of the femur, equal to the projection of the complete reaction along the implant axis on the direction of the anatomical axis of the femoral axis of the femur, attached in the point O_2;
O_2 – the point of attachment of the implant element to the upper condyle of the knee joint;
$M_{BP...2BH}$ – the torque applied to the implant element, from an external force F_{OUT} around the centre O_2;
$M_{ROT...2r}$ – reactive torque of rotation around the centre O_2;
M_{1IMP} – the moment of rotation of the LTB from external influence with respect to fixation in the ankle joint;

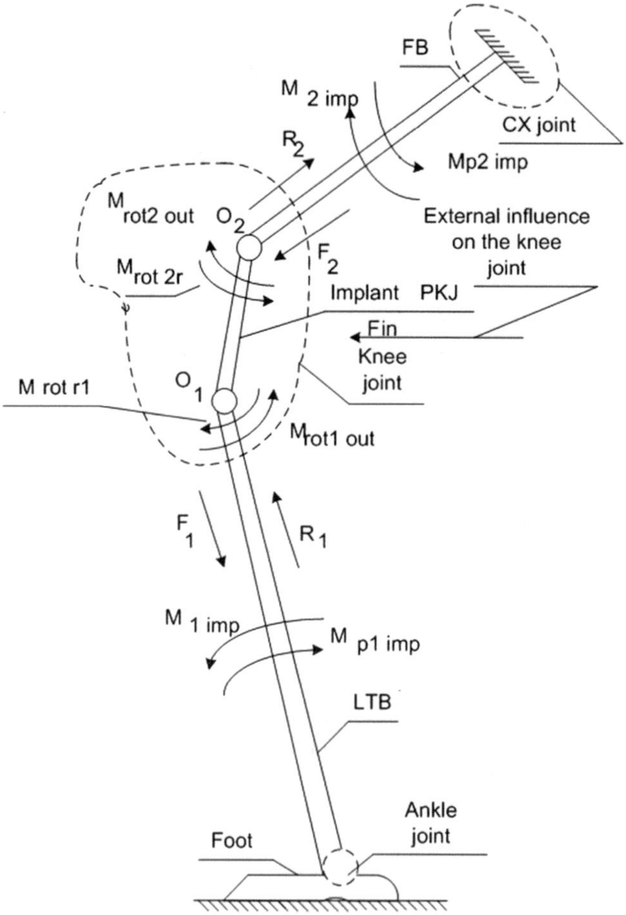

Figure 9.9. Structural model of loading of the lower limb.

M_{2IMP} – the moment of rotation of the femur from external influence with respect to fixation in the hip joint;
$M_{R1...IMP}$ – the moment of reaction with respect to the attachment of the LTB in the ankle joint;
$M_{R2...IMP}$ – the moment of reaction relative to the coxofemoral joint.

9.8 ANALYTICAL MODEL OF IMPLANT CARRYING LOADS

We took in to account the biomechanical situation represented by the structural model of limb loading (Figure 9.9) and constructed a structural model of the knee joint containing implant fixed in the body of the upper and lower joint elements (Figure 9.10). Then the algebraic loading systems under the condition of the equilibrium state of the implant (Rabotnov 1979; Timoshenko 1969) (when the stability condition is satisfied) are generally as follows:

$$\sum_i \vec{F}_{i\ nom} = 0 \quad \sum_i \vec{M}_{i\ nom} \tag{9.7}$$

or

$$\begin{cases} \sum F_{xi...nom} = 0, \\ \sum F_{yi...nom} = 0, \\ \sum F_{zi...nom} = 0. \end{cases} \quad \begin{cases} \sum M_{xi...nom} = 0, \\ \sum M_{yi...nom} = 0, \\ \sum M_{zi...nom} = 0. \end{cases} \tag{9.8}$$

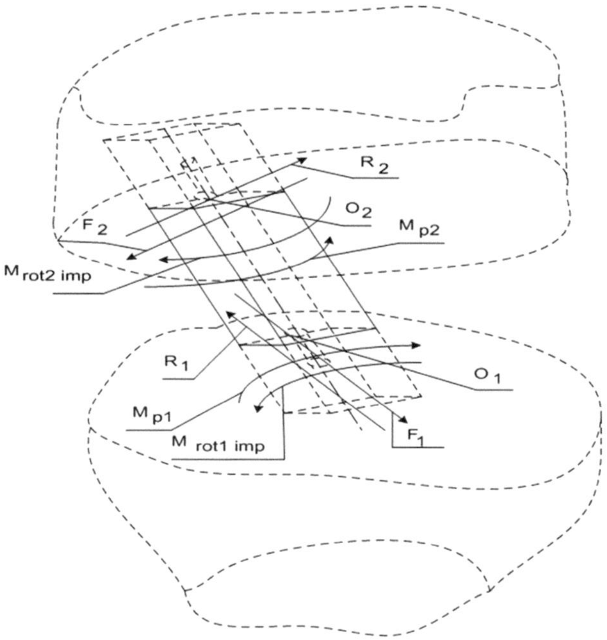

Figure 9.10. Implant Loading Scheme.

In accordance with the structural model (Figure 9.3), the systems of Equations (9.1) and (9.2) can be represented in expanded form:

$$\begin{cases} F_{x...\mathrm{OUT}} + F_{1x...nom} + F_{2x...nom} + R_{2x...nom} - R_{1x...nom} = 0, \\ F_{y...\mathrm{OUT}} + F_{1y...nom} + F_{2y...nom} + R_{2y...nom} - R_{1y...nom} = 0, \\ F_{z...\mathrm{OUT}} + F_{1z...nom} + F_{2z...nom} + R_{2z...nom} - R_{1z...nom} = 0. \end{cases} \tag{9.9}$$

and

$$\begin{cases} M_{ROT\,OUT\,x} - \mathrm{M}_{\mathrm{ROT\,R1\,x}} + \mathrm{M}_{\mathrm{ROT\,OUT\,2\,x}} + \mathrm{M}_{\mathrm{ROT\,R2\,x}} + \mathrm{M}_{1\,\mathrm{IMP\,x}} + \mathrm{M}_{2\,\mathrm{IMP\,x}} + \mathrm{M}_{\mathrm{P1\,IMP\,x}} + \mathrm{M}_{\mathrm{P2\,IMP\,x}} = 0, \\ \mathrm{M}_{ROT\,OUT\,\mathrm{y}} - \mathrm{M}_{ROT\,\mathrm{R1\,y}} + \mathrm{M}_{ROT\,OUT\,2\,\mathrm{y}} + \mathrm{M}_{ROT\,\mathrm{R2\,y}} + \mathrm{M}_{1\,\mathrm{IMP\,y}} + M_{2\,\mathrm{IMP\,y}} + \mathrm{M}_{1\,\mathrm{IMP\,y}} + \mathrm{M}_{\mathrm{P2\,IMP\,y}} = 0, \\ \mathrm{M}_{ROT\,OUT\,\mathrm{z}} - M_{ROT\,R1\,z} + \mathrm{M}_{ROT\,OUT\,\mathrm{z}} + \mathrm{M}_{ROT\,\mathrm{R2\,z}} + \mathrm{M}_{1\,\mathrm{IMP\,z}} + \mathrm{M}_{2\,\mathrm{IMP\,z}} + \mathrm{M}_{\mathrm{P1\,IMP\,z}} + M_{P2\,\mathrm{IMP\,z}} = 0. \end{cases} \tag{9.10}$$

9.9 EQUATIONS OF IMPLANT CARRYING LOADS

The loading function of the implant can be written on the basis of the system of Equations (9.10) as follows:

$$R_{1\,nom} = \pm\sqrt{R_{1x\,nom}^2 + R_{1y\,nom}^2 + R_{1z\,nom}^2}, \tag{9.11}$$

where

$$R_{1x\,nom} = F_{x\,OUT} + F_{1x\,nom} + F_{2x\,nom} + R_{2x\,nom}; \tag{9.12}$$

$$R_{1y\,nom} = F_{y\,\mathrm{OUT}} + F_{1y\,nom} + F_{2y\,nom} + R_{2y\,nom}; \tag{9.13}$$

$$R_{1z\,nom} = F_{z\,\mathrm{OUT}} + F_{1z\,nom} + F_{2z\,nom} + R_{2z\,nom}. \tag{9.14}$$

Similarly, the moment of rotation around one of the centres of rotation, for example, around, is determined. The loading torque of rotation can be defined from the system of Equations (9.11) as follows:

$$M_{ROT\,R1} = \pm\sqrt{M^2_{ROT\,R1x} + M^2_{ROT\,R1y} + M^2_{ROT\,R1z}}, \tag{9.15}$$

where

$$M_{ROT\,R1x} = M_{ROT\,OUT\,x} + M_{ROT\,OUT\,2x} + M_{ROT\,R2\,x} + M_{1\,IMP\,x} + M_{2\,IMP\,x} + M_{P1\,IMP\,x} + M_{P2\,IMP\,x}; \tag{9.16}$$

$$M_{ROT\,R1y} = M_{ROT\,OUTy} + M_{ROT\,OUT2y} + M_{ROT\,R2y} + M_{1IMPy} + M_{2\,IMPy} + M_{P1\,IMPy} + M_{P2\,IMPy}; \tag{9.17}$$

$$M_{ROT\,R1z} = M_{ROT\,OUTz} + M_{ROT\,OUT2z} + M_{ROT\,R2z} + M_{1\,IMPz} + M_{2\,IMPz} + M_{P1\,IMPz} + M_{P2\,IMPz}. \tag{9.18}$$

9.10 CONCLUSIONS

Biomechanical characteristics (kinematic, dynamic, energy) are one of the main issues of the biomechanics of the organs of motion. We can't count on success in studying and applying the estimates of the biomechanical state of the corresponding element of the organ of motion without the analysis of that biomechanical characteristics. Thus, the structurability of the information space, for example, of the knee joint, made it possible to define a set of functional elements in the system and assign relations between them so that the external function of the system remains unchanged with the independence of the choice of sets of elements and the connections between them. It is also obvious that the choice of a system parameter for analyzing the state of a certain organ is essentially determined by the effective procedure for designating the structure.

REFERENCES

Gagala, J., M. Tarczynska, & K. Gaweda. 2014. A seven- to 14-year follow-up study of bipolar hip arthroplasty in the treatment of osteonecrosis of the femoral head. *Hip International* 24(1):14–19.

Kapandji, A. I. 2009. *The Lower Limb. Functional anatomy*. Moscow: Eksmo.

Malanin D.A. 2015. The region of tibialis attachment of the anterior cruciate ligament from the position of surgical anatomy. *Bulletin of Volgograd Medical University* 1:53.

Mukha, Yu.P., Bezborodov, S.A., Malanin, D.A. & Demeshchenko, M.V. 2016. Structural and analytical model of the loading of the anterior cruciate ligament implant. *News of the South-Western state, University Ser. Management, computer facilities, informatics. Medical instr. making* 4(21): 89–96.

Mukha, Yu.P., Bezborodov, S.A. & Rusakov, S.A. 2013. The category model of the knee joint. *Bulletin of the Volgograd state. Medical University* 4: 104–106.

Rabotnov, Yu.N. 1979. *Mechanics of a deformable solid*. Moscow: Science.

Timoshenko, S.P. 1969. *Fluctuations in engineering*. Moscow: Science.

CHAPTER 10

Objective parameterisation of the load on the knee joint

S.A. Bezborodov, A.A. Vorobiev, Y.P. Mukha,
A.A. Kolmakov & A.S. Barinov
Volgograd State Medical University, Volgograd, Russian Federation

A. Smolarz & M. Plechawska-Wójcik
Lublin University of Technology, Lublin, Poland

S. Smailova
East Kazakhstan State Technical University named after D. Serikbayev, Ust-Kamenogorsk, Kazakhstan

ABSTRACT: Authors made a system analysis of the load on the knee joint, depending on the shape of the lower limbs. They developed a technique for determining the load on the knee joint, described and determined the numerical values of the load parameters for the knee joint. They described the distribution of loads in the knee joint with different forms of the lower extremities within the anatomical variants (under the conditions of the anatomical norm).

10.1 INTRODUCTION

The knee joint is the largest and most complex joint of man and many mammals, which is the result of a long evolutionary process (Dye, 2003; Makarov et al. 1999). In the last two decades, significant progress has been made in the understanding of its structure and functioning, but this knowledge of the knee joint does not yet have clear parametric characteristics (Asfandiyarov 1987; Biedert et al. 2000; Woo & Livesay 1994, 1999).

We looked through the many works on morphology, anthropology, development and variant anatomy of the lower extremities. Many authors paid so insignificant attention to the issues of concerning their shape, longitudinal, transverse and angular characteristics for healthy people. In addition, these works are mostly dated from the '60s to the '90s of the last century, and they are more often represented in the form of teaching aids.

Meanwhile, the lower limbs are not yet completely formed at the age of 17 to 20 years, and therefore, many external influences can adversely affect their further development. Only three or four forms are distinguished for this time from the whole variety of forms of the lower limbs: straight, varus, valgus and false curvature. In this case, the criteria for assessing the shape of the lower extremities are both very simple and unreliable for diagnosis, or too laborious, as, for example, the radiographic method, and are not suitable for screening preventive examinations.

The main roles of the lower limbs for man are the support and movement of the body in space, which is ensured by the functional unity of all its elements. Legs can perform three functions: to give the trunk a stable position, i.e. work statically, lengthen and shorten the longitudinal axis of the body and rotate it in different directions, and, finally, act independently. However, all this is possible only with healthy, normally developed lower limbs.

Static overloads of the external or internal condyles of the thigh and lower leg occur depending on the degree and type of frontal curvature of the knee joint. In this case, it is necessary to distinguish two types of forces acting on the knee joint: compression and tension forces. The compression forces are found on the concave side and affect mainly the bone and cartilaginous tissues. The stretching forces arise on the convex side. They predominantly affect soft tissue - the capsule, ligaments, and tendons. The resulting static overloads lead to certain structural shifts in the bone and cartilage tissues.

The compensatory bone reshaping is expressed in thickening of the cortical layer of the hip and shin diaphysis from the outside. We diagnose the valgus curvature of the knee joint when the outer halves of the hip and shin bones are under more pressure than the internal. In addition, the size of the outer half of the femur and tibia is increasing in the metaphysical area, as well as the external condyles of the thigh and lower leg with a huge accumulation of "thickened bony beams" (Albrecht 1907).

Another type of restructuring of bone tissue of compensatory character for this deformation is the thickening of the fibula. This was pointed out by Albrecht (1907), T. S. Zatsepin (1928), G. I. Turner (1906). Varus curvatures of the knee are accompanied by similar structural changes in the inner halves of the femur and tibia.

According to A. Schanz (1933), uneven force loads on the knee joint with genu valgum et genu varum lead to premature wear of the articular cartilage at the sites of greatest force application followed by the development of deforming arthrosis.

The possibility of developing deforming arthrosis of the knee joint with its lateral curvatures is indicated by a number of authors (Brusko et al. 1989; Gafarov 1983; Jackon & Waughw 1982; Leonova & Valentsev 1991; Nasonova 2003; Onoprienko et al. 1990).

The technical capabilities of most X-ray machines ensure the display of bones and joints only in two planes of the human body (frontal and sagittal). Many orthopaedic deformations are also pathological rotation or torsion, including the curving of the bones and subluxations in joints in the frontal and sagittal planes (Semizorov & Shakhov, 2002). The essence of X-ray diagnostics consists in achieving an accurate quantitative characteristic of the components of the bone-joint system that are not displayed on radiographs or displayed in a distorted form employing geometric constructions and mathematical calculations. The overwhelming number of methods in x-ray anatomy is based on the calculation of the spatial angles or the true anatomical angles with the reference to the osteoarticular system (Kosinskaya 1961; Lagunova 1951; Zedgenidze 1984). X-ray computed tomography also has a lot of limitations in the study of joints. So a low degree of contrast of images of soft tissues does not allow to make an optimal assessment of the degree of their damage (Watt 1997). Summarising the foregoing, we can conclude that X-ray computed tomography is a highly effective method in the study of intravital anatomy of a human; however, despite a number of advantages, it also has its drawbacks: it is a radiation research method that is not always harmless to the patient; the soft-tissue structures and intra-articular anatomical structures are not visualised clearly.

Specialists have proven that magnetic resonance imaging (MRI) is highly effective in diagnostic of the assessing of intra- and periarticular changes in patients with rheumatoid arthritis (Beltran et al. 1986; Beltran et al. 1987; Gilkeson et al. 1988; Koenig et al. 1990). We can get the images of inflamed synovial tissue, joint effusion and cartilage structures with a high contrast of soft tissue images on magnetic resonance tomograms (Bjorkengren, Al-Rowaih et al. 1990; Chekley et al. 1989; Waterton et al. 1990). Although MRI is less informative than conventional radiography and PCT in detecting cortical destruction, endosteal and periosteal reactions (Gagala et al. 2014; Petterson & Hamlin 1985), it can clearly identify bone changes that are not visible on radiographs (Chan et al., 1991; Cimmino et al. 1997; Foley-Nolan et al. 1991; McAlindon et al. 1991; Poleksic et al. 1993). According to M.O. Senac et al. (1988) and L.A. Verbruggen et al. (1990), essential for prognosis and therapeutic tactics in rheumatoid arthritis, can identify the earliest signs of proliferative synovitis (Senac & Deutsch 1990).

We analyzed literature data concerning the use of MRI in wide clinical practice. We understood that the MRI -method of visualisation has a high potential in the study of intravital anatomy. However, MRI also has a number of limitations in its use: it is not possible to examine patients on a tomograph who have metal structures (magnetic artificial pacemakers, metal vascular clips, traumatic and orthopaedic fixation systems) in the body; and patients suffering from claustrophobia. Solid structures are not clearly visualised using the method of magnetic resonance imaging.

We proposed a methodology, in which we use a combination of X-ray computer and magnetic resonance imaging for the optimal study of intravital anatomy of the joint. These methods complement each other and give a clear idea of the anatomy for alive person having a number of advantages and disadvantages.

10.2 FORMULATION OF THE PROBLEM

Stabilometry is the recording of the position and movements of the common pressure centre on the support plane when a person is standing. Stabilometer – specialised (one-component) dynamometric platform. We can record the position and movements of the pressure centre during the patient's standing on it. During the research we must determine:

1) The common centre of mass, which is a hypothetical point, located 2–3 cm ahead of the pelvis, corresponding to the common centre of mass of the body;
2) The pressure centre, which is a point localised on the vertical projection or the support reaction vector. In other words, the centre of pressure is the resultant, produced by the mass of the body and its movements, onto the stabilometric or dynamometric platform. Thus, the centre of pressure is the average position of the resultant body pressure on the support within the support area. The pressure centre as a whole is physically independent of the common centre of mass. Nevertheless, with a calm standing, the centre of pressure and the centre of mass lie on the same vertical. With a certain assumption, we can say that the centre of pressure is the vertical projection of the centre of mass on the plane of support. If one foot is on the support, then the pressure centre will lie within the foot area of this foot. If both feet are on the support, then it will lie in some place between the stops. And his position will depend on how much weight will be transferred to one or to the other leg.

Stabilometry is a method for studying the balance of a vertical rack and a number of transient processes by recording the position, deviations and other characteristics of the projection of the common centre of gravity on the support plane.

Maintaining balance while standing is a dynamic process as everybody knows. The body of a standing person sometimes performs almost invisible, sometimes noticeably vibrational movements in various planes around some middle position. The characteristic of the oscillations: their amplitude, frequency, direction, and also the average position in the projection on the support plane are sensitive parameters reflecting the state of the various systems involved in maintaining the balance.

Stabilometry, as a method of research in clinical practice, is used relatively recently, no more than 20 years. Nevertheless, this method is becoming increasingly important in various fields of practical medicine. This is due to the following factors:

- we use the test of motor function, the main stance, includes the action of many systems of the body (musculoskeletal, nervous, vestibular, visual, proprioceptive and others);
- the study takes relatively little time (from a few seconds to a minute);
- it does not require the installation of sensors on the body of the subject (with the exception of special techniques);
- the parameters that we obtain are very sensitive and have both diagnostic and prognostic value.

That is why stabilometry today is widely represented in the practical medicine of developed countries, especially in the US, France, Japan, Italy, and in other countries. From these countries, France should be recognised as the leader in the clinical development of this method, where a specialised institute of post-urology successfully functions.

Thus, the use of stabilometry as a method of direct evaluation of biomechanical parameters of the knee joint is impossible. But, the stabilometry is an integral method of obtaining data for carrying out calculations, constructing physico-mathematical models that allow treating the knee joint as a biomechanical system with specific parametric characteristics.

Thus, above we described some research methods, which are not sufficient for the most complete determination of the anatomical and biomechanical characteristics of the knee joint. Because we need to define a set of anatomical and biomechanical parameters of the knee joint and to create a method that allows these characteristics to be quickly and clearly defined for use in scientific and clinical purposes.

We developed a specialised software and hardware complex for the objective parametrisation of the anatomical and biomechanical characteristics of the knee joint to achieve that goal.

Table 10.1. Distribution of the sample by sex and age.

Sex	Youth age	First period of adulthood	Second period of adulthood	Elderly age	Total
male	92	103	109	65	369
female	89	98	94	70	351
TOTAL:	181	201	203	135	720

We made an analysis of the data of X-ray computer and magnetic resonance imaging to reveal the peculiarities of the individual anatomical structure of the soft-tissue and bone structures of the knee joint region. We looked through the total volume of studies on a spiral computer tomograph and magnetic resonance imaging and made the conclusion that all studies were made of the lower extremity and particularly in the knee joint region. The array of DICOM files was combined into a single database for their software analysis.

In addition, we examined 149 patients without knee pathology in the Department of Traumatology and Orthopedics (Surgery) of the Volgograd Regional Clinical Hospital of Veterans of Wars. All the subjects were divided into age groups according to the recommendations of the VII All-Union Conference on Problems of Age Morphology, Physiology and Biochemistry (Moscow 1965). The distribution of patients by sex and age was shown in Table 10.1.

We identified for all patients individual anatomical features of the structure, morphometric measurements of the lower extremities, which were performed using a millimetre ruler and atasometer. We performed the CT-scan and MRI study using virtual topographic anatomical media:

1. The distance between the superior anterior iliac spines (A).
2. The distance between the large trochanters of the femurs (B).
3. The distance between the false epicondyles of the femurs (C).
4. The distances between the medial and lateral epicondyle of the femur on the right (DD) and on the left (DS).
5. The distances between the pubic symphysis and the medial epicondyle of the femur on the right (ED) and on the left (ES).
6. The distances between the large trochanter and the lateral epicondyle of the femur on the right (FD) and on the left (FS).
7. The distances between the medial and lateral condyles of the tibia on the right (GD) and on the left (GS).
8. The distances between the lateral and medial malleolus to the right (HD) and to the left (HS).
9. The distance from the pubic symphysis to the support (I).
10. The distances between the superior anterior iliac spine and the large trochanter of the femur on the right (JD) and on the left (JS).
11. The distances between the medial epicondyle of the femoral and condyle of the tibia on the right (KD) and on the left (KS).
12. The distance from the medial condyle of the tibia to the support (L).
13. The distance between lateral condyles of tibia (M).
14. The distance between the lateral ankles (N).
15. The distance from the medial malleolus to support (O).
16. The valus and varus angles (α, β).

Morphometric data were recorded in the individual lower limb examination map, which was developed by us.

For further computer analysis and virtual visualisation of morphometry, digital photography was carried out for patients.

We implemented this method by the processing of digital photos using the Adobe Photoshop® software package. We put dermal markers when digital photography was performed to accurately visualise the topographic anatomical landmarks of the lower limb (pubic symphysis, upper anterior iliac spine, large femur spine, medial and lateral epicondyle of the femur, lateral and medial condyle of the tibia, lateral and medial malleolus) (Figure 10.1).

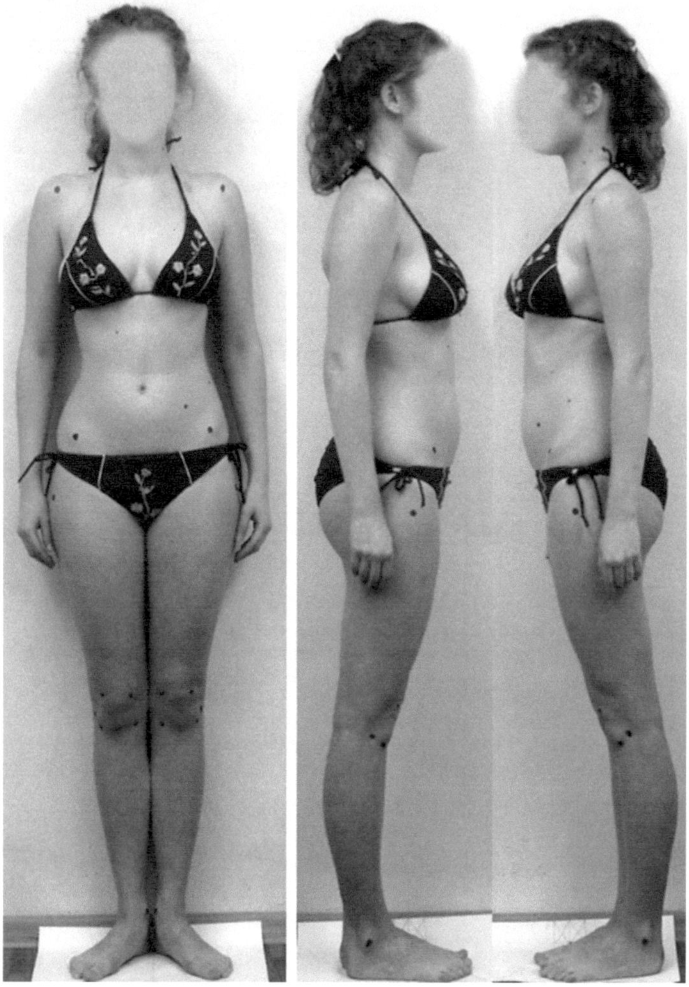

Figure 10.1. Digital photography using skin markers.

We used the "Method for determining the value of the correction of the axis of the lower extremities and the device for its implementation" to determine the magnitude of the varus or valgus angles, (application No. 2007118915/14 (020603) dated May 21, 2007). The device for determining the angles of the lower extremities (Figure 10.2) consists of a ruler 1, on which runners 3 are fixed. A ruler 2 is attached to the runners 3. It is moving on the basis to the ruler 1. A ruler 4 is attached to the runners 7 is fixed at an angle 90° by the movable yoke 5 to the ruler 1. The ruler 1 is made of wood, the remaining parts of the device are made of stainless steel. On the rulers are plotted divisions (units of measurement – mm). The reference point 8 is located on the ruler 1, the reference point 9 – on the ruler 4.

To determine the axial deformities of the lower limbs, the reference point 8 is set to the pubic symphysis of the examinee (the position of the subject is standing or lying, legs are straightened, connected). The end of the movable ruler 2 is set at the level of the medial malleolus. To determine the varus strain, ruler 4 is set at the level of the medial epicondyle of the femur using a movable clamp 5. To determine the valgus deformity of the lower extremities, the clamp 5 with the ruler 4 is set at the end of the ruler 2, that is, at the level of the medial malleolus of the examinee. By dividing the rulers 1,2,4 determine one or another type of axial deformation of the lower limbs. For this, the lengths of the legs of the right triangle ABB_1 – a and c are determined, and the angle α is determined (Figure 10.3).

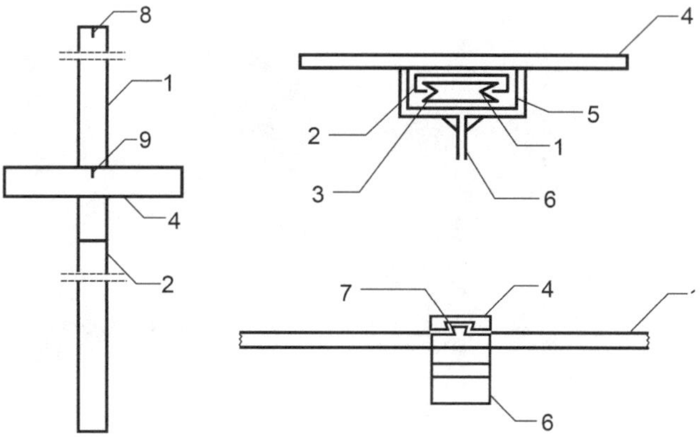

Figure 10.2. The device for determining axial deformities of the lower limbs.

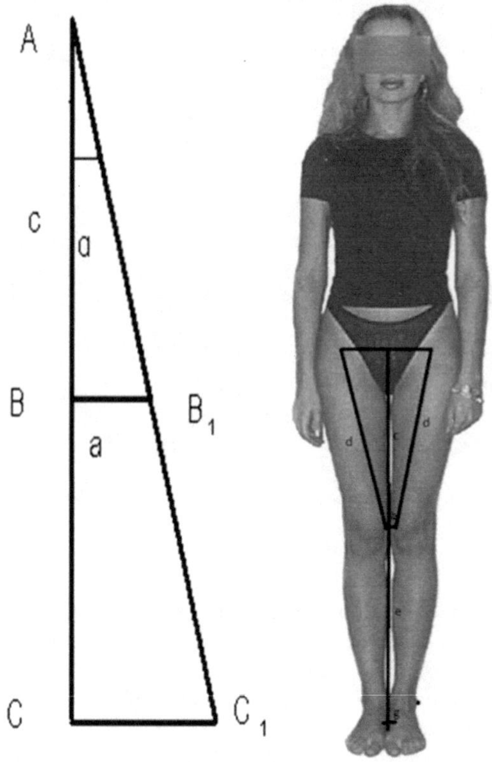

Figure 10.3. Determination of the size of the varus angle.

To determine the centre of pressure during standing, the patients underwent stabilometric examination (Romberg test). Registration and evaluation of stabilometric data were carried out using MBN-Biomechanics Version 4.00 software packages, Microsoft Office Excel 2007 (Microsoft).

When performing X-ray computed tomography, indications were:

- inconsistency of the clinical picture of the disease and data obtained by traditional radiographic diagnosis;
- marked violations of the function of the lower limb.

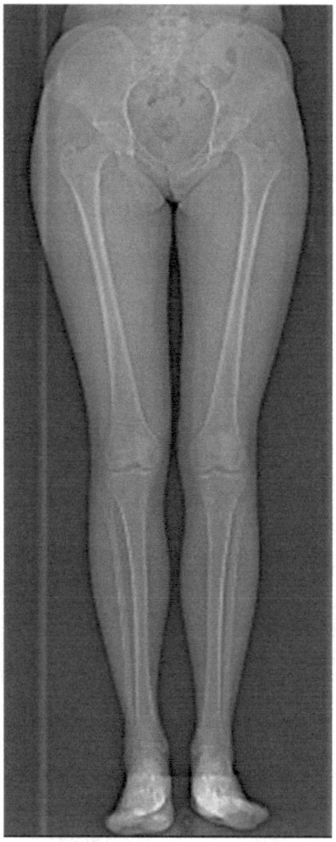

Figure 10.4. A survey digital X-ray of the lower limbs (topogram).

The study was conducted on a spiral computer tomograph Somatom plus 4 (Siemens). The study was started from the topogram (a survey digital radiograph) of the lower limb (Figure 10.4). Making the topogram before the start of the scan allowed immediate localisation of the research area (AOI) and perform its marking to determine the level of the first computer tomographic "cut" and the length of the study zone. In the course of the study, the topogram helped to control the location of the performed tomograms.

Indications for the magnetic resonance imaging were:

- inconsistency of the clinical picture of the disease and the data obtained by the traditional radiographic technique of the study;
- severe violations of the function of the lower limb;
- pronounced changes in the soft tissues of the lower limb.

The study was performed on a magnetic resonance tomograph Magnetom Vision (Siemens) with a magnetic field strength of 1.5 Tesla. To evaluate the results of the study, obtained by computer and magnetic resonance imaging, we used the eFilmLt program. Using the eFilm toolbar, it is possible to measure the anatomical formations of various anatomical objects. So, we can measure the length and breadth of bones, calculate the area of the soft tissue and bone structures of the limb, and measure the angles between planes and projections. To obtain objective characteristics of the structure of the knee joint with the help of modern methods of medical imaging (PKT and MRI), we performed the following morphometric measurements:

1. Distance between the superior anterior iliac spines (A).
2. The distance between the large trochanteres of the femurs (B).
3. The distance between the false epicondyles of the femurs (C).

4. Distances between the medial and lateral epicondyle of the femur on the right (DD) and on the left (DS).
5. Distances between the pubic symphysis and the medial epicondyle of the femur on the right (ED) and on the left (ES).
6. Distances between the large trochanter and the lateral epicondyle of the femur on the right (FD) and on the left (FS).
7. Distances between the medial and lateral condyles of the tibia on the right (GD) and on the left (GS).
8. Distances between the lateral and medial malleolus to the right (HD) and to the left (HS).
9. Distance from the pubic symphysis to the support (I).
10. Distances between the superior anterior iliac spine and the large trochanter of the femur on the right (JD) and on the left (JS).
11. Distances between the medial epicondyle of the femoral and condyle of the tibia on the right (KD) and on the left (KS).
12. Distance from the medial condyle of the tibia to the support (L).
13. Distance between lateral condyles of tibia (M).
14. The distance between the lateral ankles (N).
15. Distance from medial malleolus to support (O).
16. Valus and varus angles.
17. Area of articular surfaces of bones.

Analysis of the shape of the lower extremities was performed according to characteristic features (Figure 10.5). For the direct shape of the legs, the medial surfaces of the lower extremities touch at the level of the broad parts of the hips, the medial condyles of the hip and the medial malleolus. This form can also be referred to as "genu rectum", since there is no angle between the hip axis and the shin axis, their longitudinal axes are on the same straight line.

Valgus form of the legs is characterised by complete contact of the lower extremities at the level of the wide parts of the hips and medial condyle of the thigh. This form can be defined as "genu valgum with false curvature of the thigh", since there is complete contact of the knee joints, the femur axis is not on the same line with the shin axis, but forms an angle in the frontal plane that is open to the outside.

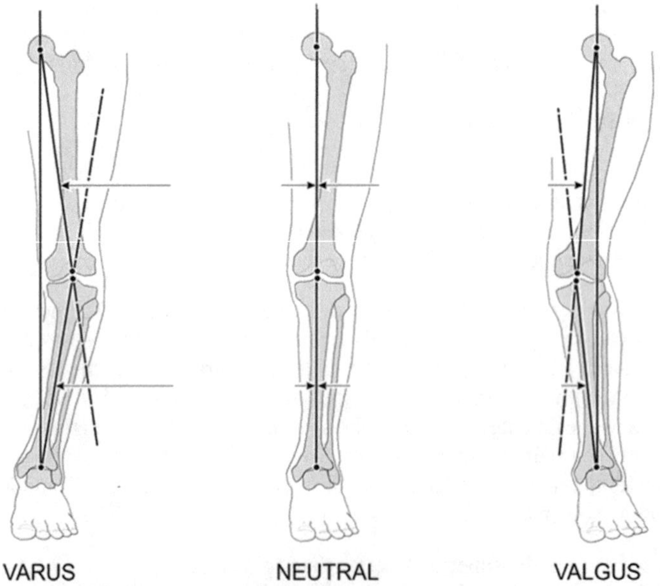

Figure 10.5. X-ray signs of the shape of the lower extremities.

Varus form is characterised by the presence of gaps between the wide parts of the thigh, knee joints and medial malleolus.

Analysis of the morphology of the condyles of the femur included the longitudinal dimensions of the medial and lateral condyles, their transverse dimensions, and on the front surface of their vertical dimensions. The longitudinal dimension was defined as the maximum distance between the anterior and posterior surfaces of the condyles, the transverse between their outer and inner lateral surfaces (Figure 10.6).

The study of the structure of the condyles of the tibia included the determination of their longitudinal and transverse dimensions. The longitudinal dimension corresponded to the maximum distance between the anterior and posterior surfaces of the condyles, and the transverse dimension corresponded to the outer and inner surfaces of the condyles (Figure 10.7).

A study of menisci included measuring their length and thickness of the projection of the anterior and posterior horns. The length of the meniscus was defined as the maximum distance between its inner and outer surface, and the thickness between the upper and lower.

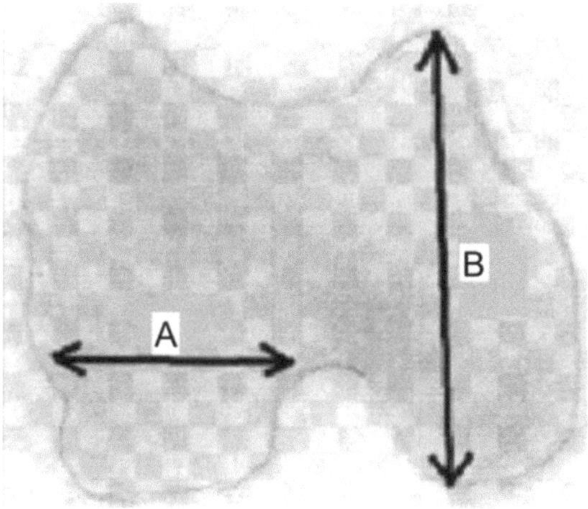

Figure 10.6. Morphometric examination of the condyles of the femur. A is the longitudinal size of the condyle, B is the transverse size of the condyle.

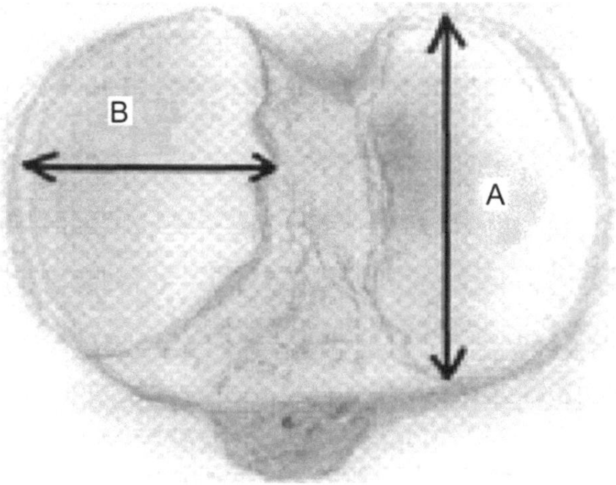

Figure 10.7. Morphometric examination of condyles of the tibia. A is the length of condyle, B is the width of condyle.

The mathematical analysis of the parameters obtained consisted of successively conducted statistical methods of investigation (Avtandilov 1990; Georgievsky 1981; Lakin 1990; Plokhinsky 1970). The following variational-statistical elements were determined: M, m, σ, t, p.

The evaluation of the statistical significance of the differences between the mean values was tested on the basis of the t-test of the Student: the null hypothesis was tested on the absence of differences between the signs. For verification, the t-statistics (ts) were calculated and compared with the tabulated value (tv), determined using the table (Lukyanova 1999, Urbakh 1964).

Software and hardware complex and methods of anatomical and biomechanical research of the human knee.

To solve the set research goal, we developed and built a software and hardware complex capable of measuring the objective biomechanical parameters of the lower limbs. The complex includes the following elements:

1. The camera;
2. Device for determining the amount of correction of the axis of the lower limbs;
3. MBN-stabilometer;
4. Magnetic resonance tomograph Siemens somatom 4 plus;
5. A computer with the installed software package for carrying out this research.

The block diagram in Figure 10.8, describes the operation of the whole complex. It includes three stages of measurements carried out using the described methods plus four units for calculating various parameters and a block for outputting data to the computer screen. The general algorithm for the operation of the complex is shown in Figure 10.9.

10.3 MAIN PART OF THE RESEARCH

Based on the processing of the obtained initial parameters in the above described steps, the developed software package determines the representation of the total static load produced by the mass of the human body using the reduced mass method, which in this study is a loading primitive used to

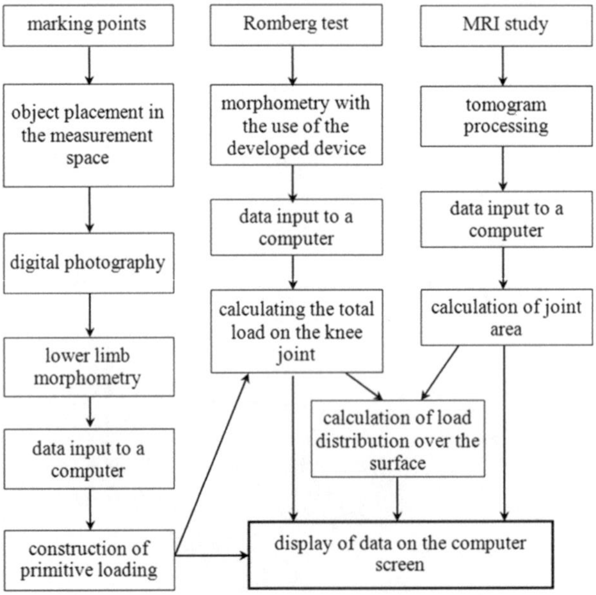

Figure 10.8. Block diagram of software and hardware for biomechanical evaluation of loads on the knee joint of a person.

determine the load on the surface of the knee joint. The result of its construction can be used not only to study loads on the surface of the knee joint, but also to study the distribution of loads at any point of the human body.

To determine the pressure centre and the reaction force of the support, a stabilometric study was carried out. During the study, the following were determined:

1) The common centre of mass is a hypothetical point, located 2–3 cm in front of the pelvis, corresponding to the common centre of mass of the body;
2) The pressure centre is a point localised on the vertical projection or vector (Winter et al. 1998) of the support reaction. In other words, the centre of pressure is the resultant, produced by the mass of the body and its movements, onto a stabilometric or dynamometric platform. Based on the data obtained in the construction of an individual model of the loading of the human body, the distribution of the total mass of the human body onto certain points of the biomechanical axes of the lower limbs is projected. The values of x and y are distances from the point of the pressure centre to the points of application of the forces of reaction of the support to the feet (Figure 10.10).

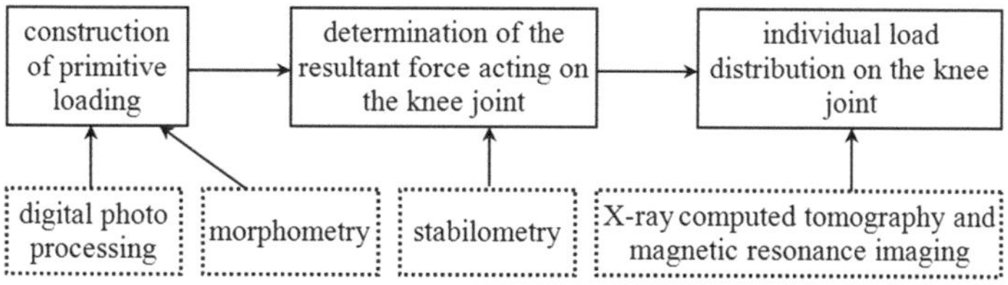

Figure 10.9. General algorithm of the software and hardware complex for determining the biomechanical characteristics of the human knee.

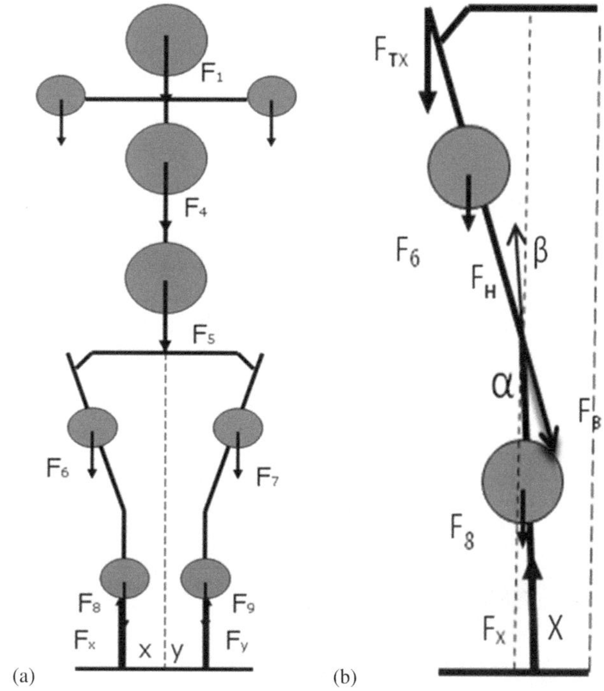

Figure 10.10. Construction of load distribution (a – total distribution, b – right lower limb).

The resulting pressure centre is used in the decomposition of the total reaction force of the support into the components Fx and Fy, which are the forces of the foot reaction to the feet. The forces Fx and Fy can be obtained from the following formulas:

$$|\vec{F_x}| = \frac{|\overrightarrow{F_{\text{р.оп}}}|}{x+y} \quad |\vec{F_y}| = \frac{|\overrightarrow{F_{\text{р.оп}}}|}{x+y} Y$$

Consider the right limb. In Figure 10.11 shows the right limb where Fmx is the force acting on the right hip joint.

$$|\overrightarrow{F_{\text{TX}}}| = |\vec{F_x}| - |\vec{F_6}| - |\vec{F_8}|$$

To determine the resultant force acting on the knee joint in the frontal plane, it is necessary to obtain the forces F_H and F_B – the forces acting on the lower and upper surfaces of the joint. The angle α is the angle between the perpendicular to the support surface and the mechanical axis of the femur, and the angle β is the angle between the perpendicular to the support surface and the mechanical axis of the tibia bones.

From the obtained model it follows that:

$$|\vec{F_{\text{B}}}| = (|\overrightarrow{F_{\text{TX}}}| + |\vec{F_6}|)\cos\beta \quad |\vec{F_{\text{H}}}| = (|\vec{F_{\text{X}}}| + |\vec{F_8}|)\cos\alpha$$

The developed software and hardware complex contains an application for determining the resultant force acting on the knee joint, the Romberg test, which is part of the MBN-Biomechanics Version 4.0 software, was conducted. After the test, the position of the pressure centre on the coordinate plane is determined (Figure 10.11). In the field of the software package, the position of the centre of mass is marked with a red dot. The distances of x and y were measured from the grid located in the program interface.

To determine the shape of the lower extremities (varus or valgus angles), we used the "Method for determining the value of the correction of the axis of the lower extremities and the device for its implementation", developed by us. The result of using the described methods and calculations is the biomechanical evaluation of the human body used in the work to determine the load distribution over the surface of the knee joint.

In the third stage of the study, the knee joints that transmit the load were determined.

The study is conducted on a spiral computer tomograph Somatom plus 4 (Siemens).

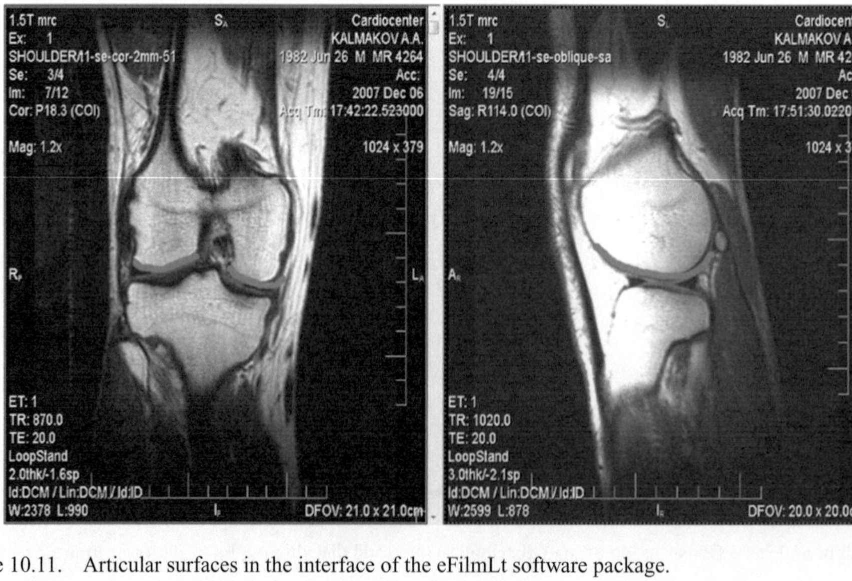

Figure 10.11. Articular surfaces in the interface of the eFilmLt software package.

The analysis of the obtained data was carried out on the main tomograph console or on the Magic View workstation. It includes the construction of multiplanar reconstructions (MPR) in the sagittal, frontal and oblique planes. Three-dimensional (3D) reconstruction of images shaded on the surface (SSD) with preservation of tissues was performed, densitometric indicators of which exceeded 150 units. N. The obtained 3D reconstructions are studied from any angle.

When studying tomograms, the control points of the surface of the knee joint are determined.

Figure 10.11 shows the interface of the eFilmLt program and the red color indicates articular surfaces, the area of which should be investigated. In the software package there is a built-in tool for determining the coordinates of any point of the surface. From these coordinates, the following points of the centre of both joint ellipsoids and the distance from the centres of the ellipsoids to the right and left boundaries are determined.

With the help of the eFilmLt software, the obtained 3D model of the knee joint may be cut into the required number of sections, both in the frontal and sagittal planes. Using the obtained cuts in the frontal plane in the (x, z) and (y, z) planes, we can compare them, obtain each one a region for discretisation and find the coordinates of the nodes of interest to us.

To do this, it is necessary to choose the point x in the (x, z) plane, then we can define the z component. To determine the y-th component, it is necessary to take a cut in the (y, z) plane corresponding to the previous slice. After that, we change x on the first slice and also find the z component for this, but the y component does not change, i.e. remains constant. As a result of this procedure, we will find all the nodes for one cut. Next, taking the following slices, we get the next value y of the component, which will be constant for the variables x and z. Thus, repeating this operation for all slices, we obtain the required coordinates of all nodes.

We can define from Figure 10.12 that if we have broken the region into quadrangular elements using the above procedure, but, as we know, any quadrilateral can always be divided into triangular elements. Thus, we have everything we need to calculate the surface area of the knee joint using the finite element method. But for this, we need to know how the area of the triangle is considered with respect to the three coordinates of all vertices. To derive the formula of interest to us, consider the segment AB in the (z, x) plane and project it onto the (y, x) plane. It can be seen from Figure 10.12 that if we apply the Pythagorean Theorem, we can find the length of the projected segment A_1B_1:

$$A_1B_1 = \sqrt{(x_B - x_A)^2 + (y_B - y_A)^2}$$

Further, assuming that the segment A_1B_1 is equal to the segment AB, that is, $A_1B_1 = AB$, then applying the Pythagorean theorem, we can find the length of the segment AB:

$$AB = \sqrt{(z_B - z_A)^2 + (A_1B_1)^2} = \sqrt{(x_B - x_A)^2 + (y_B - y_A)^2 + (z_B - z_A)^2}$$

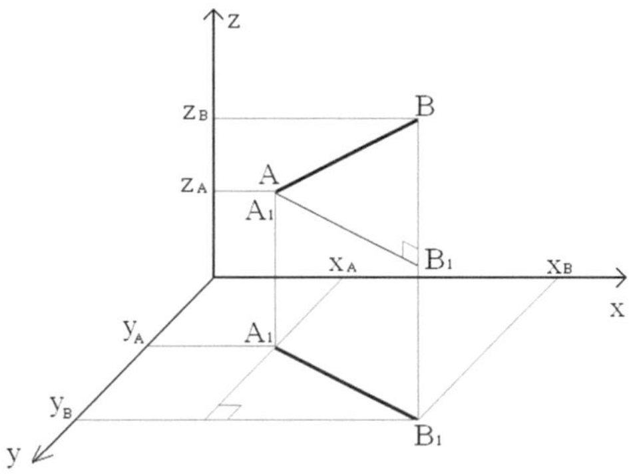

Figure 10.12. Division of the area into components.

Similarly to the above calculations one can obtain the lengths of the sides of the triangular element:

$$AB = \sqrt{(x_B - x_A)^2 + (y_B - y_A)^2 + (z_B - z_A)^2}$$
$$BC = \sqrt{(x_C - x_B)^2 + (y_C - y_B)^2 + (z_C - z_B)^2}$$
$$CA = \sqrt{(x_C - x_A)^2 + (y_C - y_A)^2 + (z_C - z_A)^2}$$

After that, we can find the area of the triangle using the Heron formula:

$$S = \sqrt{p\,(p - AB)\,(p - BC)\,(p - CA)}$$

where $p = (AB + BC + CA)/2$ is the half-diameter of a triangle.

Thus, by finding the areas of all the triangular elements, on which we have broken the knee joint region, and summing them, we get the required area of the lower surface of the knee joint. After processing, the data is entered in the program package table.

At the final (fourth) stage, the distribution of contact pressure over the surface of the knee joint was determined. To determine it, the mathematical method was chosen. The load distribution along the X and Y axes is determined by the following formulas.

$\sigma = F \cos\gamma$ – normal pressure on the surface of the knee joint at the point (x_1, y_1).

$\tau = F \sin\gamma$ – tangential pressure on the surface of the knee joint at the point (x_1, y_1)

$$|\overrightarrow{F_B}| = (|\overrightarrow{F_{TX}}| + |\overrightarrow{F_6}|)\cos\beta$$

where F is the contact pressure on the surface of the knee joint, β is the angle at which this force acts on the joint.

From the anatomy of the knee joint, it follows that the intra-articular cavity is filled with liquid, which means that the pressure on the surface will be determined according to Pascal's law.

$$F = \frac{|\overrightarrow{F_B}|}{S}$$

Proceeding from this, the load distribution over the surface of the knee joint is determined by constructing σ and τ at certain points, defining $\cos\gamma$ and $\sin\gamma$ at these points. The distribution is displayed in the program window (Figure 10.13).

Possible applications of the developed method:

- prophylaxis of diseases associated with disruption of load distribution on the knee joint;
- correction of axial deformations of the lower limbs;
- endoprosthetics, the manufacture of individual endoprostheses,
- selection of orthopaedic footwear, insoles;
- research work;
- sports medicine, the development of sports shoes;
- teaching process at the departments of medical, technical, physical education institutions.

In addition, we proposed the calculation of the following coefficients, which make it possible to perform an objective parametrization of the load on the knee joint:

the coefficient of medial – lateral load distribution:

$$C_1 = (F_{med}/S_{med})/(F_{lat}/S_{lat}),$$

where F_{med} and F_{lat} – load on the medial and lateral parts of the joint, respectively; S_{med} and S_{lat} – the areas transferring the load to the medial and lateral parts of the joint, respectively.

Thus, during the experiment, biomechanical estimates of the load on the knee joint were obtained (Figure 10.14).

At $C_1 = 1$ the joint is loaded evenly, with $C_1 < 1$ – an overload of the lateral sections, with $C_1 > 1$, an overload of the medial parts.

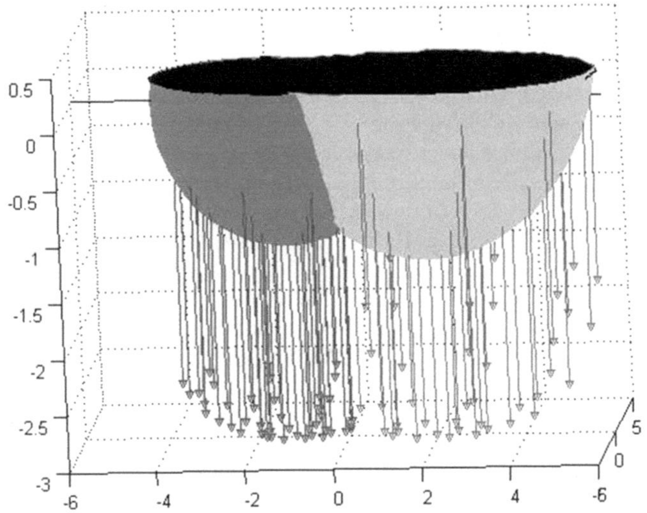

Figure 10.13. Load distribution over the knee joint surface.

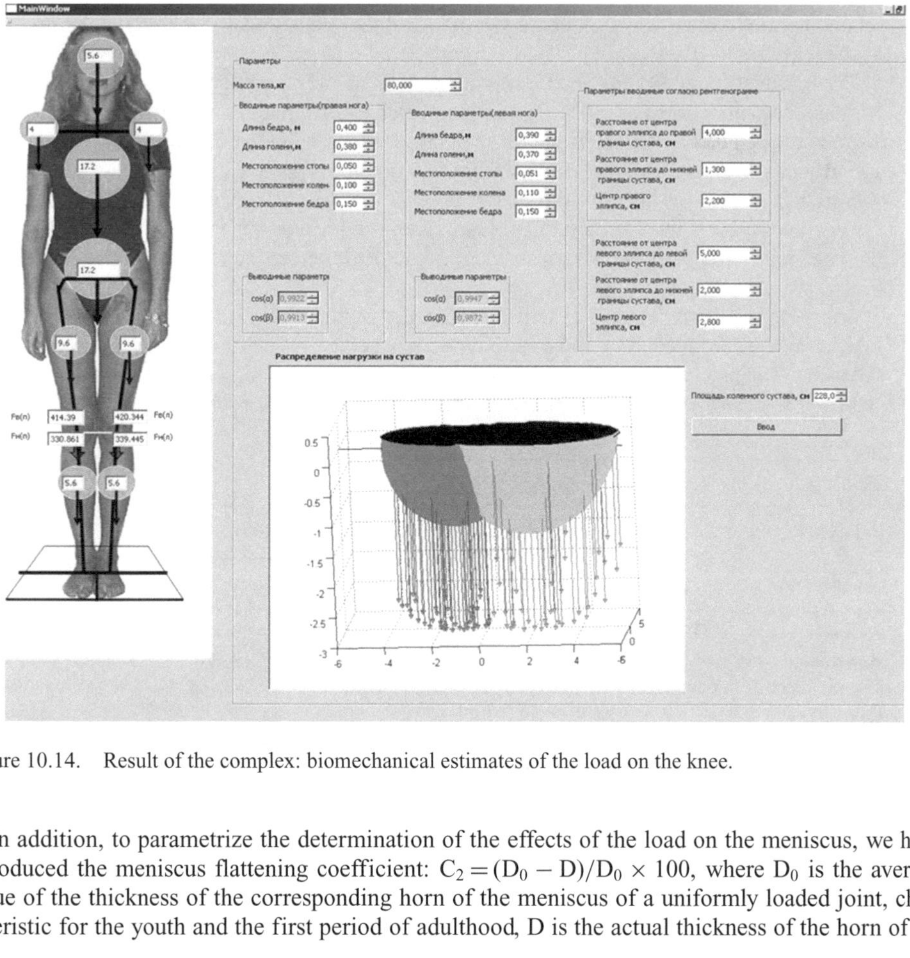

Figure 10.14. Result of the complex: biomechanical estimates of the load on the knee.

In addition, to parametrize the determination of the effects of the load on the meniscus, we have introduced the meniscus flattening coefficient: $C_2 = (D_0 - D)/D_0 \times 100$, where D_0 is the average value of the thickness of the corresponding horn of the meniscus of a uniformly loaded joint, characteristic for the youth and the first period of adulthood, D is the actual thickness of the horn of the meniscus, at $C_2 << 0$ the thickness is more typical for the youth and I period of adulthood and at $C_2 >> 0$ – the thickness decreases.

Thus, the developed method for determining the load distribution on the knee joint surface and the software and hardware complex are effective for studying a number of objective anatomo-biomechanical parameters of the knee joint of a living person, which allowed introducing new anthropometric data into clinical practice that characterize the features of the etiopathogenetic factors of the pathology development of the knee joints, contributing to the most rational approach to the choice of treatment tactics and prevention methods.

Load distribution on the surface of the knee joint in groups of people with various forms of lower limbs is of great importance for the investigation of etiopathogenesis and the development of possible methods for prevention of gonarthrosis, can be used both in virtual and in classical anthropometry, and also has practical value for orthopedics, sports medicine.

The results of the survey showed that there were no statistically significant differences in the anthropometric data of men in the juvenile and 1st periods of mature age. Males of the youth and the first stage of adulthood are tall in comparison with men of the second period of mature and elderly ages, mainly due to reliably large lengths of the body and length of the legs (Table 10.2).

The greatest length of the femur and tibia was in men of the juvenile and first stages of the mature age, in comparison with the men of the older age groups, which determined a significantly longer leg length.

The body weight of men of the second period of adulthood reached significantly high values in comparison with men of youth, I period of mature and elderly ages.

Women of the juvenile and first stages of adulthood are tall in comparison with women of the second period of mature and elderly ages, mainly due to reliably large lengths of the body and length of the legs (Table 10.3).

The greatest length of the femur was in women of the juvenile and I periods of mature age in comparison with women of older age groups, which determined their significantly longer leg length. Women of the juvenile and first stages of the mature age had an average pelvis, women of the older age groups – wide-spread. The body weight of women in the juvenile and first stages of mature age was significantly lower than in women of the second stage of the mature and elderly ages.

When comparing the biomechanical features of the knee joint, it was found that the total load on the knee joint (Table 10.4) did not have significant differences, depending on the shape of the lower limbs.

There are statistically significant differences, depending on sex and age. The total load on the knee joint in men of the second period of adulthood reached significantly high values in comparison with the men of the juvenile, I period of the mature and elderly ages, and in women of the juvenile and first stages of mature age had significantly minimal values in comparison with the women of the second

Table 10.2. Anthropometric indicators of men of different age groups.

	Anthropometric indicators in groups (M±m)		
Parameters	Men of youth and I of a mature age	Men of the second period of adulthood	Men of advanced age
Body length, cm	178.20±0.55*	172.34±0.49*	172.72±0.57*
The diameter of the pelvis, cm	28.32±0.21*	29.77±0.25*	29.33±0.21*
Case length, cm	88.80±0.41*	85.89±0.37*	86.52±0.42*
Length of trunk, cm	55.21±0.38	54.86±0.35	55.18±0.29
Length of foot, cm	94.55±0.48*	92.56±0.33*	92.37±0.28*
Thigh length, cm	45.32±0.32*	43.51±0.25*	43.84±0.37*
Shank length, cm	42.51±0.24*	41.57±0.21*	40.36±0.14*
Height of foot, cm	7.03±0.11*	7.48±0.07*	7.87±0.07*
Body weight, kg	70.29±1.14*	80.02±1.06*	76.97±0.87*

* – the differences are reliable ($p<0.05$).

Table 10.3. Anthropometric indicators of women of different age groups.

	Anthropometric indicators in groups (M±m)		
Parameters	Women of the juvenile and the first stage of adulthood	Women II period of adulthood	Women of advanced age
Body length, cm	164.77±0.32*	161.95±0.39*	159.94±0.40*
The diameter of the pelvis, cm	26.95±0.13*	29.36±0.24*	29.74±0.26*
Case length, cm	80.78±0.20*	79.53±0.27*	78.32±0.20*
Length of trunk, cm	50.97±0.19*	51.61±0.22*	50.82±0.26*
Length of foot, cm	89.33±0.25*	88.30±0.29*	86.85±0.34*
Thigh length, cm	43.07±0.18*	41.20±0.16*	41.39±0.17*
Shank length, cm	39.10±0.18*	39.41±0.19*	37.91±0.20*
Height of foot, cm	7.12±0.07*	7.64±0.06*	7.55±0.07*
Body weight, kg	57.63±0.52*	66.50±1.08*	72.47±0.96*

* the differences are reliable ($p<0.05$).

Table 10.4. The total load on the knee joint, depending on the sex, age and shape of the lower extremities.

		Total load on the knee joint (Newton)			
Form of lower limbs	Sex	Juvenile age	I period of mature	II period of mature	Elderly age
Valgus	M	324.0±10.2 d	331.3±10.1 d	369.4±12.4 d	357.0±11.3 d
		323.4±7.3 s	320.7±6.8 s	357.2±11.3 s	352.4 ± 9.1 s
	F	267.6±10.8 d	277.8±11.7 d	303.7±10.2 d	341.3±13.4 d
		256.2±9.2 s	272.3±12.1 s	295.3±10.7 s	335.2±12.2 s
Straight	M	320.3±12.3 d	330.2±11.2 d	364.7±14.1 d	350.8±13.9 d
		318.1±11.2 s	322.7±11.8 s	358.4±13.7 s	352.4±11.5 s
	F	262.6±9.8 d	281.1±11.0 d	303.0±12.7 d	330.3±14.9 d
		256.2±9.2 s	278.3±11.1 s	297.3±12.8 s	328.2±12.9 s
Varus	M	319.1±10.3 d	327.8±11.2 d	365.9±13.7 d	350.8±12.7 d
		314.2±10.2s	324.1±11.8 s	358.4±11.2 s	347.2±10.7 s
	F	268.2±7.9 d	284.1±10.1 d	310.3±11.2 d	339.3±14.8 d
		258.4±8.9 s	277.5±10.6 s	304.7±9.9 s	332.8±12.7 s

d (dextra) – right, s (sinistra) – left.

period of mature and elderly ages. In general, the total load on the knee joint in men was significantly greater than in women. There was a non-uniformity in the transfer of the load to the right and left knee joints: the right joint was loaded more than the left one, at the same time, the discrepancy was statistically insignificant.

The total area of the knee joints that transmit the load (Bezborodov 2011), did not have significant differences depending on age, as a result of which the dependence on sex and the shape of the lower extremities was compared. There are significant differences in the size of the area, depending on sex. In men, the area of the knee joint was significantly larger than in women (Table 10.5). In general, with the varus form of the lower limbs, there is an increase in the lower extremities in men, in women this indicator did not have significant differences.

When studying the coefficient of load distribution, it was found that with the varus form of the lower extremities, a large load is exerted on the medial parts of the articular surfaces of the knee joint, with the valgus form of the lower limbs, the load is directed to the lateral sections. At the same time, the straightest shape of the lower extremities is optimal from the point of view of uniform distribution of the load.

This fact is confirmed by a comparative study of the flattening coefficient of meniscuses of the knee joint, which from the point of view of mechanics are on the one hand elastic members working on compression (shock absorbers). On the other hand menisci are adapters of mating surfaces that distribute the load. Obviously, with the same elasticity coefficient, both meniscus functions will be performed the better, the larger its thickness. On the other hand, the elastic element, which is subjected to a longer load for a long time, undergoes flattening over time, which reduces its functional capabilities. Since the study of the load distribution coefficient has revealed that the most direct form of the lower limbs is optimal, there were no age changes in the juvenile and I periods of adulthood, the average values of the corresponding indicators were taken into account for normative ones taking into account gender differences.

When studying the flattening coefficients of the horns of the medial and lateral meniscuses, it was found that in men and women the flattening coefficients of the anterior and posterior horns of the medial meniscus (Tables 10.6, 10.7, 10.8, 10.9) did not have significant differences in adolescence. The negative value of this coefficient (on the verge of statistical errors) indicates the presence of some "stock" in the thickness of the elastic element. At the same time it was found that with the varus form of the lower limbs, starting from the first period of adulthood, the values of this coefficient increase significantly, reaching intermediate values characteristic of the straight and valgus forms of the lower limbs in the second period of mature and elderly ages.

At the given group of people at the profound inspection in 49% of cases signs of beginning signs of dystrophic changes in knee joints were noted. Subchondral sclerosis of the condyles of the tibia was noted along the medial side, which also indicated an overload of the internal parts of the knee joint. In addition, the decrease in the height of the joint gap along the medial side, which is caused by the "deformation" of the meniscus is another factor contributing to the development of arthrosis of the

Table 10.5. The area of the surfaces transmitting the load and the coefficient of medial-lateral load distribution.

		Form of lower limbs		
Parameters	Sex	Valgus M±m	Straight M±m	Varus M±m
Area of surfaces transferring the load (cm^2)	M	27.29±1.8	28.84±1.6	31.35±1.5*
	F	23.31±1.7	22.62±1.5	23.42±1.6
The coefficient of medial-lateral load distribution	M	0.70±0.024*	1.07±0.091*	1.62±0.037*
	F	0.74±0.021*	1.15±0.139*	1.81±0.042*

* – the differences are reliable (p<0.05).

Table 10.6. The coefficient of flattening of the anterior horn of the medial meniscus in men of different age groups, depending on the shape of the lower limbs.

Form of lower limbs	Youthful age	I period of adulthood	II period of adulthood	Elderly age
Valgus	−3.87±1.97	−1.93±1.54	1.29±1.03	16.12±3.90*
Straight	−1.29±1.65	1.29±1.03	3.22±1.58	18.06±3.45*
Varus	2.58±1.64	7.74±1.94*	13.54±2.84*	27.74±3.19*

* – the differences are reliable (p<0.05).

Table 10.7. The coefficient of flattening of the horn of the medial meniscus in men of different age groups, depending on the shape of the lower limbs.

Form of lower limbs	Youthful age	I period of adulthood	II period of adulthood	Elderly age
Valgus	−0.88±1.06	0.34±1.15	2.20±1.64	9.25±3.11*
Straight	−0.44±1.05	0.44±1.05	3.08±2.37	10.57±2.26*
Varus	1.32±1.58	3.96±1.47*	12.33±2.48*	14.53±2.74*

* – the differences are reliable (p<0.05).

knee joints. The increase in body weight with age (or unrelated to it) also aggravates the situation, further increasing the load on the knee joint.

On the other hand, in men and women, the coefficients of flattening of the anterior and posterior horns of the lateral meniscus (Tables 10.10, 10.11, 10.12, 10.13) did not have significant differences in adolescence. The negative value of this coefficient (on the verge of statistical errors) indicates

Table 10.8. The coefficient of flattening of the anterior horn of the medial meniscus in women of different age groups, depending on the shape of the lower limbs.

Form of lower limbs	Youthful age	I period of adulthood	II period of adulthood	Elderly age
Valgus	−2.93±1.16	2.28±1.01	4.23±1.45	21.17±2.64*
Straight	−1.62±1.86	1.62±1.66	1.62±1.64	20.52±2.11*
Varus	2.28±1.01	8.14±1.33*	14.00±2.65*	28.33±3.87*

* – the differences are reliable ($p<0.05$).

Table 10.9. The coefficient of flattening of the horn of the medial meniscus in women of different age groups, depending on the shape of the lower limbs.

Form of lower limbs	Youthful age	I period of adulthood	II period of adulthood	Elderly age
Valgus	−1.55±1.21	−0.66±1.51	2.88±1.24	9.53±1.43*
Straight	−0.66±1.51	0.66±1.45	3.76±1.94	12.19±2.51*
Varus	0.66±1.58	3.76±0.94*	6.87±1.36*	15.74±2.27*

* – the differences are reliable ($p<0.05$).

Table 10.10. The coefficient of flattening of the anterior horn of the lateral meniscus in men of different age groups, depending on the shape of the lower limbs.

Form of lower limbs	Youthful age	I period of adulthood	II period of adulthood	Elderly age
Valgus	−1.66±1.13	4.31±1.89*	8.97±1.01*	17.60±2.79*
Straight	−0.99±0.66	0.99±1.66	3.65±1.44	13.62±2.12*
Varus	−2.99±1.03	−0.99±1.68	0.99±1.78	12.29±2.23*

* – the differences are reliable ($p<0.05$).

Table 10.11. The coefficient of flattening of the horn of the lateral meniscus in men of different age groups, depending on the shape of the lower limbs.

Form of lower limbs	Youthful age	I period of adulthood	II period of adulthood	Elderly age
Valgus	0.99±0.66	4.24±1.52*	8.01±1.88*	17.45±2.28*
Straight	−0.94±1.34	0.94±1.33	2.35±1.84	12.73±2.58*
Varus	−2.35±1.84	1.32±1.45	1.88±1.67	11.32±2.07*

* – the differences are reliable ($p<0.05$).

Table 10.12. The coefficient of flattening of the anterior horn of the lateral meniscus in women of different age groups, depending on the shape of the lower limbs.

Form of lower limbs	Youthful age	I period of adulthood	II period of adulthood	Elderly age
Valgus	−1.32±1.45	3.31±1.12*	10.59±1.60*	17.88±2.07*
Straight	−1.32±1.45	1.32±1.45	4.63±1.57	13.24±2.50*
Varus	−1.98±1.67	0.66±0.62	3.97±1.35	11.92±2.05*

* – the differences are reliable ($p<0.05$).

Table 10.13. The coefficient of flattening of the horn of the lateral meniscus in women of different age groups, depending on the shape of the lower limbs.

Form of lower limbs	Youthful age	I period of adulthood	II period of adulthood	Elderly age
Valgus	0.47±0.41	4.71±1.69*	11.79±2.45*	17.92±2.45*
Straight	−0.47±0.46	0.47±0.45	3.30±1.18	13.67±2.92*
Varus	−1.88±1.67	−0.47±0.41	1.41±1.25	12.73±2.58*

* – the differences are reliable ($p<0.05$).

the presence of some "stock" in the thickness of the elastic element. At the same time, it has been established that with the valgus form of the lower limbs, beginning with the first period of adulthood, the values of this coefficient increase significantly, reaching intermediate values characteristic of the straight and varus forms of the lower extremities of the second period of mature and elderly ages.

10.4 CONCLUSIONS

With the varus form of the lower extremities, a large load is exerted on the medial parts of the articular surfaces of the knee joint (the medial-lateral load distribution coefficient is 1.62 ± 0.037 and 1.81 ± 0.042), contributing to flattening of the medial meniscus over time (flattening coefficient from 14, 53 ± 2.74 to 28.33 ± 3.87); with the valgus form of the lower extremities, the load is directed to the lateral sections (the coefficient of medial lateral load distribution is 0.70 ± 0.024 and 0.74 ± 0.021), contributing to flattening of the lateral meniscus with the course of time (flattening coefficient in the range of 17.45 ± 2.28–17.92 ± 2.45). In addition, a factor such as the age-related increase in body weight leads to a significant increase in the total load on the knee joint from 320.3 ± 12.3 H to 369.4 ± 12.4H in men and from 262.6 ± 9.8 H to 350 , 8 ± 13.9 H in women, which, along with the uneven distribution of load on the surface of the knee, are one of the anatomical risk factors for the development of gonarthrosis.

So, in order to prevent diseases associated with disrupting the distribution of loads on the knee joint, as well as in case of correction of axial deformities of the lower limbs, surgical interventions to increase growth, in endoprosthetics, the manufacture of individual endoprostheses, in some cases, the selection of orthopedic footwear and insoles Studies of load distribution on the components of the knee joint.

REFERENCES

Albrecht G.A. 1907. *To the pathology and therapy of lateral curvature of the knee*. St. Petersburg: Diss.

Asfandiyarov R.I. 1987. Factors determining the dysplasia of articular joints. *Proc. XVI Symposium of the European Society of Osteoarthrologists "Joint Destruction"*: 13.

Avtandilov G.G. 1990. *Medical morphometry*. Moscow: Medicine.

Beltran J., Caudill J.L., Herman L.A. et al. 1987. Rheumatoid arthritis: MR imaging manifestation. *Radiology* 165: 153–157.

Beltran J., Noto A.M., Mosure J.C. et al. 1986. The knee: surface coil MR imaging at 1.5 T. *Radiology* 159: 747–751.

Bezborodov S.A. 2011. *Program-technical complex for biomechanical assessment of the load on the human knee joint: Author's abstract.* Dissertation for Candidate of Medical Science. Volgograd.

Biedert R., Lobenhoffer C., Latterman C. 2000. Free nerve endings in the medial and posteromedial capsuloligamentous complexes: occurrence and distribution. *Knee Surg., Sports Traumatol., Arthrosc.* 8: 68–72.

Dye S.F. 2003. Functional morphologic features of the human knee: an evolutionary perspective. *Clin Orthop.* 410: 19–24.

Gagala, J., M. Tarczynska, & K. Gaweda. 2014. A seven- to 14-year follow-up study of bipolar hip arthroplasty in the treatment of osteonecrosis of the femoral head. *Hip International* 24(1):14–19.

Gilkeson G., Polisson R., Sinclair H. et al. 1988. Early detection of carpal erosions in patients with rheumatoid arthritis: a pilot study of magnetic resonance imaging. *J.Rheumatol.*15:1361.

Kapanji A.I. 2010. *Lower limb: functional anatomy.* Moscow: Eksmo.

Koenig H., Sieper J., Wolf K.J. 1990. Rheumatoid arthritis: evaluetion of hypervascular and fibrous pannus with dynamic MR-imaging enhanced with Gd-DTPA. *Radiology* 176:473–477.

Kolmakov A.A. 2013. *The relationship of intravital anatomical and biomechanical parameters of the knee joints with various forms of the lower extremities: Author's abstract.* Dissertation for Candidate of Medical Science. Volgograd.

Kosinskaya N.S. 1961. *Degenerative-dystrophic lesions of the osteoarticular apparatus.* Leningrad.: Medgiz.

Lagunova I.G. 1951. *The basics of the general X-ray diagnosis of bone and joint diseases.* Moscow: Medicine.

Lavrishcheva G.I. & Onoprienko G.A. 1996. *Morphological and clinical aspects of reparative regeneration of supporting organs and tissues.* Moscow: Medicine, 149–174.

Makarov A.N., Mironov S.P., Lisitsyn M.P. et al. 1999. Embryonic development and primary differentiation of the cruciform complex of the human knee. Proc. of the III Congress of the Russian Arthroscopic Society, Moscow: CITO: 4–5.

Mukha Yu.P., Vorobiev A., Bezborodov S.A., Kolmakov A.A. 2009. Method for calculating the surface of the knee joint. *Bulletin of the Volgograd Scientific Center of the Russian Academy of Medical Sciences and the Administration of the Volgograd Region* 1: 54–57.

Mukha Yu.P., Kolmakov A.A., Bezborodov S.A., Barinov A.S., Chekanin I.M., Alborov A.Ts. 2015. Possibilities of using the categorical model as an anatomical and functional characteristic of the human knee joint. *Modern problems of science and education* 5: 356.

Pitkin MR, 2006. Biomechanics of articular moments in the design of lower limb prostheses. *Bulletin of the All-Russian Guild of Orthopedic Prosthetists* 1(23): 27–33.

Semizorov A.N. & Shakhov B.E. 2002. *Radiodiagnosis of diseases of bones and joints.* Nizhny Novgorod: Publishing House NGMA.

Vorobiev A.A., Mukha Yu.P., Barinov A.S., Bezborodov S.A., Kolmakov A.A. & Egin M.E. 2008. Methodology for determining the individual distribution of load on the knee joint. *Biomedical electronics* 4: 54–59.

Waterton J.C., Chekley D. & Johnston D. 1990. Supression of signal from extracellular fluid and from fat in T2-weghted MRI on inflammatory arthritis. *Abstracts of the 9th Annual Meeting Of the Society Of Magnetic Resonance in Medicine.* Berkley, CA: SMRM:1184.

Wegener O.H. 1992. *Whole body computed tomography.* Springer.

Winter D A., Patla A E., Prince F, Ishac M. & Gielo-Perczak, K. 1998. Stiffness Control of Balance in Quiet Standing. *The Journal of Neurophysiology* 80(3): 1211–1221.

Woo S. L.Y. & Livesay G.A. 1994. Kinematics of the knee. In: Fu F.H., Harner C.D., Vince K.G. (Eds.). *Knee Surgery.* – Baltimore: Williams and Wilkins, 155–173.

CHAPTER 11

Anatomical parameterisation as the basis for effective work of a passive exoskeleton of the upper limbs

A.A. Vorobiev & F.A. Andryushchenko
Volgograd Scientific Medical Center, Volgograd, Russian Federation

W. Wójcik, M. Maciejewski & M. Kamiński
Lublin University of Technology, Lublin, Poland

A. Kozbakova
Institute of Information and Computational Technologies CS MES RK, Almaty, Kazakhstan;
Almaty University of Power Engineering and Telecommunications, Kazakhstan

ABSTRACT: Authors investigated the possibility of the anatomical parameterization of the passive exoskeleton of the upper limb, EXZAR. It was used for habilitation and rehabilitation of patients with upper flaccid couple (mono) paresis.

11.1 ANALYTICAL REVIEW OF THE PROBLEM

Hands play a big role in human activities. Neither an independent life nor a full mastery of the world are possible without them. It is especially the case with children. A lot of mobility aids (walkers, strollers, vehicles) have been developed for people with disabilities of the lower limbs. Their supply is prescribed by law. At the same time, despite numerous attempts, no systemic technical solution has as yet been submitted for patients with upper limb (mono)paresis.

Interest in exoskeletons for handicapped people is dictated by practical necessity. The exoskeletons have recently been moved to the field of medicine from the military area, where all developments are strictly classified, and both active and passive varieties are used. For all their innovative components, active exoskeletons have a number of disadvantages: high cost, dependence on power sources, high weight, low mobility. We use the residual muscle force in passive exoskeletons. A number of various elements are used to strengthen them (rubber thrusts, springs, etc.). These elements often cease to work or even further violate the function of the affected limbs with abnormal anatomical and mechanical correlations (Budziszewski 2013; Iqbal et al. 2014). In view of the absence of this problem in the literature, we attempt an original explanation of it in this study.

Anatomical-mechanical correspondences between the various anatomical characteristics of the structure of the human body and the parameters of a mechanical device determine the optimal work of a biomechanical system such as a passive exoskeleton. The method of reasonable selection of such correspondences was expediently called anatomical parameterisation.

We turned our attention to the creation of a passive exoskeleton of the upper limbs according to the principles developed by a group of researchers and their leader, Professor Tarik Rahman (USA) (Rahman et al. 2006). We formed the clinical-anatomical requirements for our design and determined a list of indications for its use (Vorobiev et al. 2014; Vorobiev et al. 2016) in our earlier scientific works. In particular, the exoskeleton of the upper limbs should:

- have a volume of movements close to the indicators of a healthy person;
- mimic the structure of the upper limb of a person;
- have a light and strong construction, adaptable to the anatomical parameters of the limb;
- be made of biologically inert materials;

Table 11.1. The amplitude of the movements of man and apparatus (in degrees).

	Joint norm	Apparatus joint	Movements deficiency
Shoulder			
bending	180	155	25
rectification	60	+20	80
lead	180	155	25
reduction	0	20	20
Elbow			
bending	40	45	5
rectification	0	0	0

– have the possibility of replacing elements of the exoskeleton design as the child grows up;
– financially available for a mass consumer;
– be mobile and independent of power supplies.

We determined more than 20 nosological forms in our list of pathologies serving as an indication for the use of the passive exoskeleton of the upper limbs and found it more convenient to use the concept of a complex of symptoms of the flaccid upper limb (mono) paresis. This diagnosis is characterised by a decrease in the strength of the muscles of the upper limbs; restriction of the velocity, volume (amplitude) of movements in the proximal and distal parts of the upper limbs with predominant deterioration in the proximal parts; decreased muscle tone in the proximal and distal parts of the upper limbs, or the presence of a mixed tone, with a predominance of hypofunction; decrease or absence of tendon reflexes from the hands (flexor-ulnar, extensor-ulnar, carporadial).

The purpose of our investigation is the determination of the anatomical parametrisation for the EXZAR (**EX**oskeleton for h**A**bilitation and **R**ehabilitation) passive exoskeleton on the basis of the anatomical and mechanical correlations, and the composition of an individual's optimal technical parameters for the apparatus, which would allow to replace the functions lost with upper paraparesis.

11.2 MATERIALS AND METHODS

We have created two stationary and one mobile version of the EXZAR exoskeleton to achieve our practical goal. Stationary versions are designed for patients with upper and lower extremity lesions. Stationary version number 1 was linked to the patient's chair or wheelchair. Stationary version number 2 was fixed to the chair-lodgment. The mobile version of the EXZAR exoskeleton was attached to a special jacket placed on the patient's body. Exoskeleton EXZAR is a proprietary product (Vorobyov & Andryuschenko 2017). It was aimed at people with flaccid upper limb symptom of (mono)paresis of extremities. It is a mobile system of supporting connections, which is set to the child's active joints and muscles and forms a passive exoskeleton. The limb movement is rquires little force. The lost strength of muscles and the volume of movements are compensated by the system of levers and the simplest elastic elements. Our construction allows for motion with limited amplitude in three dimensions.

The main part of our research was carried out on a mobile version of the exoskeleton. We can formulate the advantages of our investigation in a few words: the child could move freely during the study, actively use the device and compensate for all the lost functions. We have taken into account the possibility of maximally full reproduction of normal movements of the upper limb in the design of the device and construction of its hinges. Understandably, we cannot achieve the complete replacement of all the movements. (Table 11.1).

We can conclude from this table that the amplitude of movements allows the patient to fully fill in the lost functions, in spite of some deficit of the movements, which was demonstrated in the EXZAR apparatus.

Tests of the device were carried out in accordance with the bioethical norms in 21 patients with a syndrome of flaccid upper limb (mono)paresis caused by various diseases, their age ranging from

Table 11.2. The distribution of patients by weight, age, sex, cause of disease and version of exoskeleton used.

Disease resulting in flaccid upper limb (mono)paresis	Age	Sex	Weight	Approved version of the device
Arthrogryposis	5	Female	17	Mobile version
Traumatic rupture of the brachial plexus	21	Male	64	Mobile version
Ischemic stroke in the right hemisphere in the form of left-sided hemiparesis with a low muscular tone	72	Female	79	Mobile version
Mucolipidosis, type 3. Flaccid upper limb (mono)paresis.	12	Female	17	Mobile version
Mucolipidosis, type 3. Flaccid upper limb (mono)paresis.	10	Female	18	Mobile version
Generalised myopathy: proptosis, bulbar disorders, flaccid tetraparesis with predominance on the left.	25	Female	49	Mobile version
Progressive muscular dystrophy, Erba-Landusi-Dezherina syndrome	29	Female	51	Stationary version 2
Arthrogryposis with a lesion of upper and lower extremities. Condition after surgical treatment.	6	Female	17	Mobile version
Dushen's muscular dystrophy	23	Male	104	Fixed version 1
Becker's progressing muscular dystrophy	21	Male	53	Fixed version 2
Motor neuron disease	61	Male	82	Mobile version
Motor neuron disease	67	Male	96	Mobile version
Arthrogryposis (generalised form)	10	Female	42	Fixed version 2
Personone-Turner syndrome on the right (neurologic amyotrophy, idiopathic shoulder plexopathy of the upper fascicles)	10	Male	37	Mobile version
Arthrogryposis (generalised form)	7	Male	19	Mobile version
Cerebral palsy, right-sided hemiparesis, condition after botulinum therapy	7	Male	23	Mobile version
Duchenne-Erba Paralysis	33	Male	77	Mobile version
Duchenne-Erba Paralysis	7	Male	23	Mobile version
Duchenne-Erba Paralysis	9	Female	37	Mobile version
Duchenne myodystrophy	17	Male	54	Fixed version 2
Werdnig-Hoffmann spinal amyotrophy of the second type	3,5	Male	15	Fixed version 2

3.5 to 72 years. The experimental protocol was coordinated with the regional independent ethical committee (PI Volgograd Medical Scientific Centre. The registration number is 1KB 00005839 SKO 0004900 (OCB) The distribution of patients by weight, age, sex, cause of disease and the use of different versions of the exoskeleton are presented in Table 11.2.

The criteria for patient exclusion from the study and contraindications for using the device were:

1. Age under 3 years.
2. Children with mental retardation.
3. Adults with severe cognitive impairment.
4. Patients with spastic hypertension of the muscles of the upper limbs.
5. Patients with contractures in large joints of the upper limbs.
6. Oncological diseases in the inoculated stage.

The effectiveness of using the EXZAR exoskeleton was determined by comparing the amplitude of the active movements of the upper limbs without the apparatus (the initial level taken by us for control) and immediately after putting the exoskeleton on the patient's body (comparison group). The technique for using the EXZAR exoskeleton for the upper limbs was experimental. Thus, the duration of sessions was determined individually according to the principle of subjective detection of the minimum load and its constant increase, taking into account the individual portability under the control of physical therapy doctors.

We had some safety criteria for approving our device:

- lack of electric drives;
- restriction of freedom of movement within the physiological norm of movements;
- absence of sharp angles and cutting edges in the design;
- absence of additional load on the joints;
- implementation of structural details that contact the body of the patient from materials approved for medical use in the Russian Federation.

11.3 RESULTS

The initial attempts to fit the device empirically were unsuccessful. It was not possible to achieve stable construction for a long period of time. Therefore, the necessity for the implementation of anatomical parameterisation arose.

Basically, the problems consisted in the lack of the opportunities to fill in the lost functions totally, the inadequate use of the technical capabilities of the device, and in the breakdown of concrete elements of the construction, which was associated with uneven distribution of the forces. Certain inconveniences and an insignificant risk of a trauma were due to the contact of the mobile parts of the exoskeleton and the skin of the patient. Scuffs and maceration of the skin were often formed in these places after prolonged use.

When the patient was placed in a wheelchair, it was impossible for us to exclude the displacement of the patient's body relative to the EXZAR exoskeleton fixed on the details of the chair. An optimal relationship between the patient and the anatomically dependent parts of the exoskeleton was violated when the patient's body moved, slipped, turned, tilted forward (Figure 11.1). Therefore, it was possible to achieve optimal design performance only for a short period, which served as the reason for abandoning the stationary version No. 1 of the device, and the stationary version 2, fixed on the lodgement chair (Figure 11.2), or the mobile version of the EXZAR exoskeleton (Figure 11.3).

The armchair lodgment in stationary version 2 and the carrying jacket in the mobile version of the EXZAR exoskeleton carry some additional functions apart from its basic functions: they carry out correction and prevention of curvature of the spine, which necessarily accompanies the myopathy. We produced them from the high-temperature plastics made on matrices taken from a form of a concrete patient. This approach allowed us to provide a tight and comfortable fixation of the patient in a chair-lodgment or a carrying jacket. That is how we achieved the anatomical parameterisation.

We have developed a step-by-step method of the anatomical parameterisation of the apparatus.

Stage 1. Determination of the anatomical attachment points on the patient (T).
Stage 2. Determination of the linear anatomical dimensions, useful for further design calculation (a).
Stage 3. Determination of anatomically dependent parameters of the apparatus which affect the ability of the device to replace the lost functions of the upper limb. (R)
Stage 4. Determination of the optimal constructive relationships which are necessary for the normal work of the device in replacing the lost functions of the upper limb.

We identified 7 points of an anatomical anchorage to implement the first stage of the study. We used the skeletotopic landmarks for their choice, because they are the most constant and may be easily determined by palpation. (Table 11.3). We recommended marking all points with a flushable marker for the convenience of measurements during the implementation of the second stage.

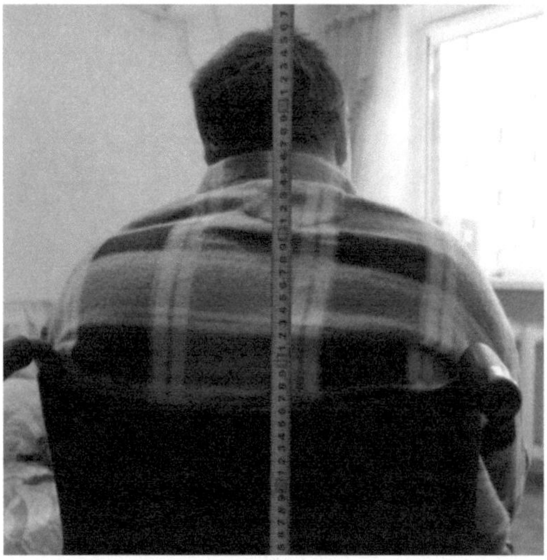

Figure 11.1. It is impossible to achieve an ideal anatomical parameterisation in fixing the wings of the EXZAR exoskeleton to the handles of a wheelchair (stationary version 1).

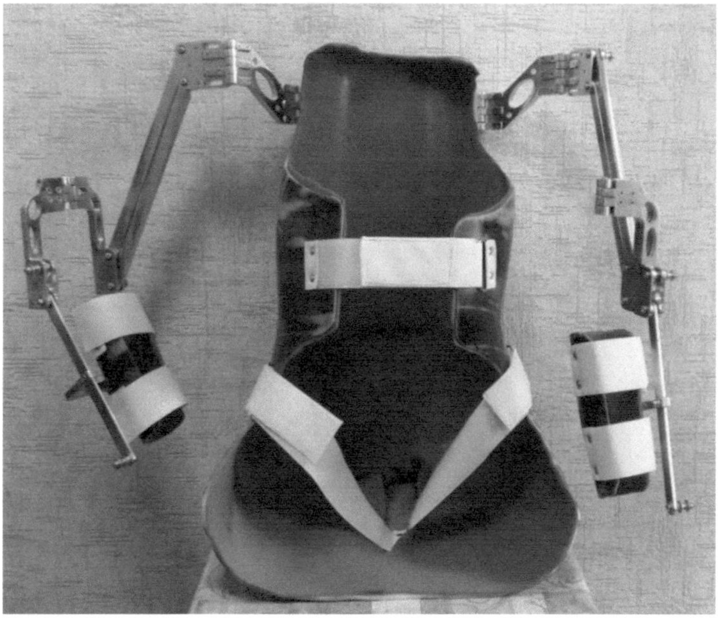

Figure 11.2. Stationary version 2 fixed on the lodgment seat, which allowed us to achieve the necessary anatomical parameterisation.

It was possible to proceed with the second stage after identifying the points. We determined the linear anatomical dimensions which were useful for further design calculation. We proposed 8 parameters for this stage. (Table 11.4).

We proposed to isolate 6 anatomically dependent parameters (P 1-6) of the EXZAR apparatus (Figures 11.4, 11.5) for the implementation of stage 3. These parameters determine the ability of the device to replenish the lost functions of the upper limb and allow the adaptation of this apparatus to

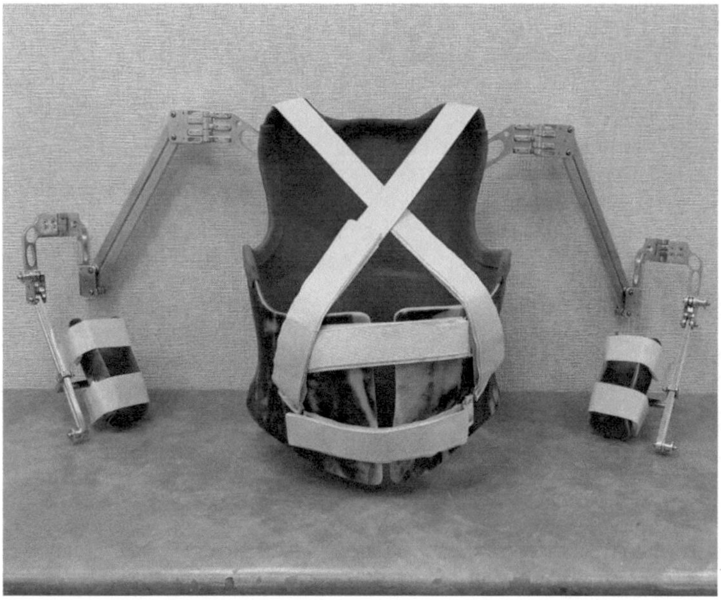

Figure 11.3. Mobile version of the EXZAR exoskeleton fixed on a special armchair-vest. We can achieve the necessary anatomical parameterisation also in this case.

Table 11.3. The points of anatomic attachment of the EXZAR exoskeleton on the patient.

Name of the point	Anatomical landmark
T1	The acute process of protruding vertebrae (C VII) – processus spinosus vertebra prominens (C VII)
T2	Acromion angle – Angulus akromii
T3	Large tuberculum of humerus – tuberculum majus os humerus
T4	Lateral epicondylitis – epicondylus lateralis
T5	Elbow process – olecranon
T6	The styloid process of the radius – processus stiloideus radii
T7	Medial epicondylitis – epicondylus medialis

Table 11.4. Anatomical parameters for calculating of the exoskeleton EXZAR.

Name of anatomical parameter	Method for determining the anatomical parameter
a1	Distance between T1-T2 (cm)
a2	Distance between T3-T4 (cm)
a3	Distance between T5-T6 (cm)
a4	Distance between T2-T3 (cm)
a5	Height of the perpendicular constructed from the middle of the line between T4-T7 to T5 in process of bending the elbow joint at an angle of 90°
a6	Length of the circumference of the forearm when it is determined through points T4-T7
a7	Horizontal plane drawn through T1
a8	Sagittal plane through median-clavicular line

Table 11.5. Anatomically dependent parameters of the EXZAR exoskeleton.

Option	Description
p1	Distance between the centreline of attachment to the supporting corset and the inner wing rotation axis
p2	Distance between the inner and outer axes of the wing rotation
p3	Distance between the axes of rotation of the upper (lower) shoulder strap
p4	Distance between the axis of rotation of the forearm flap and the hooking axis for the installation of elastic elements of the forearm located at the other end of the forearm flap
p5	Length of the support langettes
p6	Distance between the axis of rotation of the forearm flap and the plane passing through the lower part of the fastening of the axis of rotation of the elbow joint

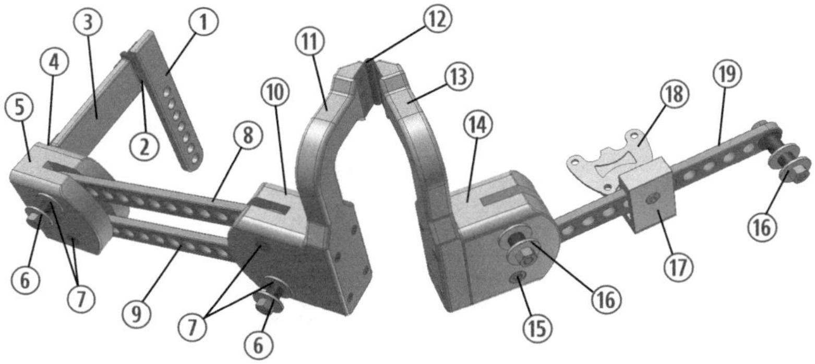

Figure 11.4. Construction scheme of the EXZAR exoskeleton for the upper extremity. The scheme does not list features protected by KNOW-HOW. 1. Bracing to the carrying jacket. 2. Inner axis of wing rotation. 3. Wing of the exoskeleton. 4. Outer axis of wing rotation. 5. Movable shoulder connected to the wing. 6. Hooks for installing the elastic elements of the shoulder. 7. Axes turning the upper (lower) shoulder straps. 8. Upper shoulder strap. 9. Lower shoulder strap. 10. Shoulder bearing element, rigidly connected to the elbow joint. 11. Shoulder segment of the elbow joint. 12. Axis of rotation of the elbow joint. 13. Forearm segment of the elbow joint. 14. Forearm support element, rigidly connected with the elbow joint. 15. Axis turning the brace of a forearm. 16. Hooks for installing the elastic elements of the forearm. 17. Slider of the supporting langet. 18. Attachment of the supporting langet. 19. Strap of the forearm.

a specific person. (Table 11.5). The other constructive elements of the EXZAR exoskeleton can be unified into the adult and child versions of the device.

Then we implemented the 4th stage of the study. We determined the optimal relationships between the allocated sizes of the upper limb and the construction of the EXZAR exoskeleton which are necessary for its effective work to replace the lost functions.

1. P1 must correspond to the point of intersection of a7 and a8. Especial attention must be paid to the exact observance of this parameter for orthoses patients with monoparesis.
2. P2 = a1 + 3 cm in children, P2 = a1 + 5 cm in adults. Deviation from these dimensions may be about 1 cm. With a further decrease in P2, we cannott rule out the possibility of contact and friction of the mobile parts of the exoskeleton with the clothing or the skin of the patient. The EXZAR exoskeleton may be disrupted in the horizontal plane with an increase in size.
3. P3 = a2 + 2 cm in children, P3 = a2 + 3 cm in adults. Deviation from these dimensions may be about 1 cm. The elbow of the exoskeleton will touch the skin of the patient's forearm with a further decrease in P3. There may be a violation of flexion in the elbow joint with an increase in size.
4. P4 = a3 + 2 cm. The apparatus does not work at full strength, limiting the raising of the arm with a decrease in P4 by more than two centimetres. With an increase in size, it is possible to contact the

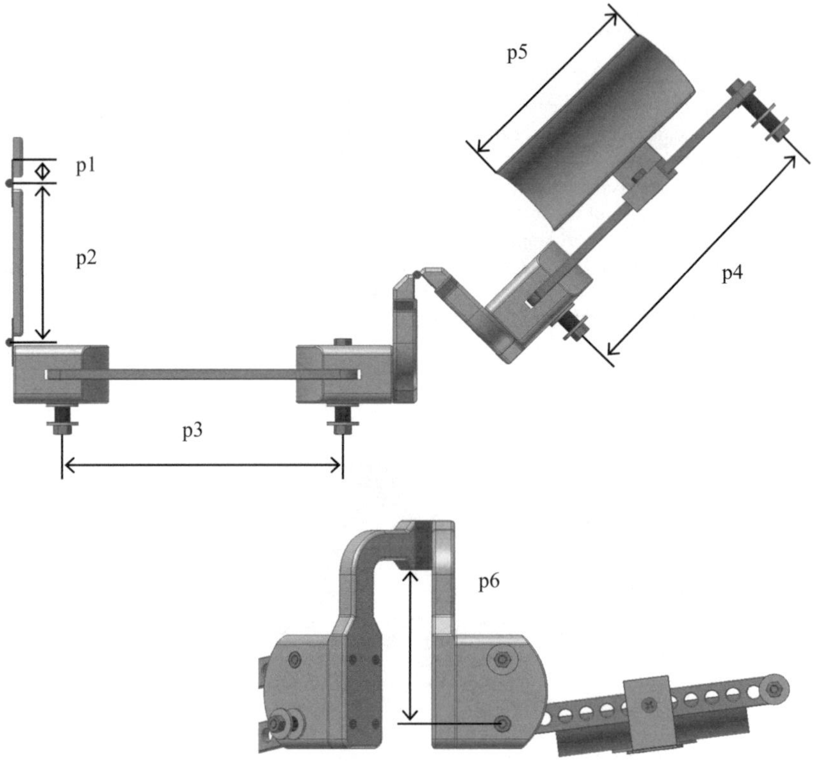

Figure 11.5. Scheme of the anatomically conditioned parameters of the EXZAR exoskeleton.

skin of the outer surface of the brush with the parts of the EXZAR exoskeleton and limit lateral movements in the wrist joint.

5. P5 = 2 a3 + 1 cm. Longure of forearm is made individually from low-temperature self-curing plastics such as "Polyvik" or "Turbocast".
6. P6 = a6/2. With a decrease in P6, it is impossible to raise the upper limb to the planned 155 degrees. With an increase in P6, the weight and dimensions of the structure increase. In this case, the axis of the elbow joint (12) should correspond to the axis between T6 and T7, which is achieved by a certain arrangement of the forearm in the longus.

With the correct implementation of the anatomical parameterisation, we achieved the following effects, to be described further:

1. the effect of increasing the amplitude of movements,
2. the effect of habilitation,
3. the effect of increasing muscle strength,
4. the effect of rehabilitation,
5. the effect of preventing posture disorder.

The effect of increasing the amplitude of movements in the shoulder and elbow joints is the key in the operation of the apparatus. We found that in all cases there is a significant increase in the amplitude of movements in the elbow and shoulder joints when using the EXZAR exoskeleton. To a certain extent, the working amplitude of the possible movements in EXZAR in the absence of contractures is determined before putting on the apparatus by detecting the difference between the residual active and passive movements of the upper limb. It is possible to fully calculate the increase in the amplitude

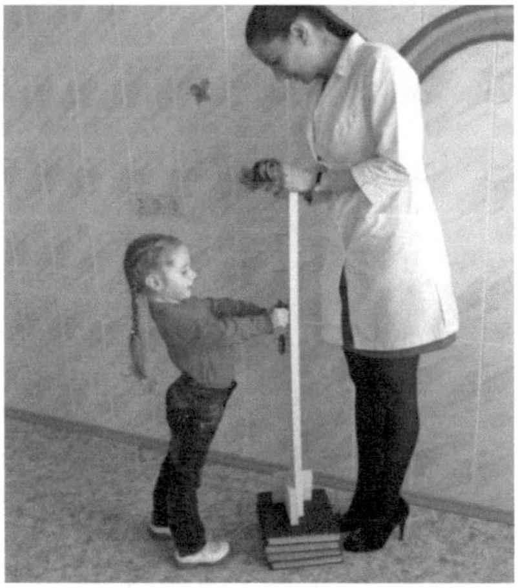

Figure 11.6. An initial level of amplitude of movements of the upper extremities in a patient with arthrogryposis.

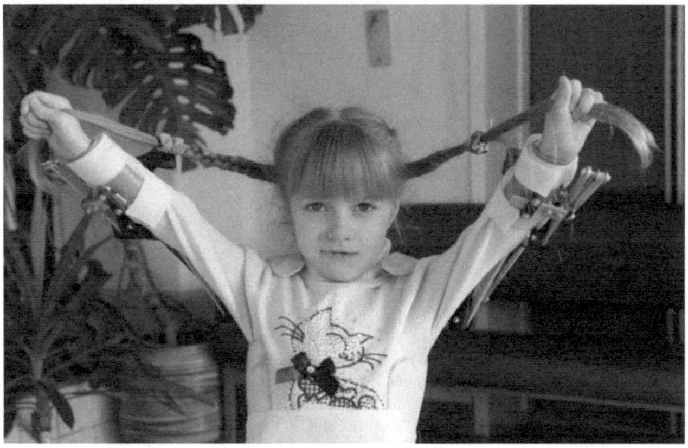

Figure 11.7. The increase in the amplitude of movements in a patient with arthrogryposis immediately after the correctly performed anatomical parametrisation of the EXZAR passive exoskeleton.

of the movements of the limb(s) to the amplitude of the movements of the passive exoskeleton in the absence of muscle and joint stiffness (Figures 11.6 and 11.7) (Figures 11.8 and 11.9).

The effect of increasing muscle strength. It is achieved with the use of elastic elements of the construction, helping to overcome the force of gravity. Thus, if the patients could not raise their hands even to the height of the upper shoulder girdle without using the device, then in the exoskeleton they had an opportunity to lift not only their hands but also the loads in them (Figures 11.10 and 11.11).

The effect of rehabilitation has not yet been adequately studied and is still the subject of our prospective study. We need to select a sufficient period of observation (2 years or more) for a full response to it and to take into account the characteristics of the course of the disease that led to paresis of the upper limbs. At the same time, a long period of observation of a patient with arthrogryposis (patient No. 1 in Table No. 1) inspired some optimism. The dynamics of the amplitude of movements of the upper limb of the patient under test when using the EXZAR exoskeleton is presented in Tables 11.6 and 11.7.

The effect of preventing posture disorder is bounded with the use of a supporting corset or a chair-lodgment. In addition to its basic function, this construction contributes to the correction of posture

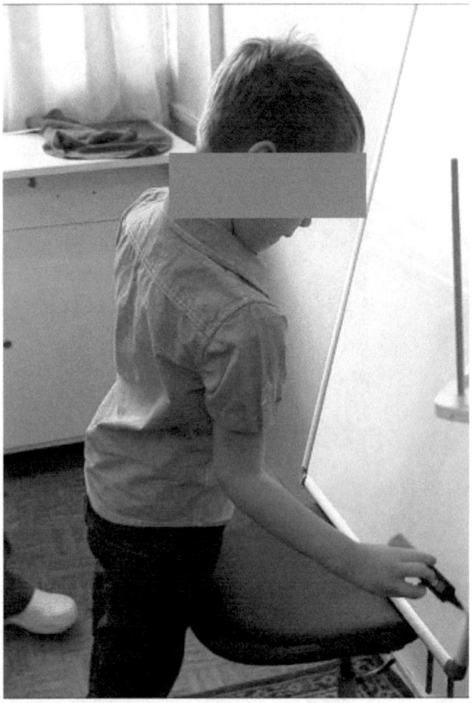

Figure 11.8. An initial level of movements of the upper limb in a patient with an upper limp monoparesis caused by the Persononeja-Turner syndrome on the right.

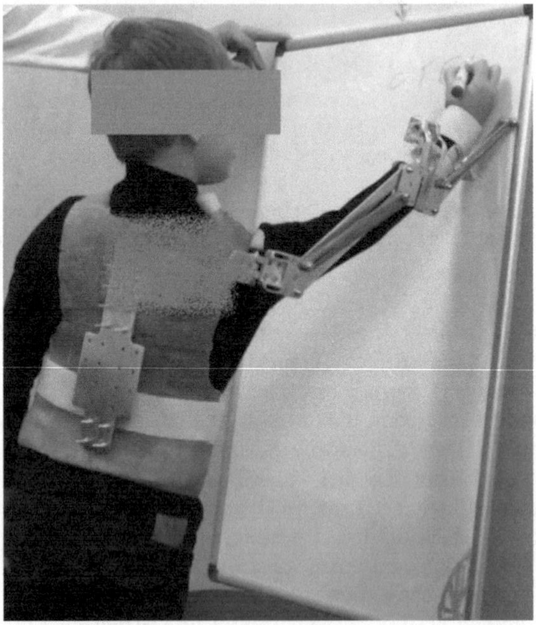

Figure 11.9. The effect of habilitation in the same patient immediately after using the EXZAR exoskeleton (shaded face and original exoskeleton node).

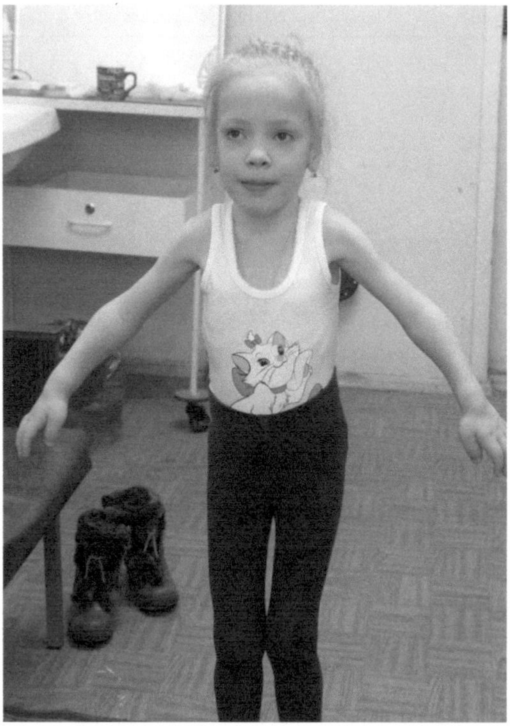

Figure 11.10. Maximum lifting of hands in a patient with mucolipidosis of type 3.

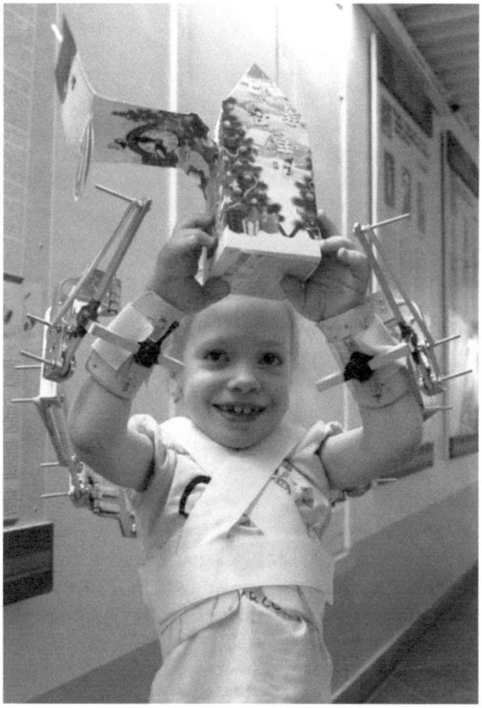

Figure 11.11. Increase in the lifting of hands holding an object to a level above the head.

Table 11.6. Amplitude of movements in the shoulder joint of the patient under test using the EXZAR exoskeleton.

Element of movements of the shoulder (straight upper limb)	Norm	Parameters of the initial state: right arm without apparatus	Parameters of the initial state: left arm without apparatus	The data after putting on the apparatus: right/left hand	Data after 12 months of using the device: right/left hand
1. Active flexion in the sagittal plane	180°	85	65	155/155	100/100
2. Passive flexion in the sagittal plane	180°	140	110	155/155	155/170
3. Active extension in the sagittal plane	40°	50	50		50/40
4. Passive extension in the sagittal plane	60° (40°)	85	75		75/70
5. Active leading off in the frontal plane	180°	85	70	155/155	105/95
6. Passive leading off in the frontal plane	180°	150	110	155/155	170/165

Table 11.7. An amplitude of movements in the elbow joint of the patient using the EXZAR exoskeleton during the test.

Element of movement in the elbow joint	Norm	Normals at the initial state, right hand	Initial state parameters, left hand	Data after putting on the apparatus, right/left arm	Data after 7 months, right/left hand
1. Active flexion	40^0	60	60	50/50	40/60
2. Passive flexion	40^0	30	30	45	30/30
3. Active extension	00^0	(0) 180	(0) 180	180	180
4. Passive extension	00^0	(0) 180	(0) 180	180	180

disorder by preventing hyperlordosis caused by the inclusion of additional back muscles in the arm lift and preventing deformity of the spinal column caused by various types of myopathy.

11.4 DISCUSSION OF THE RESULTS

In our opinion, the effect of rehabilitation is based on the mechanism of biological feedback (in English literature – biofeedback). We have proved the rationality of the treatment with the help of the biofeedback method in the activation of adaptive brain systems against the backdrop of the forming of pathological processes in the central nervous system. The flaccid paresis of the upper limbs is the core of the clinical picture of the diseases which we are researching. The main pathogenetic factor of their development is the defeat of the nervous system of various genesis leading to disruption of direct action and the feedback between its central and peripheral divisions. It is logical to include the mechanisms for their recovery in our investigation. The medical treatment of these pathologies is mainly aimed at restoring direct relations between the central nervous system and periphery. And the restoration of feedback between the peripheral and central nervous systems is a task that can be solved, mainly, with the help of physiotherapy procedures, massage, and physiotherapy exercises. From our point of view, the exoskeleton is an ideal way to restore feedback, in which an absolutely harmless effect on the classical reflexogenic receptor zones of the muscles and tendons of the upper extremities is performed. We clinically proved the effectiveness of this method in restoring the activity of reflex arcs delivering information about movements to the corresponding segments of the spinal cord. At the same time, the spinal cord activates the "silent" motor zones of the cerebral cortex along the ascending paths. We contribute to the improvement of direct CNS influence on the peripheral nervous system, self-regulation mechanisms by the restoring the biological feedback between the peripheral and central parts of the nervous system according to neurophysiological laws. Tus, we carried out the non-drug correction of the pathological structure of the nervous system, increasing the volume, speed and amplitude of movements in the upper limbs. It is also an undeniable fact that in the presence of full-fledged movements in the joints of the upper limb the likelihood of the formation of muscle and joint contractures is reduced.

11.5 CONCLUSIONS

Anatomical parameterisation of the EXZAR passive exoskeleton includes a sequential determination in 4 stages of the patient's anatomical anchor points; his/her linear anatomical dimensions necessary for further design calculation; the anatomically dependent parameters of the apparatus, influencing its ability to replace the lost functions of the upper limb; and finally the determination of the optimal design relationships, which are necessary for the normal work with replacing all lost functions.

From our point of view, it is possible to achieve the optimal possibilities for the full operation of the apparatus and the rehabilitation of the patient by using the anatomical parameterisation of the exoskeleton of the upper limb.

It is possible to achieve the following effects of using the EXZAR exoskeleton with the correct implementation of anatomical parameterisation:

- increasing the amplitude of movements in the shoulder and elbow joints,
- habilitation,
- increasing muscle strength,
- rehabilitation,
- preventing posture disorders.

REFERENCES

Budziszewski P. 2013. A low cost virtual reality system for rehabilitation of upper limb. *Virtual, Augmented and Mixed Reality. Systems and Applications*. Springer: 32–39.

Iqbal J., Khan H., Tsagarakis N.G. & Caldwell D.G. 2014 A novel exoskeleton robotic system for hand rehabilitation – Conceptualization to prototyping. *Biocybern. Biomed. Eng.* 34(2): 79–89.

Kapandji, A. I. 2014. *Upper limb. Physiology of the joints*. Moscow: Eksmo.

Rahman, T., Sample, W., Jayakumar, S., King, M. M., Wee, J. Y., Seliktar, R., Alexander M., Scavina, M. & Clark, A. 2006. *Journal of rehabilitation research and development* 43(5): 583–590.

Vorobiev, A. A., Andryushchenko, F. A., Ponomareva, O. A., Solovyova, I. O. & Krivonozhkina, P. S. 2016. Development and clinical approbation of the passive exoskeleton of the upper extremities "EXZAR". *Modern technologies in medicine* 8(2): 90–97.

Vorobiev, A. A., Petrukhin, A. V., Zasypkina O. A. & Krivonozhkina P. V. 2014. Clinical and anatomical requirements for active and passive exoskeletons of the upper extremity. *Volgograd Scientific Medical Journal* 1: 56–61.

Vorobyov A. A., Andryuschenko F. A. 2017. Patent no. 2629738 Russian Federation, IPC7 A61H 1/00, A61H Exoskeletus of upper extremities/Vorobyov A. A., Andryuschenko F. A.; applicant and patent owner. Vorobiev A. A., Andryushchenko F. A., No. 2016109511; claimed. 03/16/2016; publ. August 31, 2017, Bul. No. 25. 15.

CHAPTER 12

Application of quantum-mechanical methods in biotechnical research

Yu.P. Mukha
Volgograd State Medical University, Volgograd, Russian Federation
Volgograd State Technical University, Volgograd, Russian Federation

A.M. Steben'kov
Volgograd State Medical University, Volgograd, Russian Federation

N.A. Steben'kova
Volgograd State Technical University, Volgograd, Russian Federation

W. Wójcik & M. Chmielewska
Lublin University of Technology, Lublin, Poland

A. Kalizhanova
Institute of Information and Computational Technologies CS MES RK, Almaty, Kazakhstan
University of Power Engineering and Telecommunications, Almaty, Kazakhstan

ABSTRACT: The possibilities of an application of the quantum-mechanical methods for the development of a technology of an efficient osteo-integration were considered for bone – implantable interaction. We made an exact analysis for energy, frequency and length of the communication of the atoms forming the surface communications. We were able to assess the external influence of the high-pitched laser on a surface of a material, and take into account the metrological aspects of the process of an efficient merging of an implant and a bone tissue. Our investigated will form the base for improvement of quality of life of the patient.

12.1 INTRODUCTION

We usually understand the concept of biotechnical researches as a wide range of methods and models from various branches of modern science and technology. We look through the passport of educating of the specialists in "Biotechnical systems and technologies", and find that the graduate student has to be able to develop and project new methods and technologies. We offered a method of using the apparatus of a quantum mechanics for the solution of a big class of problems of an atomic-molecular scale. Generally supposing, we can simulate any process in an alive organism by means of the apparatus of a quantum mechanics. In our opinion, this is a very perspective direction of preclinical researches. We are capable to essentially reducing the actual number of expensive experiments. We knew common information: many scientists allow preclinical researches on average only 250 medicines from 10000 of the new medicines, and only 5 of them will be selected for performing clinical trials. We also must find an effective computer model operation to prevent some possible ghost effects, which usually arise only after the long clinical trials. Methods of quantum mechanics are well proved as the potent tool for prediction of structure and synthesis of new difficult connections. They are used in experimenters of various branches of science and techniques as a preliminary stage.

The possible spheres of the preclinical researches:

1. interaction of a medicinal preparation with a virus/bacterium;
2. choice of the most efficient way of medical intervention to an organism;

3. interaction of several medicines among themselves in the system of the complex treatment (the synergism and the antagonism);
4. transformation of the medicines under the influence of various salts and liquids before their getting into the field of the direct application;
5. interaction of the medicines with all types of body tissues (an indirect action of medicine on an organism);
6. definition of optimum dosage of medicines, and research of an effect of shortage or surplus of the medicine.

The purpose of our research is a consideration of the possibility of application of the quantum mechanical methods for the development of technology of an efficient osteointegration in a bone – implantable interaction.

Earlier at the start of the development, the main problem for every specialist in a sphere of dental implantation as a method of restitution was the improvement of the ability of engraftment of an implant during the removal or loss of teeth. Violation of an osteointegration was the most often bound to violations of the protocol of operation, care of the established implant, discrepancies of a design of an implant to the volume of bone tissue or to the chosen implantation method.

One of the main factors significantly influencing engraftment of implants is the quality of their surface, which adjoins immediately to cells of bone tissue All experiences of an application of different implants and also numerous researches confirm that deposition of an implant having high biocompatibility considerably raises the degree of their survival. Because of the contact of bone tissue with a surface of an implant is more intimately in this case. Therefore, various technologies of changing the properties of a surface by drawing coverings on implants were developed. Different coverings gave to the implants the roughness and porosity for increasing of an osteointegration.

Such surfacing of an implant is the final procedure for its production. At the moment there is no technology, which will be capable of choosing the frequency of laser radiation for surfacing of an implant for each patient. That frequency considerably influences the process of survival of bone tissue and an implant.

The reliability of this work is in the concentration on a problem of survival of implants with bone tissue. We made a lot of new conclusions despite the development of the new technologies of drawing biocompatible coverings on implants. We allowed reducing the risk of a casting-off of an implant by selection for each patient of the frequency of laser radiation for surfacing of an implant. That is the main idea of an application of our technology.

An implant is covered with special dusting, which possesses high biocompatibility with bone tissue of a person. This dusting will make an implant better accustomed. We know that the structure of a bone is various for every person.

So, the covering must correspond to the structure of bone tissue of the person. To satisfy that condition, it is necessary to put a covering by using the laser with a particular impact frequency for surfacing of an implant. That is why we decided to develop a computer technology for simulating of an implant covering, which would consist of the necessary components, and to investigate the possibility of choice of the frequency of laser radiation for surfacing of an implant for each patient. Our main goal was to promote high biocompatibility of bone tissue and an implant and to reduce the risk of its casting-off.

The complexity of this development is caused by a synthesis of the various scientific directions, such as technique, medicine, chemistry, and physics. However, we carry it to the category of the biotechnical systems because of this complexity.

12.2 CREATION OF THE MODEL

The researcher usually solves the following problems in the process of creation of a model for quantum chemical analysis:

1. As a rule, the atomic-molecular structure of the investigated objects (viruses, DNA, different types of fabrics, new medicinal preparations) is insufficiently precisely known;

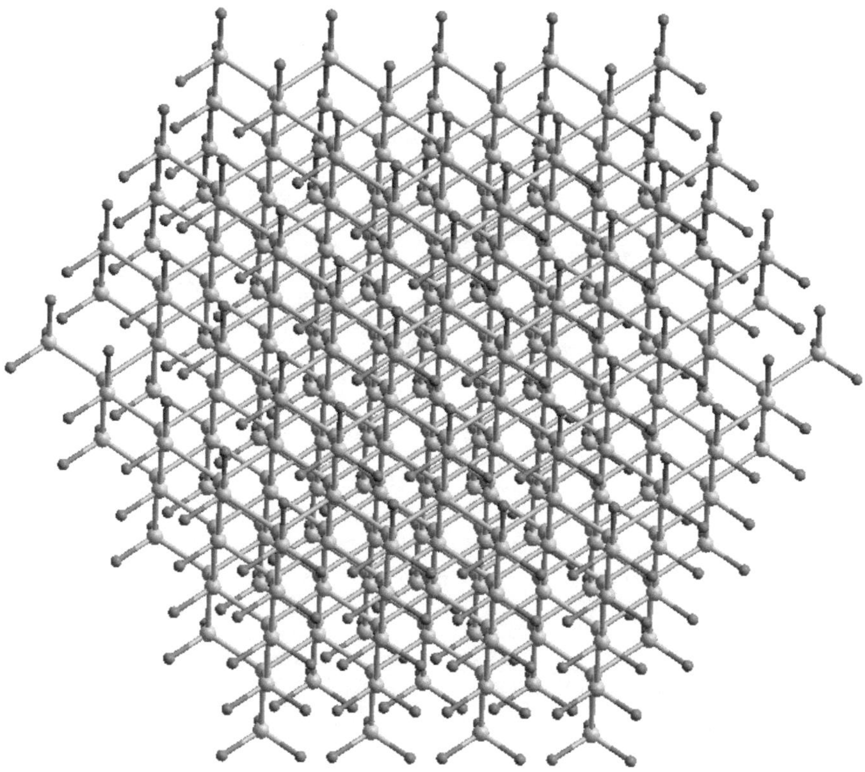

Figure 12.1. Molecular model of a tetrahedral crystal.

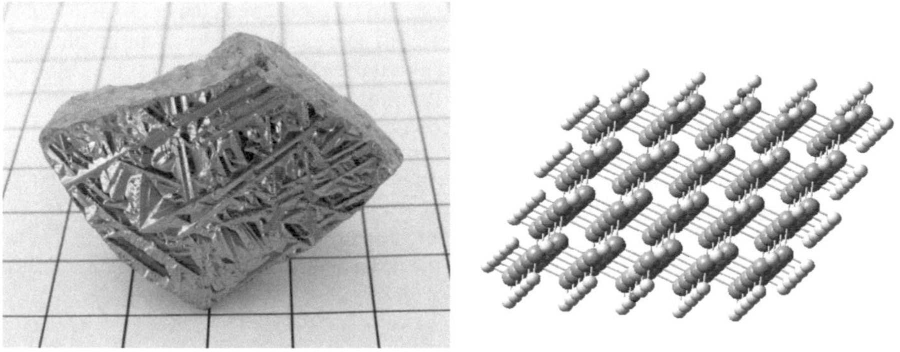

Figure 12.2. Crystal of silicon and its molecular model.

2. The second problem is in case of the possibility of simulation of the completely studied object: the model will contain a large number of atoms, so it will be difficult for us to calculate and find a computer inventory for this object at this stage of the development of a technology (Figure 12.1), the more atoms contain in the model, the especially simpler methods of a quantum mechanics have to be used.

Therefore we use several simplifications in the practice of creation of the model:

1. We use characteristically or surface structures, which will influence on adsorption processes. We will take a crystal of silicon and its model as an example (Figure 12.2).

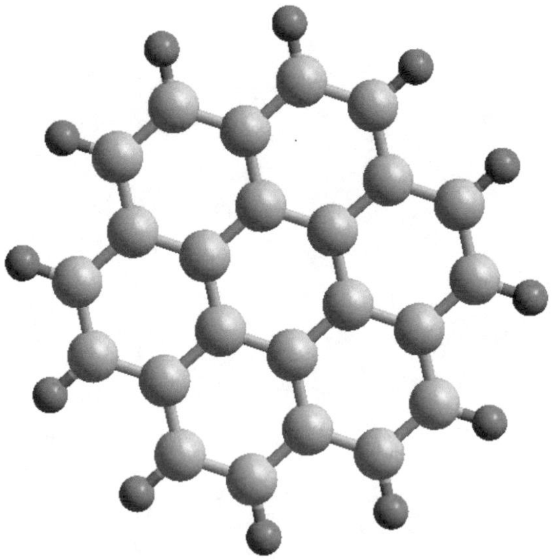

Figure 12.3. Molecular model of graphene with boundary atoms of hydrogen.

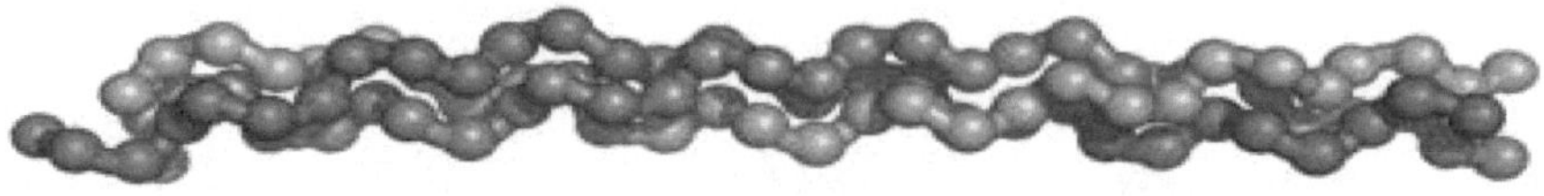

Figure 12.4. Molecular model of collagen.

2. We replace all other atoms with the pseudo-atoms. It is convenient to choose hydrogen atoms in the role of the pseudo-atoms. As an example, we will consider the model of the graphene consisting of 7 cells of hexogen. It will be quite enough as a model for researching a simple atom in the centre of hexogen. Other cells are replaced with atoms of hydrogen (Figure 12.3).
3. We use the models with cyclic boundary conditions.

For example, collagen is a part of bone tissue. It is fibrillary protein, which molecular mass is about 300 kDa (kilo Dalton), the length is 300 nanometers, the thickness is 1,5 nanometers. We analysed that it is very problematic to create a molecular structure on a base of such protein. Therefore, it was possible to consider as a first approximation the groups of several dozens of atoms, which repeat the infinite number of times (Figure 12.4).

12.3 THE QUANTUM AND CHEMICAL RESEARCH TECHNIQUES

12.3.1 *The restricted method of Hartree-Fock-Roothan*

We carried out a calculation of electronic and power characteristics of the cluster (quasimolecular) models by various semiempirical and not empirical methods. For example, we got good results with the calculated scheme based on the Hartree-Fock-Rootan method (Stepanov 2001, Minkin 1997, Hehre et al. 1986) – the procedure at the core of which the isentropic approximation and one-electron approach are applied to the multielectronic system.

Let us look at a molecule with N cores and n electrons. The Hamiltonian contains the terms of the kinetic energy of electrons, the potential energy of an attraction of the electrons to the cores, the terms for the causation of an interelectronic repulsion, and also the term of electrostatic repulsion of the kernels and their kinetic energy:

$$\hat{\mathrm{H}} = -\frac{\hbar^2}{2}\sum_{\alpha=1}^{N}\frac{1}{M_\alpha}\nabla_\alpha^2 - \frac{\hbar^2}{2m_e}\sum_{i=1}^{n}\nabla_i^2 + \sum_{\beta}^{N}\sum_{>\alpha}^{N}\frac{Z_\alpha Z_\beta e^2}{R_{\alpha\beta}} - \sum_{\alpha}^{N}\sum_{i}^{n}\frac{Z_\alpha e^2}{R_{i\alpha}} + \sum_{i}^{n}\sum_{>j}^{n}\frac{e^2}{r_{ij}}, \quad (12.1)$$

where indexes α and β belong to the atomic cores, and indexes i and j are for the electrons, and concrete designations are injected: $R_{\alpha\beta} = \left|\mathbf{R}_\alpha - \mathbf{R}_\beta\right|$, $R_{i\alpha} = |\mathbf{r}_i - \mathbf{R}_\alpha|$ and $r_{ij} = \left|\mathbf{r}_i - \mathbf{r}_j\right|$.

Apparently from (12.1), the Hamiltonian of a molecule depends on the coordinates of the electrons and the kernels. Therefore, the complete wave function of the system has to contain both electronic, and nuclear coordinates: $\Psi(r, R)$.

The nuclear mass considerably exceeds the electronic mass. Respectively, the travelling speed of the kernels is smaller in comparison with the travelling speed of electrons. As a result, sluggishly moving cores form an electric field, in which the electrons move with much larger speed. Therefore, it is possible to consider that the atomic nuclei are fixed, and only electrons are moving. Therefore, we represented the complete wave function of a molecule $\Psi(r, R)$ in the form of multiplication of the electronic $\Psi_E(r, R)$ and the nuclear $\Psi_N(R)$ function:

$$\Psi(r, R) = \Psi_E(r, R)\Psi_N(R). \quad (12.2)$$

The Schrodinger's equation for a molecule with a Hamiltonian (12.1) and a wave function (12.2) converted into a form:

$$\left(-\frac{\hbar^2}{2}\sum_{\alpha=1}^{N}\frac{1}{M_\alpha}\nabla_\alpha^2 - \frac{\hbar^2}{2m_e}\sum_{i=1}^{n}\nabla_i^2 + V_{NN} + V_{NE} + V_{EE}\right) \times \Psi_E(r, R)\Psi_N(R) = E\Psi_E(r, R)\Psi_N(R) \quad (12.3)$$

where V_{NN} is the energy of repulsion of the nuclear, V_{NE} is the energy of an attraction of the electrons to the nuclear, V_{EE} – the energy of repulsion of the electrons.

We used such designations:

$$\hat{H}_E = -\frac{\hbar^2}{2m_e}\sum_{i=1}^{n}\nabla_i^2 + V_{NN} + V_{NE} + V_{EE}, \quad (12.4)$$

$$\hat{H}_E = -\frac{\hbar^2}{2}\sum_{\alpha=1}^{N}\frac{1}{M_\alpha}\nabla_\alpha^2, \quad (12.5)$$

and then got an equation (12.3) in a form of:

$$\left(\hat{H}_N + \hat{H}_E\right)\Psi_E(r, R)\Psi_N(R) = E\Psi_E(r, R)\Psi_N(R). \quad (12.6)$$

We developed then an idea of a method of the molecular orbitals (MO), in which the complete wave function of a molecule may be constructed from the functions describing the behavior of separate electrons in the field created by other electrons, and all atomic cores, which form a molecular basis.

We can represent the method of MO by a single-electron function (i.e. depending obviously on coordinates of only one electron), which includes space and spin components – a spin-orbital:

$$\varphi(\mathbf{r}_1, \sigma_1) = \varphi(\mathbf{r}_1)\chi(\sigma_1) \quad (12.7)$$

All electrons of a molecule settle down pairwise (two spins on MO, $\chi_1(+1) = \alpha(1)$ and $\chi_1(-1) = \beta(1)$, are for one space function). They fill in a molecule as their energy increases.

For the molecule containing $2n$ electrons on n pairwise of the filled MO, the complete wave function is described by a Slater's determinant:

$$\Psi = [(2n)!]^{-1/2}\begin{vmatrix} \varphi_1(\mathbf{r}_1)\alpha(1)\varphi_1(\mathbf{r}_2)\alpha(2)...\varphi_1(\mathbf{r}_{2n})\alpha(2n) \\ \varphi_1(\mathbf{r}_1)\beta(1)\varphi_1(\mathbf{r}_2)\beta(2)...\varphi_1(\mathbf{r}_{2n})\beta(2n) \\ \cdots\cdots\cdots\cdots\cdots\cdots\cdots\cdots\cdots\cdots \\ \varphi_n(\mathbf{r}_1)\beta(1)\varphi_n(\mathbf{r}_2)\beta(2)...\varphi_n(\mathbf{r}_{2n})\beta(2n) \end{vmatrix}. \quad (12.8)$$

Expression (12.8) considers the requirement of antisymmetry of a wave function in relation to the shift of any couple of the electrons.

The total energy of a molecule with a wave function (12.8) is determined by a ratio $E = \left\langle \Psi | \hat{H} | \Psi \right\rangle$, where the Hamiltonian undertakes in an approximation (12.4) and can be written down as

$$E = 2\sum_{i=1}^{n} \varepsilon_i - \sum_{i=1}^{n}\sum_{j=1}^{n}(2J_{ij} - K_{ij}) + \sum_{\alpha}^{N}{}_{>}\sum_{\beta}^{N}\frac{Z_\alpha Z_\beta e^2}{R_{\alpha\beta}}, \quad (12.9)$$

where ε_i is the energy of MO, $J_{ij} = e^2 \iint \Psi_i^2(i) r_{ij}^{-1} \Psi_j^2 d\tau_i d\tau_j$ – Coulomb' integral (represents average energy of a coulomb repulsion of the electrons on orbitals Ψ_i and Ψ_j), and $K_{ij} = \iint \Psi_i^*(1)\Psi_j^* \frac{e^2}{r_{12}} \Psi_i(2)\Psi_j(2) d\tau_1 d\tau_2$ – exchange integral.

Thus, a primal problem of the MO-method is finding of the MO space functions φ_i, on the basis of which expression (12.9) is formed.

One of the best approximations which can be applied to the creation of MO is a representation of MO in the form of the linear combination of atomic orbitals (MO LCAO). In this approximation we register each MO φ_i in the form of the linear combination of the atomic orbitals (AO) χ_ν of the atoms forming a molecule:

$$\varphi_i = \sum_{\nu=1}^{N} c_{i\nu}\chi_\nu. \quad (12.10)$$

The index ν is for numbers of the atomic orbitals (AO) of all atoms in the system. The set of all χ_ν represents a basic set of atomic orbitals. We use the variation principle for minimization of the total energy of the multielectronic system (12.9) with the equations:

$$\sum_{\nu=1}^{N} c_{i\nu}\left(F_{\mu\nu} - \varepsilon_i S_{\mu\nu}\right) = 0; \quad \mu = 1, 2, \ldots, N, \quad (12.11)$$

where matrix elements are:

$$F_{\mu\nu} = H_{\mu\nu} + \sum_{j}^{\text{occupied}}\sum_{\lambda}\sum_{\sigma} c_{j\lambda}c_{j\sigma}[2(\mu\nu|\lambda\sigma) - (\mu\lambda|\nu\sigma)]; \quad (12.12)$$

$$S_{\mu\nu} = \int \chi_\mu(1)\chi_\nu(1)d\tau_1; \quad (12.13)$$

$$H_{\mu\nu} = \int \chi_\mu(1)\left[-\frac{\hbar^2}{2m_e}\nabla_1^2 - \sum_{\alpha=1}^{N}\frac{Z_\alpha e^2}{r_{1\alpha}}\right]\chi_\nu(1)d\tau_1; \quad (12.14)$$

$$(\mu\nu|\lambda\sigma) = \iint \chi_\mu(1)\chi_\nu(1)r_{12}^{-1}\chi_\lambda(2)\chi_\sigma(2)d\tau_1 d\tau_2. \quad (12.15)$$

Summarizing in (12.12) is conducted only on not empty MO. The matrix $S_{\mu\nu}$ is called a matrix of the integrals of an overlap of the AO, χ_μ and χ_ν. $(\mu\nu|\lambda\sigma)$ – are integrals of an interelectronic interaction. The equations (12.11) are called by the name of the American physicist S.S.J. Roothan. He received them for the first time.

Roothan's equations (12.11) are non-linear homogeneous equations with the unknown quantities $c_{j\lambda}$. We used such designation:

$$P_{\lambda\sigma} = 2\sum_{j=1}^{occup} c_{j\lambda}c_{j\sigma}, \tag{12.16}$$

where the summarizing is conducted on all occupied electrons on MO. $P_{\lambda\sigma}$ is a matrix of the orders of the relations between the AO, χ_λ and χ_σ. Then we found an expression (12.12) in a form of:

$$F_{\mu\nu} = H_{\mu\nu} + \sum_{\lambda}\sum_{\sigma} P_{\lambda\sigma}\left[(\mu\nu|\lambda\sigma) - \frac{1}{2}(\mu\lambda|\nu\sigma)\right]. \tag{12.17}$$

The total electronic energy may be defined by an expression:

$$E_{el} = \frac{1}{2}\sum_{\mu}\sum_{\nu} P_{\mu\nu}\left(H_{\mu\nu} + F_{\mu\nu}\right). \tag{12.18}$$

We described the calculation scheme for the closed electronic shell, in which *n*/2 lower on the energy of MO is filled on two electrons (with opposite directional spins) on each MO. This scheme was called the restricted (by spin) method of Hartree-Fock-Roothan.

12.3.2 *The unlimited method of Hartree-Fock-Roothan*

The equations of a restricted method of Hartree-Fock-Rootan cannot be applicable for multielectronic systems, in which a complete spin is other than zero. We assumed that the *m* of MO is filled with two electrons and the *n* of MO are filled with one electron in the system. According to the Hund's rule, the wave function of a ground state has to have the maximal multiplicity and, therefore, we can write it down in the form of a Slater's determinant:

$$^{n+1}\Psi_{res} = |\varphi_1\bar{\varphi}_1\varphi_2\bar{\varphi}_2 \ldots \varphi_m\bar{\varphi}_m\varphi_{m+1}\varphi_{m+2} \ldots \varphi_{m+n}|, \tag{12.19}$$

The multiplicity of this function is equal to $n+1$, that is the number of electrons with a spin wave function α are one *n* more than the number of electrons with a spin-wave function β.

The wave functions of this kind, which are written down in the form of one Slater's determinant (12.19), possess an essential shortcoming: the coupled electrons with the different spin-wave functions α and β are also described by the same space part of a spin-orbital (one MO). But the number of the α-electrons in our case is more than the number β-electrons. Therefore, the electrons with α-spin in twice filled MO will suffer a larger repulsion from not coupled α-electrons than the electrons with β-spin in twice filled MO. This effect has to be reflected by the particular differences in the space functions for α- and β-electrons in the filled MO. If we set the same space part for α- and β-electrons, then we do not impose quite a reasonable restriction for a wave function, and consequently on the spatial distribution of the electrons. To lift that noted limit, it was necessary for us to set for α- and β-electrons the various forms of space functions $\varphi_1^\alpha, \varphi_2^\alpha, \ldots, \varphi_{m+n}^\alpha$ and $\varphi_1^\beta, \varphi_2^\beta, \ldots, \varphi_m^\beta$, where $\varphi_1^\alpha \neq \varphi_1^\beta; \varphi_2^\alpha \neq \varphi_2^\beta$ etc. Then we got the complete wave function of the considered system in a form:

$$\begin{aligned} ^{n+1}\Psi_{un\,\lim} &= \left|\varphi_1^\alpha\alpha\varphi_1^\beta\beta\varphi_2^\alpha\alpha\varphi_2^\beta\beta \ldots \varphi_m^\alpha\alpha\varphi_m^\beta\beta\varphi_{m+1}^\alpha\alpha\varphi_{m+2}^\alpha\alpha \ldots \varphi_{m+n}^\alpha\alpha\right| \\ &= \left|\varphi_1^\alpha\bar{\varphi}_1^\beta\varphi_2^\alpha\bar{\varphi}_2^\beta \ldots \varphi_m^\alpha\bar{\varphi}_m^\beta\varphi_{m+1}^\alpha\varphi_{m+2}^\alpha \ldots \varphi_{m+n}^\alpha\right| \end{aligned} \tag{12.20}$$

The wave function $^{n+1}\Psi_{\lim}$ is a special case of the function $^{n+1}\Psi_{un\,\lim}$. As appears from the variation theorem, the use of the function $^{n+1}\Psi_{un\,\lim}$ has to lead to a decrease in the total energy of the system. We can prove it in the equation:

$$E = \left\langle ^{n+1}\Psi_{un\,\lim}|\mathrm{H}|^{n+1}\Psi_{un\,\lim}\right\rangle \leq \left\langle ^{n+1}\Psi_{\lim}|\mathrm{H}|^{n+1}\Psi_{\lim}\right\rangle. \tag{12.21}$$

Thus, the function ${}^{n+1}\Psi_{un\,\mathrm{lim}}$ is more precise wave function, than ${}^{n+1}\Psi_{\mathrm{lim}}$. The method based on using of $\Psi_{un\,\mathrm{lim}}$ was called an unlimited method of Hartree-Fock-Roothaan. The equations of Hartree-Fock-Rootan for open envelopes are:

$$\sum_{\nu=1}^{N} c_{i\nu}^{\alpha}\left(F_{\mu\nu}^{\alpha} - \varepsilon_i^{\alpha} S_{\mu\nu}\right) = 0; \quad \sum_{\nu=1}^{N} c_{i\nu}^{\beta}\left(F_{\mu\nu}^{\beta} - \varepsilon_i^{\beta} S_{\mu\nu}\right) = 0. \tag{12.22}$$

We took the matrix elements $F_{\mu\nu}^{\alpha}$ and $F_{\mu\nu}^{\beta}$ in these equations in a form of:

$$\begin{aligned} F_{\mu\nu}^{\alpha} &= H_{\mu\nu} + \sum_{\lambda\sigma}\left[P_{\lambda\sigma}(\mu\nu|\lambda\sigma) - P_{\lambda\sigma}^{\alpha}(\mu\sigma|\lambda\nu)\right]; \\ F_{\mu\nu}^{\beta} &= H_{\mu\nu} + \sum_{\lambda\sigma}\left[P_{\lambda\sigma}(\mu\nu|\lambda\sigma) - P_{\lambda\sigma}^{\beta}(\mu\sigma|\lambda\nu)\right], \end{aligned} \tag{12.23}$$

where

$$P_{\lambda\sigma}^{\alpha} = \sum_{i}^{m+n} c_{i\lambda}^{\alpha} c_{i\sigma}^{\alpha}; \quad P_{\lambda\sigma}^{\beta} = \sum_{i}^{m} c_{i\lambda}^{\beta} c_{i\sigma}^{\beta},$$

and matrix elements of the complete density matrix

$$P_{\lambda\sigma} = P_{\lambda\sigma}^{\alpha} + P_{\lambda\sigma}^{\beta}. \tag{12.24}$$

12.3.3 *The semiempirical MNDO-method*

We often neglect some integrals for a simplification of the computing procedures in the calculating matrix elements in a method of Hartree-Fock-Roohtan. Then we calculate the remained items proceeding from the experimental data (potentials of ionization, enthalpies of education, dissociation energies). So, we accelerate significantly the calculation in such a way, however accuracy of the results at the same time goes down. All methods, in the core of which the partial neglect in electronic integrals takes place, were called semiempirical. We usually realize the semiempirical methods within a valence approximation. So, we consider a wave function only of valence electrons, describing basis electrons by an efficient potential.

The MNDO-method (modified neglect of diatomic overlap) (Evarestov 1982, Bliznuk & Voytyuk 1986, Dewar & Thiel 1977, Thiel 1988) represents a semiempirical method, which is suitable for calculations of the molecules consisting of *s*- and *p*-elements.

We represented electrostatic energy of interaction of two electronic distributions around atoms A and B by the integral (12.15) in a Fock's matrix $F_{\mu\nu}$ (12.12) of the Rootan's (12.11) equation. In an approximation of MNDO (12.15) the multipole – multipolar interaction may be substituted by an amount:

$$(\mu\nu|\lambda\sigma) = \sum_{l}\sum_{k}\sum_{m}\left[\mathbf{M}_{lm}^{A}, \mathbf{M}_{km}^{B}\right], \tag{12.25}$$

where $\mathbf{M}_{lm}^{A}$ is the multipolar moment of the atom A, with 2^l charges, size $e/2^l$ and orientation of m. We calculated $\left[\mathbf{M}_{lm}^{A}, \mathbf{M}_{km}^{B}\right]$ by a summarizing of the interactions of two charges in each multipole:

$$\left[\mathbf{M}_{lm}^{A}, \mathbf{M}_{km}^{B}\right] = \frac{e^2}{2^{l+k}}\sum_{i}\sum_{j} f(\mathbf{R}_{ij}), \tag{12.26}$$

where $\mathbf{R}_{ij}$ – a distance between charges of i and j in configurations of charges of the atoms A and B, and $f(\mathbf{R}_{ij})$ – an empirical function which has to satisfy the following boundary conditions: it will be equal to zero on infinity, and at small distances ($\mathbf{R}_{ij} \to 0$) it will reflect an interaction of electrons in a diatomic molecule. Two model functions, the DSK-function (the Dewar-Sabelli-Klopmen) and MN-function (Mataga - Nishimoto), satisfy these requirements (Dewar & Thiel 1977, Minkin 1997):

$$\text{DSK:}f(\mathbf{R}_{ij}) = \left[\mathbf{R}_{ij}^2 + (\rho_l^A + \rho_k^B)^2\right]^{-\frac{1}{2}}, \text{MN:}f(\mathbf{R}_{ij}) = \left[\mathbf{R}_{ij} + \frac{1}{\rho_l^A + \rho_k^B}\right]^{-1},$$

ρ_l^A, ρ_k^B are the charge density on the atom A and the atom B respectively.

As a result, we approximated an interaction of electronic density of two atoms by electrostatic interaction of the corresponding multipoles (it is a point charge, a dipole or a quadrupole, depending on a type of orbitals).

We calculated the scheme MNDO. It represents a modification of an approximation of the zero differential overlap (ZDO) (Dewar & Thiel 1977, Minkin 1997). The integrals, which contain the multiplication $\chi_\mu(1)\ \chi_\nu(1)$, $(\mu \neq \nu)$, in ZDO-approximation for a Coulomb's repulsion of electrons are equal to zero. The main integrals $H_{\mu\nu}$ are not equal to zero, they are considered as the varied parameters. We presented the equations of Hartree-Fock-Roothaan in this approximation in a form of:

$$\sum_\nu c_{i\nu}(F_{\mu\nu} - \varepsilon_i \delta_{\mu\nu}) = 0, \tag{12.27}$$

where $\delta_{\mu\nu}$ is a Kronecker's delta and Fock's matrix elements are equal to:

$$F_{\mu\mu} = H_{\mu\mu} - \frac{1}{2}P_{\mu\mu}(\mu\mu|\mu\mu) + \sum_\nu P_{\nu\nu}(\mu\mu|\nu\nu),$$

$$F_{\mu\nu} = H_{\mu\nu} - \frac{1}{2}P_{\mu\nu}(\mu\mu|\nu\nu), \mu \neq \nu.$$

Considering all that we told above, we defined Fock's matrix elements in an approximation of MNDO (Dewar & Thiel 1977, Minkin 1997):

$$\begin{aligned}
F_{\mu\mu} &= U_{\mu\mu} + \sum_B V_{\mu\mu,B} + \sum_\nu^A P_{\nu\nu}[(\mu\mu|\nu\nu) - \frac{1}{2}(\mu\nu|\mu\nu)] + \sum_B \sum_{\lambda,\sigma}^B P_{\lambda\sigma}(\mu\mu|\lambda\sigma), \\
F_{\mu\nu} &= \sum_B V_{\mu\nu,B} + \frac{1}{2}P_{\mu\nu}[3(\mu\nu|\mu\nu) - (\mu\mu|\nu\nu)] + \sum_B \sum_{\lambda,\sigma}^B P_{\lambda\sigma}(\mu\nu|\lambda\sigma), \\
F_{\mu\lambda} &= \beta_{\mu\lambda}^{AB} - \frac{1}{2}\sum_\nu^A \sum_\sigma^B P_{\nu\sigma}(\mu\nu|\lambda\sigma),
\end{aligned} \tag{12.28}$$

where $U_{\mu\mu}$ are the diagonal elements of a Hamiltonian (energy of an electron in the condition χ_μ in atom A); $V_{\mu\nu,B} = -Z_B(\mu\nu|s_B s_B)$ is the energy of gravity of an electron of the atom A to an atomic nucleus of the atom$B$; $(\mu\mu|\nu\nu) = g_{\mu\nu}$ are two-centred, two-electronic integrals of a Coulomb's repulsion (are defined from the spectroscopical data); $(\mu\nu|\mu\nu) = h_{\mu\nu}$ – one-centre exchange integrals (are defined from the spectroscopical data); $P_{\mu\nu} = \sum_{i=1}^m n_i C_{\mu i} C_{\nu i}$– a density matrix ($n_i$ – population of i-MO); $\beta_{\mu\lambda}^{AB} = \frac{1}{2}(\beta_\mu^A + \beta_\lambda^B)S_{\mu\lambda}$, and$\beta_{\mu\lambda}^{AB}$, β_μ^A are one-electron (two - and one-centre) basis parameters of the communication of the atoms); $S_{\mu\lambda} = \int \chi_\mu^A(1)\chi_\lambda^B(1)\,d\tau_1$ are the integrals of an overlap of the basic atomic orbitals.

Then we concluded an equation for the energy of the electrons E_{el} and Coulomb's interaction of the atomic basis E_{AB}^{basis} in the MNDO-scheme:

$$E_{el} = \frac{1}{2}\sum_\mu \sum_\nu P_{\mu\nu}(H_{\mu\nu} + F_{\mu\nu}) \tag{12.29}$$

$$E_{AB}^{basis} = Z_A Z_B (s_A s_A | s_B s_B)[1 + \exp(-\alpha_A R_{AB}) + \exp(-\alpha_B R_{AB})]. \quad (12.30)$$

The matrix elements from an equation of a Hamiltonian in (12.29), (12.30) may be presented through the equalities:

$$H_{\mu\mu} = U_{\mu\mu} - \sum_B Z_B (\mu\mu | s_B s_B),$$

$$H_{\mu\nu} = -\sum_B Z_B (\mu\nu | s_B s_B),$$

$$H_{\mu\lambda} = \beta_{\mu\lambda} = \frac{1}{2}(\beta_\mu^A + \beta_\lambda^B) S_{\mu\lambda},$$

where s_A and s_B are s-orbitals of the atoms A and B respectively, and α_A and α_B are the empirical parameters.

We would not be able to investigate the hydrogen bridges, the properties of ionic connections and molecules in an electron excited states using the MNDO-method. Therefore we used the more efficient method – MNDO-PM/3 [8, 9] (Stewart 1989a, Stewart 1989b). It was based on the MNDO-method. But it is different from MNDO-approaching in the fact that expression for the energy of repulsion of the atomic basis A and B is approximated by the expression:

$$\begin{aligned} E_{AB}^{bas} &= Z_A Z_B (s_A s_A | s_B s_B)[1 + \exp(-\alpha_A R_{AB}) + \exp(-\alpha_B R_{AB})] \\ &+ \frac{Z_A Z_B}{R_{AB}} \left\{ \sum_{i=1}^{2} a_i^A \exp\left[b_i^A (R_{AB} - c_i^A)^2\right] + \sum_{i=1}^{2} a_i^B \exp\left[b_i^B (R_{AB} - c_i^B)^2\right] \right\} \end{aligned} \quad (12.31)$$

in which an author injected the additional empirical monoatomic parameters a_i, b_i, c_i.

The MNDO-PM/3 procedure is suitable for calculation of the hyper valence connections and molecules containing transition elements. Within the MNDO-PM/3-scheme, it is possible to receive power characteristics of the studied objects to a closer approximation, than when using the MNDO procedure.

12.3.4 *The computing circuits on the basis of the density functional theory*

The schemes based on the density functional theory (DFT) are the most widely used in applied calculations and universal methods of the electrophysical characteristics of the systems of many particles. DFT is the alternate approach to the theory of electronic structure in which the major role is played by not a multielectronic wave function, but the distribution of electronic density (Game, 2002).

According to this theory, all properties of an electronic structure of a system in a nondegenerate main state is completely defined by its electronic density (Kohn & Hohenberg 1964, Kohn & Sham 1965):

$$\rho(\mathbf{r}) = \sum_m^{occup} |\psi_m(\mathbf{r})|^2, \quad (12.32)$$

where the sum on N was made on the lowest occupied states, $\psi_m(\mathbf{r})$ is the wave function of an electron.

The system of N electrons in an adiabatic approximation is described by a Hamiltonian:

$$\mathrm{H} = \sum_i^N \left(-\frac{\Delta_i}{2}\right) + \sum_{i<j}^N \frac{1}{r_{ij}} - \sum_{i=1}^N \sum_k \frac{Z_k}{r_{ik}} \quad (12.33)$$

The main state of energy is defined by minimization of a functional of energy $E[\psi]$:

$$E[\psi] = \frac{\langle\psi|\mathrm{H}|\psi\rangle}{\langle\psi \mid \psi\rangle} \quad (12.34)$$

The term $\sum_k \frac{Z_k}{r_{ik}} = V_{ex}(r_i)$ (defining an external potential of the atomic kernels) and quantity of N electrons completely define all properties of the system for the main state (only such state will be considered further). The number of electrons can be defined from a condition:

$$N = \int \rho(\mathbf{r})d\mathbf{r}. \tag{12.35}$$

We received a reliable theoretical justification of DFT using the theorems of Hohenberg-Kohn. In their first theorem authors, Hohenberg and Kohn claim that density $\rho\,(\mathbf{r})$ of a ground state of the related system of the interacting electrons in some external potential $V_{ex}\,(\mathbf{r})$ uniquely determinates this potential (Kohn & Hohenberg 1964).

The second theorem represents the variation principle of a quantum mechanics formulated for a functional of density: the energy of an electronic subsystem, which is written down as a functional of an electronic density, has the minimum equal to an energy of a ground state.

According to the DFT-method, MO valence (or any) electrons $\varphi_j(\mathbf{r})$ may be found from the solution of a one-electron Schrodinger's equation (in atomic units)

$$(-\frac{1}{2}\nabla^2 + \upsilon_{eff}(\mathbf{r}) - \varepsilon_j)\varphi_j(\mathbf{r}) = 0, \tag{12.36}$$

where $-\frac{1}{2}\nabla^2$ is the operator of kinetic energy of an electron, ε_j - the energies of MO φ_j, $\upsilon_{eff}(\mathbf{r})$ - an efficient potential:

$$\upsilon_{eff}(\mathbf{r}) = \upsilon(\mathbf{r}) + \int \frac{n(\mathbf{r}')}{|\mathbf{r} - \mathbf{r}'|}d\mathbf{r}' + \upsilon_{xc}(\mathbf{r}), \tag{12.37}$$

$\upsilon(\mathbf{r})$– the potential caused by an attraction of electrons to bases (or to nuclear), without the interaction of electrons; the second member in (12.37) is a Coulomb's interaction of an electron in a condition $\varphi(\mathbf{r})$ with other electrons; $\upsilon_{xc}(\mathbf{r})$ – the exchange and correlative potential which is functionally depending on the complete distribution of the electronic density $\tilde{n}(\mathbf{r})$ according to an expression:

$$\upsilon_{xc}(\mathbf{r}) = \frac{\delta \mathrm{E_{xc}}[\tilde{n}\,(\mathbf{r})\,]}{\delta\,(\tilde{n}\,(\mathbf{r}))}\Big|_{\tilde{n}(\mathbf{r})=n(\mathbf{r})}, \tag{12.38}$$

$$n(\mathbf{r}) = \sum_{j=1}^{N_\upsilon} |\varphi_j(\mathbf{r})|^2, \tag{12.39}$$

(N_υ – valence number (or all) electrons, $\mathrm{E}[\tilde{n}\,(\mathbf{r})]$ – a functional of exchange-correlative energy. The equations (12.36)–(12.39) of MO $\varphi_j(\mathbf{r})$ in the self-consistent equations of DFT are presented in the decomposition form on the AO of all atoms of the system:

$$\varphi_j(\mathbf{r}) = \sum_A \sum_\mu{}^A C_{\mu j}\chi_\mu^{(A)} \tag{12.40}$$

The AO $\chi_\mu^{(A)}$ is localized on atom A. Therefore, the equation (12.36) is equivalent to a task on the own functions (matrix $C_{\mu j}$) and own values ε_j of the operator of Hartree-Kohn-Shem

$$\mathrm{F} = -\frac{1}{2}\nabla^2 + \upsilon_{eff}, \sum_\mu C_{\mu j}(F_{\mu\nu} - \varepsilon_j S_{\mu\nu}) = 0, \tag{12.41}$$

where $F_{\mu\nu} = \langle\chi_\mu|\hat{F}|\chi_\nu\rangle$ are the matrix elements of an operator F in a basis of the AO χ_μ, $S_{\mu\upsilon} = \langle\chi_\mu\,|\,\chi_\nu\rangle$ - the integrals of an overlap of the AO χ_μ and χ_ν.

Nowadays, the DFT-method is one of the most widely applicable methods, both in physics and in biology. It was called the "reference model" for the periodic solid objects. Walter Kohn, one of the ideologists of DFT, who got the Nobel Prize in chemistry in 1998, made some conclusions in his

Nobel lecture about his model. He told that he had expected that the theories on the basis of the wave functions and on the basis of the electronic density, supplementing each other, will allow receiving more precise quantitative responses in the future, and will make a contribution to deepening of our ideas of an electronic structure of substance (Game 2002).

12.4 CONCLUSIONS

Scientists proved long ago that methods of a quantum mechanics give an efficient way of a research of the electronic and power characteristics of the molecular structures. Therefore, their use for studying a process of merging of an implant with bone tissue is represented as a relevant problem of the modern biotechnical systems and technologies. We need to make an exact analysis for energy, frequency and length of the communication of the atoms forming the surface communications. Only in this way, we will be able to assess the external influence of the high-pitched laser on a surface of a material and take into account the metrological aspects of the process of an efficient merging of an implant and a bone tissue. That will be the way of improvement of quality of life of the patient.

REFERENCES

Bliznuk, A.A. & Voytyuk, A.A. 1986. The MNDO-85 system of programs for calculating the electronic structure, physicochemical properties, and reactivity of molecular systems by the MDNO, MNDOC, and AM1 semiepirical methods. *Journal of Structural Chemistry* 27(4): 674–676.

Dewar, M. J. S. & Thiel W. 1977. Ground states of molecules. 38. The MNDO method. Approximation and Parameters. *Journal of American Chemical Society* 99(15): 4899–4906.

Evarestov, R.A. 1982. *Quantum-mechanical methods in the theory of a solid body*. L.: LIE publishing house.

Game, V.E.K. 2002. Electronic structure of substance – wave functions and functionals of density. *Achievements of physical sciences* 172(3): 336–348.

Hehre, W. J., Radom, L., Schleyer, P.v.R. & Pople, J.A. 1986. *Ab initio molecular orbital theory*. New York: J. Wiley.

Kohn, W. & Hohenberg P. 1964. Inhomogeneous electron gas. *Phys. Rev.* 136B: 864–871.

Kohn, W. & Sham, J. 1965. Self-consistent equations including exchange and correlation effects. *Phys. Rev.* 140A: 1133–1138.

Minkin, V.I. 1997. Theory of a structure of molecules. Rostov-on-Don: Phoenix.

Stepanov, N. F. 2001. *Quantum mechanics and quantum chemistry*. Moscow: Mir.

Stewart, J .J. P. 1989a. Optimization of parameters for semiempirical methods. 1. Methods. *J. Comput. Chem.* 10(2): 209–220.

Stewart J. J. P. 1989b. Optimization of parameters for semiempirical methods. 2. Methods. *J. Comput. Chem.* 10 (2): 221–264.

Thiel, W. 1988. Semiempirical methods: current status and perspectives. *Tetrahedron* 44(24): 7393–7408.

CHAPTER 13

A system of the processing, monitoring of results and biofeedback training

T.V. Istomina, E.V. Petrunina, A.E. Nikolsky & V.V. Istomin
Moscow State University of Humanities and Economics, Moscow, Russian Federation

Z. Omiotek & M. Dzieńkowski
Lublin University of Technology, Lublin, Poland

B. Amirgaliyev
Astana IT-University, Nur-Sultan, Kazakhstan

ABSTRACT: The study considers the problem of increasing the efficiency of diagnosis and prevention of the development of nervous, musculoskeletal and cardiovascular diseases, diseases that often lead to disability, especially at a young age. An analysis is made of approaches to solving this problem, associated with the need to process a large pool of unstructured data that requires the use of modern intellectual methods. An integrated approach is proposed which includes the theoretical study of the problem and the practical implementation of research, the creation of methods for finding interdependent factors and the development of special equipment and software. The chapter details the problems associated with the lack of a theoretical study describing the process of biofeedback functioning. A model of biofeedback is presented with elements of the theory of automatic control. A software is developed for the implementation of experimental research of the proposed model of biofeedback. Methodologically, a three-level ontological structure is used to examine analytical decision models of an inclusive process. Based on the ontological description of the process of inclusion, a generalised structure of the information-analytical system was developed, the core of which is the knowledge base, built on the databases on the physical and psychological characteristics of students. A practical implementation of the analysed approach to building an intelligent information system of support for the educational process will allow creation of individual learning paths for students, which will improve the quality of the educational process and prevent the risk of developing nervous, musculoskeletal and cardiovascular diseases.

13.1 INTRODUCTION

In Russia, as well as worldwide, ischemic heart disease remains the main cause of health loss, the next cause is a stroke. Nervous, musculoskeletal and cardiovascular diseases are a major barrier to sustainable human development. In 2011, the United Nations formally recognised non-communicable diseases, including nervous and cardiovascular ones, as a major concern for global health. Determination of effective methods for biomarking such diseases, development of a system of precision medicine and fuzzy pathological zone recognition belongs to an extreme class of Artificial Intelligence (AI) for which there are no traditional solutions. There are many studies which reflect the integration of AI in medicine.

Despite the fast development of computing technology, utilisation of Data Mining methods in intelligent analytical systems for cardiovascular and nervous disease predictors is still at its beginning. This difficulty can be reduced by introducing effective scientific approaches and developing computer decision-making support systems utilising the creative professional capabilities of an interdisciplinary team of specialists in the fields of medicine, big data, mathematics, and computer technology.

To date, domestic and foreign mathematical methods of modelling processes of nervous and cardiovascular disorders, which lead to one or more of the associated diseases (diabetes, overweight, reduced physical and mental activity) represent various techniques for adequately reproducing numerous experimental and clinical data dynamics of cardiovascular predictors. Cardiovascular and nerve predictors are complex and heterogeneous in nature, as they are caused by multiple genetic and behavioural factors. Many more advancements and developments in Data Mining need to be made to predict outcomes accurately and effectively. These studies are focused on the creation of an intelligent information-analytical environment for preventive medicine, providing an individual approach and increasing the information content of data presentation and the effectiveness of prevention and prediction of the risk of nervous diseases with the cardiovascular system.

Adaptation of modern cognitive approaches to the processing of biomedical data in the intelligent information-analytical system (IAS) will allow to create individualised methods of disease prevention, in particular to solve problems of reducing their impact on people with disabilities in the education process. To address this issue, it is necessary to apply an integrated approach, which includes the theoretical elaboration of the problem and the practical implementation of research in developing computer decision-making support systems.

Early comprehensive prevention of diseases of the nervous and CVD includes a combination of motor, cognitive, and emotional-personal correction methods. Thus, it is necessary to develop preventive methods, individually adapted for the characteristics of people with different disabilities. Diagnostic and prevention the effects of nerve, musculoskeletal and CV disabilities requires the development of Data Mining methods and creating intelligent information and analytical systems that provide an individual approach to the person and increase the effectiveness of visualisation and analysis of data.

13.2 METHODOLOGY

To date, domestic and foreign mathematical methods for modelling processes of nerve and cardiovascular disorders represent various techniques, including the following approaches:

- classical statistical methods;
- game theory and fuzzy set theory;
- theory of Artificial Intelligence, and artificial neural networks;
- semantic and cognitive technologies.

The most effective approaches are based on the theory of fuzzy sets, Artificial Intelligence and artificial neural networks, as well as semantic and cognitive technologies.

The task of the inclusive process is to ensure the interaction of the V bio-object B with the system S in a single control loop with the overall objective efficiency function E:

$$B\,(x_1, x_2, \ldots, x_n) \rightarrow V \rightarrow S\,(y_1, y_2, \ldots, y_n) \rightarrow E, \tag{13.1}$$

where $x_1, x_2, \ldots, x_n$ are the values of the parameters of bio-object B and $y_1, y_2, \ldots, y_n$ are the values of parameters of the control system S on bio-object B.

In this study, a student with disabilities is considered as a biological component of an inclusive process. These disabilities include nervous, musculoskeletal and cardiovascular diseases, as well as problems with vision, hearing and speech dysfunctions. As a technical component of the biotechnical system considered, various devices can be presented for temporary, partial or full restoration of lost functions. Operator V is determined on set $G\,(g_1, g_2, \ldots, xg_n)$, where g_i is a complex of operations, which include medical, technical, material, informational, educational, economic and psychological tools for compensation of impaired body functions and working capacity and determining in general the diagnostics, correction, adaptation and development of cognitive abilities and rehabilitation students with disabilities. Operator V determines the relationship between objects B and S by converting the values of the parameters of the biological object $B\,(x_1, x_2, \ldots, x_n)$ into values that do not contradict the parameters of the object $G(g_1, g_2, \ldots, xg_n)$. The result is estimated by the efficiency function E.

To represent an inclusive process, it is necessary to build an ontological domain model as an information system to accompany the inclusion process (Nikolskiy 2017). Thus, it is required to create an information structure that describes the values of the elements of an inclusive process in the form of concepts, rules and statements about these concepts, with the help of which it is convenient to form and describe relations, classes and functions of inclusion (Nikolskiy & Petrunina 2018).

Formally, the ontology of inclusion is defined as:

$$\mathrm{O} = <\mathrm{I}, \mathrm{R}, \mathrm{F}>, \tag{13.2}$$

where $I(XY)$ is a finite set of concepts of the subject area of inclusion, R is a finite set of relationships between concepts, F is a finite set of interpretation functions defined on inclusive processes and relationships.

The ontological model of the system in the form:

$$\mathrm{MO} = <\mathrm{V}, \mathrm{K}, \mathrm{W}>, \tag{13.3}$$

where V is top-level ontology, includes common concepts and relationships; K is a variety of subject ontologies tailored to specific tasks and user requirements; W is set of rules for the ontological model of the system.

The ontological model of an intelligent information-analytical system is based on the proposed ontological description of the process of inclusion, which allows describing the relationship of inclusion at different functional levels. The level of metaontology contains general such concepts as "object", "property", "value", etc. The level of the ontology of the subject contains concepts that represent a specific subject domain and relationships that are semantically meaningful for a given subject domain. The level of the ontology of tasks and methods contains as concepts the types of tasks to be solved, as well as the decomposition of tasks into subtasks. The level of the network ontology allows describing the results of actions performed by the domain objects and tasks, as well as control actions.

The process of inclusion is presented in the form of an ontological information structure that describes the values of the elements of an inclusive process in the form of concepts, rules and statements. This allows to form relationships, classes and functions of inclusion and assess the degree of compatibility of the professional capabilities of a person who has physical and functional limitations in the functional requirements of society.

The ontological model of an intelligent information-analytical system allows to reveal the interaction of information and technical means for diagnosing deviations in the physical parameters of persons with disabilities and means of compensation for lost functions. In addition, it allows to describe the relationship of deviations of psychophysical parameters and indicators of the correction of cognitive functions, which is of great importance in the information process of the formation of professional knowledge and skills of persons with disabilities.

A generalised model of the ontological approach to the creation of an intelligent information-analytical system of inclusion is presented in Figure 13.1 and contains three levels of detail:

- the first level includes sensors measuring physical and psychophysiological parameters, as well as means of compensating for lost functions;
- the second level includes diagnostic tools (algorithms, databases, and knowledge in the field of diagnostics, interactive tools of the researcher, allowing to generate control actions on the examined persons with disabilities);
- the third level takes into account information and technical means of rehabilitation (algorithms, databases, and knowledge in the field of rehabilitation and correction of cognitive functions, interactive tools of the examined persons, including means of managing biofeedback training of various types).

The ontological model of the first level includes compensation for physical deviations, such as impaired speech, vision, mobility of hands and fingers, as well as other means of information technology:

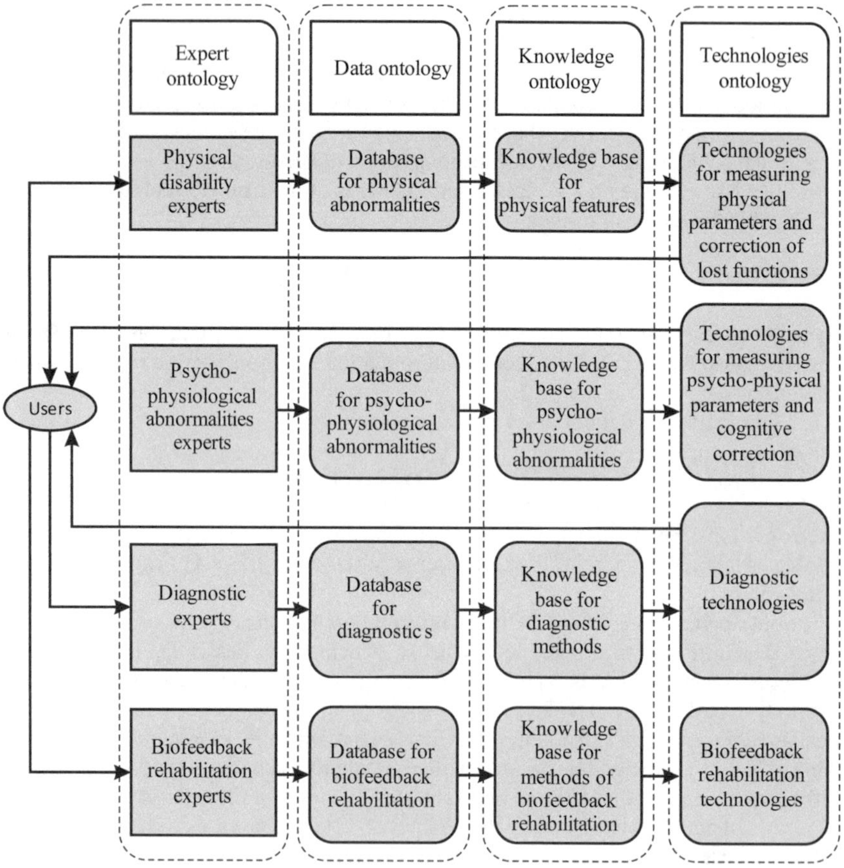

Figure 13.1. Generalised model of the ontological approach to the creation of an intelligent information-analytical system of inclusion.

speech-text-speech converters, robotic devices, etc. The ontological model of the second level includes compensation of psychophysical features, such as low concentration of attention, naivety, alienation, constraint, etc. The ontological model of the third level includes the normalisation and stability of the psyche, the activation of behaviour and disability, the restoration of students' cognitive functions. The ontological model is the basis of an intelligent information-analytical system, represented as an expert system that implements reflexive-active self-developing technology for perceiving situations of the external environment and effective actions to support the harmonious functioning of professional educational organisations in the field of inclusive education for people with disabilities.

The model of intelligent IAS monitoring, biofeedback training and support activities for persons with disabilities for educational organisations in the field of inclusive education includes the presentation of the functional structure of the information-analytical system in the class of ontological databases, knowledge base, methods, tools, technologies, as well as the user interface.

In the process of ontological modelling, regularities are identified and the information flow of the developed system is increased. The development of models is carried out following the main objectives of the intelligent system, namely to solve the problem of planning the educational process of students with nosological features, choosing assistance equipment during the educational process, building an intermediate control system or choosing individual learning paths (Rybina 2017). The information system of the educational process is considered as a complex dynamic system that should give a complete description of the process of the formation of knowledge and skills, taking into account the aspects caused by the nosological features of students.

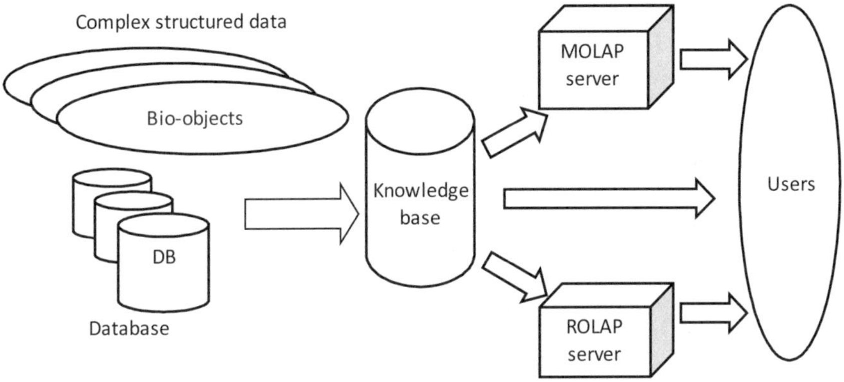

Figure 13.2. Generalised structure of the information-analytical system.

During the research, a heterogeneous data structure is formed:

- multidimensional data for medical analytics;
- medical analytical data that may appear as a result of clinical analytics;
- average statistics on norms and pathologies;
- infrastructure data – analytics, algorithms, registers, estimated points, monitoring tools.

The use of intelligent prognostic methods and the integration of heterogeneous information resources based on the results of functional diagnostics (Efremov et al. 2019; Kiselev et al. 2019 is proposed.

The developed IAS is implemented within the framework of the concept of an integrated information space, which is characterised by the use of various microservice architectures (Chedvik et al. 2013), which will allow for the dynamic exchange of content. It is necessary to solve the following tasks:

- provide a homogeneous ontological representation of knowledge;
- organise the allocation of joint resources and their management.

Based on the ontological description, a generalised structure of the information-analytical system has been created which general structure is shown in Figure 13.2.

The basis of the information-analytical system is a knowledge base, based on the databases on the physical and psychological characteristics of students. This system allows to track the dynamics of the current physical, psychological and emotional state of students with disabilities using the monitoring subsystem based on the testing system. The work uses the methods of visually oriented and object-oriented software design and database design, and the proposed architecture forms the basis of the developed system of complex intelligent analysis of biomedical data in the IAS. The monitoring subsystem is designed to track the dynamics of the psychological and emotional state of students, as well as the effectiveness of rehabilitation activities. The processing of the received volume of Big Data is performed using the OLAP and ROLAP data processing technologies. The proposed approach includes the representation of the functional structure of the information-analytical system in the class of ontological database, knowledge base, methods, tools and user interface.

The main functions of the subsystem for monitoring the status of students with disabilities:

- identification of the parameters of individual norms;
- passing examinations;
- processing of results;
- tracking the dynamics of results;
- development of recommendations for training;
- analysis of the dynamics of the results.

It is known (Sarkisyan 1999) that the inclusive educational process places special demands on the development of measures aimed at improving the efficiency of teaching people with disabilities and adapting the educational process for various categories of students.

One of the effective methods for solving this problem is the development and implementation of computer cognitive tools (Bayramov 2018; Nikolskiy 2017) during diagnosis and rehabilitation, aimed at modifying and developing cognitive skills in persons with disabilities. Despite the development of modern tools for the implementation of biofeedback for training, their use as a means of improving the quality of the educational process has significant features.

Biofeedback can be defined as a group of non-pharmacological therapies, which use electronic instruments for measuring, processing and provision of information to patients on the functioning of physiological systems (Greenhalgh et al. 2009). The idea of biofeedback (BFB) has wide practical application are described and successfully operate a variety of biofeedback techniques. Experiments using BFB can be traced to the late 1950s – early 1960s (Horowitz 2006). However, in the scientific literature, there is no theoretical description of processes occurring in the operation of BFB, due to the complexity and nonlinearity of biological objects and their structural elements.

Using biofeedback allows controlling the body's biological processes that occur involuntarily, such as heart rate (HR), blood pressure (BP) or muscle tension, while maintaining the vertical position of the body, skin temperature, and others. Application of BFB gives results in solving several problems such as high levels of stress, headache, migraine, postural disorders (PD), high blood pressure, urinary incontinence and others (Holten 2009). Biofeedback is also known to be used for rehabilitation after illness (Nelson 2007) describes the role played by the BFB in the process of rehabilitation after stroke, in (Meuret et al. 2001) biofeedback is used for breathing exercises to avoid panic attacks, and in (Alvarez et al. 2013) for rehabilitation chemotherapy.

One of the problems to be solved in medicine using biofeedback correction techniques is human PD (Gopalai et al. 2012). However, to date, no approach has been implemented for the creation of rehabilitation equipment and the diagnosis and correction of PD that would provide a combination of non-invasive (imaging-based action BFB) and nano-level attempts to solve this problem. Therefore it is necessary to justify the scientific and technical solutions in this area, based on the use of perspective directions of the technology industry – medical nanorobotics (Istomin 2013). This important creation of effective algorithms of swarm robotics systems based on the theory of artificial swarm intelligence for the application of high-tech medicine in the field of remote micro diagnostics and therapy. The most significant data in the analysis of PD are stabilographic parameters which adequately describe the healing process (Gaje & Weber 2008). However, to obtain a reliable forecast of the outcome of the treatment and the possibility of timely correction based on biofeedback therapy is often required when changes-diagnostic methods such as ECG, EEG and EMG (Gusev et al. 2001).

Thus, for the objectification of control throughout the recovery of patients multidiagnostic remote systems based on biofeedback synchronous recording biosignals should be used (Istomina et al. 2014). Using biofeedback allows regulating the physiological processes that are amenable to training. Based on the positive experience accumulated in the course of biofeedback training, a set of priorities actions was established. The presence of an adequate model of the functioning of BFB would bring effective training based on it to a new level and identify the underlying mechanisms of its occurrence.

Customisation of the patient treatment program according to the type and intensity of biofeedback training will move from the empirical to the reasonable requirements of the recommendations based on multivariate analysis of physiological data. The method of remote assessment of patients with PD, implemented on the basis of the formation of integrated indicators, describing the process of biofeedback therapy, provides highly informative survey results, as well as their medical justification.

There are two types of biofeedback: direct and indirect. Direct biofeedback is based on the conscious physiological functions such as muscle contraction; indirect one corresponds to the unconscious functions of the body, such as heart rate or breathing. The barrier between direct and indirect biofeedback can be overcome, for example, when a user has awareness of the parameters of his or her breath and begins to consciously control it. Inside there is an emotional indirect BFB (Emotional/Affective Biofeedback), where a variety of involuntary signals are simultaneously interpreted to assess the impact on the emotional state of the user (Rodrigues 2013). An example of using direct biofeedback muscle rehabilitation is given in (Lyons et al. 2003). To organise biofeedback training modes of relaxation or stress are used.

Systems based on BFB should be attributed to the class of tracking systems when the reference variable represents a previously unknown function of time. The number of adjustable parameters determines the number of output vectors, respectively; the system can be one-dimensional and multidimensional. If we look at BFB from the perspective automatic control theory (ACT), it is necessary to select a control object (or a set of them that is controlled by the system) and a control system, forming a total control system. A control system, in this case, is the physiological parameters of the body and it acts by managing the central nervous system. In operation, the biotechnical system (BTS) effects occur, leading to what is desired and the actual values of the controlled variable are different. In the ACT it is a mistake of the automatic control. The case of BFB also has a similar error, as external factors can serve as stress or lead to a significant deviation of physiological parameters. Due to the presence of feedback, possible with the use of hardware – sensors and imaging devices, a biological object has at its disposal an error signal representing the difference between the set exposure and feedback.

The scientific and methodological basis of the work is the application and a description of the principle of multi-channel multiparametric BFB. Implementation of the health care decisions in the course of further research is supposed to take into account the anatomical, biomechanical, social and household characteristics of the patient. Besides, these data will also be used for the selection of individual therapeutic biofeedback training for the patient.

For a description of the BFB from ACT's position, let us use the following groups of variables:

- state variables $s_1(t), s_2(t), \ldots s_m(t)$, which represent their generalised coordinates. The number of generalised coordinates, in turn, represents the number of the system's degrees of freedom;
- control variables $u_1(t), u_2(t), \ldots u_m(t)$, i.e. exposure to managed objects that are created by the control system;
- external variables or disturbance variables $v_1(t), v_2(t), \ldots v_k(t)$, generated in the environment (the emotional impact of atmospheric pressure, temperature, load, and other various types.);
- observed variables $n_1(t), \ldots n_l(t)$, which are those of the generalised coordinates of the controlled system, the information about the change that comes to the control system.

In this case, the parameters are derived for the patient, for example, on the monitor screen.

The state vector can coincide with the vector of observation. The condition of the managed system at any given time is determined by the initial state at time t_0 and the vectors r and f:

$$s_i(t) = F_i\{s(t_0), u(t, t_0), n(t, t_0)\} \tag{13.4}$$

The control problem is to find the control vector $u(t)$, at which the extremum of a function *Ex* (the extremum – management objective) is:

$$E_x\{s(t), u(t), v(t)\} = \text{extreme (high or low)} \tag{13.5}$$

In the process of creating a model of the biotechnical system, it is necessary to ensure a balance between complexity and quality. In general, the control algorithm is represented as follows:

$$u(t) = U\{\varepsilon(t), t\} \tag{13.6}$$

As a reference variable *d(t)* is the allowable value of physiological parameters such as heart rate (the rate of private individuals in the normal state). The block comparator comes to the current recorded values of these parameters (Figure 13.3), which are transmitted by the subject, for example, in graphical form. Based on these data the error *å(t)* is calculated, from which in turn, taking into account external influences *v(t)* a control vector *u(t)* is constructed as a function of the error and external influences.

Analysis of the biofeedback mechanisms have shown that the sudden change in the input variable output does not change immediately, but there is an inertial component. In this context, modelling the

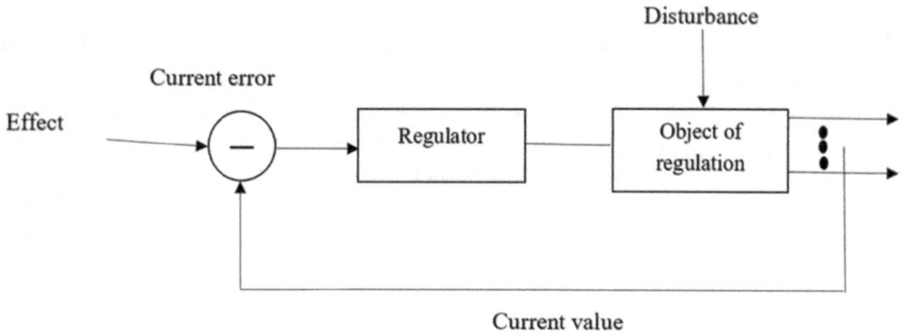

Figure 13.3. Feedback model.

mechanisms of biofeedback as a model of the control object can be used as a model of an approximate delay element 1st order with the inertial component:

$$W\,(p) = \frac{K}{T_1 p + 1} e^{-\tau p}, \tag{13.7}$$

where K – static coefficient of transmission link, T – the time constant, τ – time constant of the transient, p – Laplace operator.

In the presence of a mismatch, an applicable model of the second-order is used:

$$W\,(p) = \frac{K}{(T_1 p + 1)\,(T_2 p + 1)} e^{-\tau p} \tag{13.8}$$

To describe the operation of a multi-parametric BFB it is also advisable to use this approach.

In the absence of a comprehensive information management system, to adjust the PID controller can be done by using non-parametric methods. The most famous among them is the method of Ziegler-Nichols (Ziegler & Nichols 1942) and Astrom and Hagglund (Aström & Hägglund 1995; Ho et al. 2001; Ho et al. 2003) describe the self-tuning PID controllers, which always get the specified performance and avoid the disadvantages of classical methods. To describe the operation of a multi-parametric BFB is also advisable to use this approach.

At present, an electronic portal has been developed for the study of biofeedback of various types, which implements the software part of the system functional diagnostics web server. Using this web interface allows you to provide research with a sufficient amount of empirical data to build an adequate functioning model of the BFB. Thus, a simplified description of the functioning of the BFB based on the ACT has been proposed, and a software environment has been created that allows for the simulation of the BFB to assess the adequacy of this description.

An important result of the research is also the development of a remote access system that provides the ability to remotely monitor the progress of the process of diagnosis and therapy of postural deficit based on the advantages of multi-channel biofeedback combined with original user techniques.

13.3 RESULTS

At this stage of the research, the stabilometric platform and the Kolibri telemetry system are used as peripheral equipment for taking physiological parameters with the possibility of conducting various biofeedback training. Let us consider them in more detail. Stabilometry is a method using biofeedback: the patient himself can control deviations of the body position displayed on the computer screen during various tests, which makes it possible to correct the position in the rack.

A prerequisite for a standard job using BFB is to keep the pressure centre control mark in the specified zone. Using various visualisation tools, the most suitable options are created for solving the required tasks of static motor-cognitive tests with biofeedback according to the support reaction. An

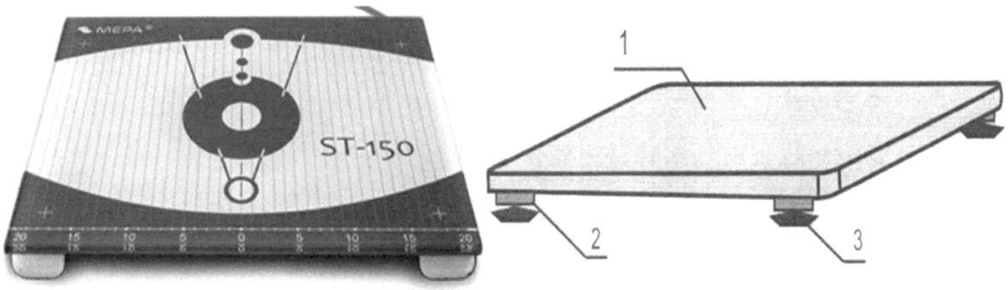

Figure 13.4. The layout of the standard stabilometric platform ST-150: 1 – the supporting surface of the platform; 2 – analogue-to-digital converters; 3 – pressure sensors.

important aspect of the use of biofeedback in studies of the equilibrium function is the combination of stabilometric tests with visual-acoustic feedback, which creates a greater number of signals for the subject. This allows increasing the likelihood of a "response" to the instruction in the "inhibited" subjects. This suggests that there are opportunities for studying biofeedback from a psychological point of view.

A stabilised platform is an electronic device for recording fluctuations in the centre of pressure, signal transformation and real-time transmission of measurement data for interpretation and analysis into a computer, to obtain objective information about the state of the motor coordination system. We used the domestic stabilometric platform ST-150. The measuring part of the stabilometric system is represented by a force-measuring platform, consisting of a supporting surface, an electronic signal converter and force sensors. Sensors sensitive to the force exerted vertically on them are fixed on a rigid base. A rigid plate is installed on top of the sensors. The calculation of the resultant force applied to the platform can be made using its value on each of the sensors. When the patient is calmly standing on the platform, the resultant will show a vertical projection onto the platform of the subject's centre of gravity. Figure 13.4 shows the layout of the stabilised platform series ST-150.

The supporting platform is made in the form of a rectangular plate of rigid material with markings applied to the supporting surface (to coordinate the installation of the feet of the subject). The signal processing circuit is implemented as a microprocessor module containing four synchronised analogue-to-digital converters that receive measuring signals from each of the load cells, normalise and transform these signals into information ones. The signal contains data on the mass of the investigated object and the coordinates of its centre of pressure on the platform relative to the coordinate system associated with the platform. The transmission of the received information signal is carried out through the serial interface to the control computer.

Thus, the principle of operation of the stabilometric device is based on measuring the vertical forces applied to the force sensors, calculating the mass of the object and the coordinates of the point of application of the resultant force acting from the side of the object. The digital signal from the stabilometric platform enters the computer, where a special program, based on the measurement data, analyses the obtained coordinates of the centre of pressure of the person on the supporting surface during the study.

Consider the test of computer stabilometry most widely used in practice – the Romberg test. The practical meaning of this test is to compare the indicators of the equilibrium function with the participation of vision and eyes closed, which allows evaluating the contribution of proprioceptive and visual systems to maintaining a given position. Note that the normal reaction to closing the eyes is an increase in the oscillations of the centre of pressure. If the subject has significant degrees of change in the field of vision, impaired eyes or other pathologies, then vision will not play a role in maintaining balance in the main stance. In this case, it is possible to observe fluctuations in the centre of pressure of smaller amplitude than with open eyes. Stability increases because the subject maintains equilibrium mainly due to proprioception, the action of vision, in this case, is only a disturbing factor.

Thus, when conducting the Romberg test, it is necessary to take into account the state of vision, the side of the preferential development of the subject, as well as the individual characteristics of athletes in whom the difference between various indicators and normal can be caused not by pathology, but by physical specialisation.

Given the specifics of the Romberg stabilometric test, some additional conditions are used for its implementation. Thus, when conducting a stabilometric examination in people with significant motor pathology, when there is a risk of a patient falling, protection systems are used: hand supports and safety belts.

The Romberg test has two modes: a mode with open and closed eyes. This circumstance affects the output results for two modes that have their own characteristics, which makes their joint analysis difficult. Therefore, to search for deviations and pathologies, it is advisable to compare the results of two examination modes with some norms separately.

In 1985, French researchers obtained normative data that made it possible to compare the results with normal indicators. The paper considers interesting parameters for clinical analysis obtained during the passage of the Romberg test: the position of the centre of pressure, the velocity of the centre of pressure, area of the statokinesiogram, LFS coefficient, Romberg coefficient.

The scope of BFB therapy using the Hummingbird telemetry system is quite wide. It allows to ensure the use of BFB according to an electromyogram, according to indicators of the cardiovascular system, and BFB training using an electroencephalogram (the so-called neuro-biofeedback, which is now of particular interest to researchers in light of intensified development of brain-computer interfaces).

If the basic principles and mechanisms of BFB therapy remain unchanged, the muscle-effectors on which EMG is recorded can be anywhere from the muscles of the neck and upper shoulder girdle to the muscles of the pelvic floor and legs.

In BFB training on indicators of the cardiovascular system, the most frequently monitored parameters are heart rate, respiratory arrhythmia of the heart and stress index, which is also the Baevsky index. These indicators are calculated by a cardiointervalogram.

EEG-BOS training is usually divided into types based on which rhythm is used as a controlled parameter. There are alpha, beta, theta and gamma types of training, training on super slow brain activity, as well as on narrower frequency sub-bands and any indices calculated on the basis of the EEG signal. The most common type of EEG training is alpha rhythm training. It is used for the correction of various types of anxiety disorders, as well as for the correction of secondary disorders that occur against the background of increased anxiety: psychosomatic pain, sleep disturbances and decreased work productivity. Alpha training is necessarily included in the training scenarios for general relaxation and increase stress resistance; it is used to increase performance, to correct attention deficit disorder in people with hyperactivity, etc.

At this stage of work, the team developed an IAS to study the possibilities of adjusting the work of the nervous, cardiovascular, and musculoskeletal systems of students with disabilities and the development of cognitive abilities of students with disorders of the musculoskeletal system. BFB-trainings are applied in this system, using EEG, EMG, heart rate and stabilogram based on the Kolibri and ST-150 equipment.

Using the WinPatientExpert software and the ST-150 stabilographic platform, the Romberg test was conducted on 30 healthy students and 30 students with various pathologies of the functions of the musculoskeletal system. When conducting balance studies, the main stand was used for removal, and the EEG, EMG and heart rate studies were conducted on the same groups of subjects using the Kolibri system. Figure 13.5 shows an example of conducting a survey of a student with a violation of the musculoskeletal system using the Kolibri telemetry system.

The most important task is to choose for each student the type of training that will help solve his problem. A controlled parameter is an indicator that underlies the student's feedback, and which he learns to manage. The choice of a controlled parameter depends on what physiological parameters your equipment can record (or calculate).

Our system currently uses BFB training in five groups of indicators: EEG (alpha and beta rhythms), EMG (an indicator of muscle activity), a cardiointervalogram (indicators of the cardiovascular system) and respiration indicators.

The set of controlled parameters that can be trained is very different for different manufacturers of equipment for BFB training and even for one manufacturer in different configurations of devices. In addition to the above, there are also pieces of training on indicators of blood circulation, skin-galvanic reaction, temperature, and many others. Our equipment provides a space of options from which controlled parameters for training can be chosen. Making the right choice is necessary

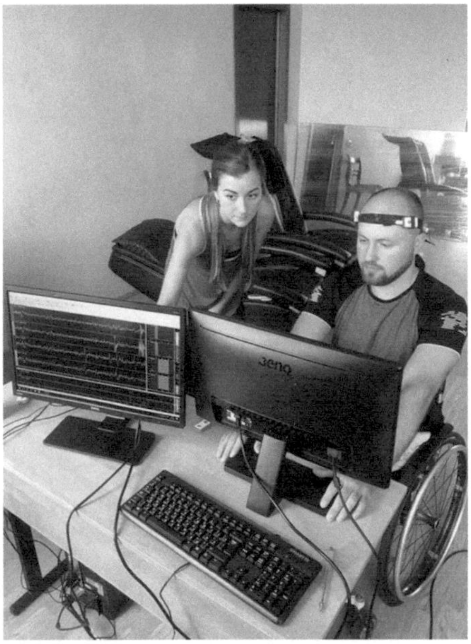

Figure 13.5. An example of a survey using the Kolibri system.

based on the following basic prerequisites: student complaints, assessments of teachers and the results of diagnostic procedures.

It is also important to understand what thresholds (upper and lower) to set for each particular student and when it can be considered that the result of training has already been achieved.

Thresholds in BFB training are the values of controlled parameters, within which the student learns to hold the trained parameter. There are also two approaches to the question of determining thresholds – physiological and psychological.

From a physiological point of view, the thresholds are determined by the upper and lower values of the norm for this indicator. If the statistical norm for the desired controlled parameter has a very large spread, then you need to reduce the interval on the basis of the results of the diagnosis. Most of the hardware and software systems for biofeedback therapy determine specific threshold values based on the student's indicators, measured immediately before the training (usually this is an average value plus or minus some value). For EMG training to increase contraction force, the upper threshold can be calculated from the maximum strength demonstrated by the student in the preparatory phase. Some programs allow setting specific numerical threshold values for controlled parameters manually. Automatic calculation of thresholds based on the current state of the student before the training is used much more often. It allows to take into account the natural lability of indicators and automatically complicates the training by the progress made. Manual setting of threshold values is sometimes needed in isolated cases, for example, if a student demonstrates a pronounced stress response at the beginning of the training or intentionally tries to lower the thresholds at the stage of statistics collection.

From a psychological point of view, setting a threshold is a setting of the complexity of a task. It happens that the control of a given parameter is given to the student with great difficulty. In this case, it makes sense to reduce the interval between thresholds so that even a minimal change in the controlled parameters during training is noticeable. You can do this either by manually adjusting the threshold value or by changing the threshold calculation formula in the script for this student. How exactly this will be done will depend on the particular device used, but the principle is similar everywhere.

For example, if by default the threshold is calculated as the average value of the plus or minus standard deviation parameter, then to reduce the interval (and therefore facilitate the task), you need to change the formula and calculate the threshold as the average value of the plus or minus 0.5 parameter from the standard deviation. Conversely, if the control of the parameter is given to the student easily,

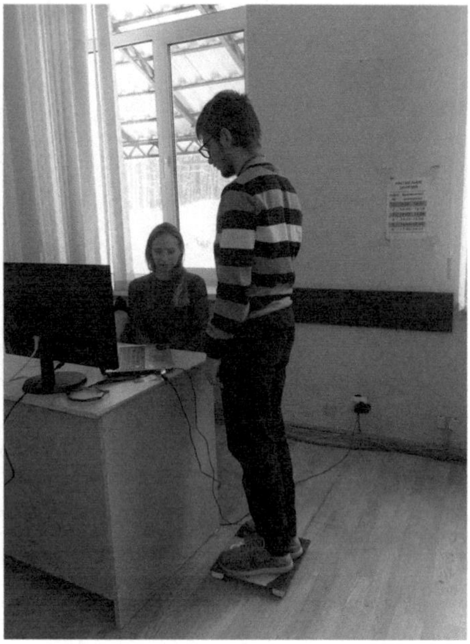

Figure 13.6. An example of a stabilometric survey.

then a simple training may soon bore him. In this case, it is worth complicating the task, either by increasing the interval between thresholds or by moving it on a scale in the right direction.

To assess the actual ability to form the skill of managing one's state, it is better to use relative indicators for the session. In our system, this is the number of successful attempts, i.e. the number of cases (in percent) of the total number of measurements when the monitored parameter was within the specified thresholds. This approach to assessment allows us to say how much the student can arbitrarily adjust the physiological parameter being trained, but cannot give an understanding of the dynamics of the indicator. That is, the student can show the result in 15% of successful attempts in the first session and 80% of successful attempts in the last. However, if at the same time the thresholds practically did not change, then there was no real change in the level of the controlled indicator. Therefore, this indicator alone can be used only to assess the ability for arbitrary self-regulation. To assess the practical significance of the use of biofeedback training to correct a particular problem, in addition to the number of successful attempts, it is necessary to indicate the threshold values at the first and last session.

Figure 13.6 shows an example of a stabilometric diagnostic of a student without musculoskeletal disorders. Examples of signals obtained in the process of monitoring the parameters of the musculoskeletal system are shown in Figure 13.7. Examples of the results of examinations and training of ECG, EEG, and EMG are shown in Figures 13.8–13.10, respectively.

A stabilograph (Holten 2009), an electrocardiograph, an electroencephalograph, and an electromyograph are combined on the basis of specialised hardware and software into a single complex that performs remote research in conditions with limited possibilities of rendering highly skilled medical care. Thus, this study is based on the application of a systems approach for a comprehensive analysis of interdependent functional characteristics, as well as their dynamics and correction of changes associated with non-invasive effects (Istomina et al. 2011). The scientific and methodological basis of the system is the application of the principle of multi-channel biofeedback (Istomina et al. 2019).

The mobile recorder includes a set of diagnostic equipment for multi diagnostics. The data are transmitted via the antenna by the telemetry method to a personal computer on which special software is installed.

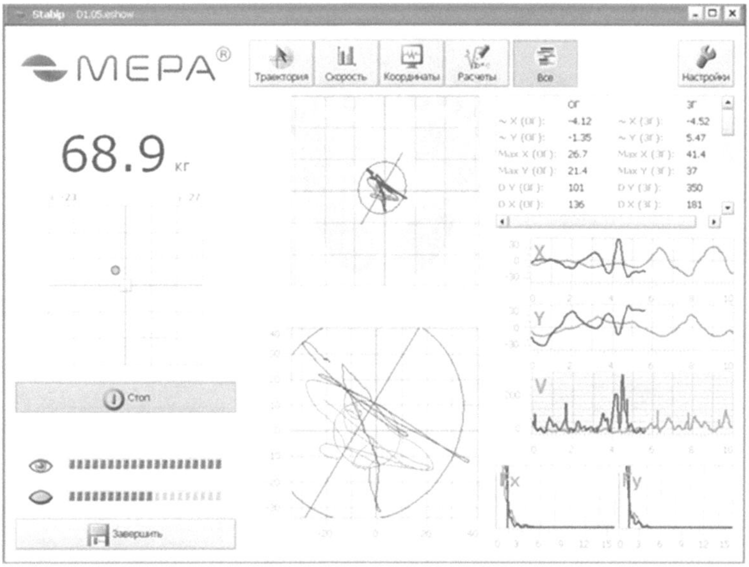

Figure 13.7. Stabilographic monitoring results.

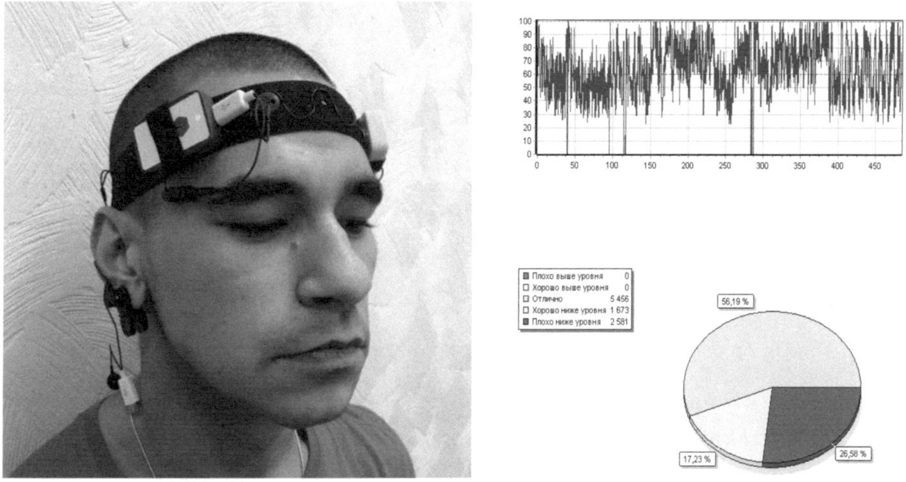

Figure 13.8. EEG monitoring and BFB-training.

After installing the channels and setting up the system, an examination is performed. The results are automatically sent to the Web-server. The installed software automatically reads data from the Web server and associates it with the registration card of the subject. The IAS includes a set of equipment for multi diagnostics and biofeedback training. The information support of the IAS includes a database of patients, software for selecting and executing examination methods, software for the rehabilitation process and game BFB training. After installing the channels and setting up the equipment, the patient is examined, the results are automatically sent to the Web server. The preinstalled software automatically reads data from the Web server and links it to the patient's registration card. The software implements the process of setting up, installing measurement channels, recording signals, transmitting multi diagnostics data to a Web server, downloading data from a Web server and automatically associating it with a patient card in a database, preparing a report and documenting it.

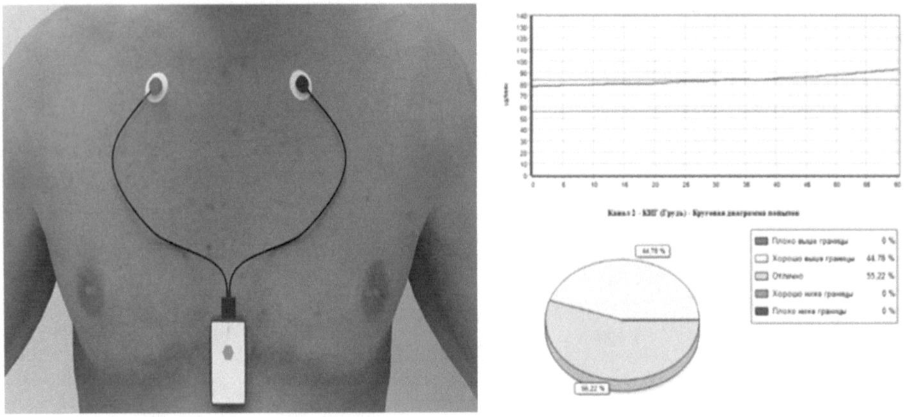

Figure 13.9. ECG monitoring and BFB-training of the heartbeat rate.

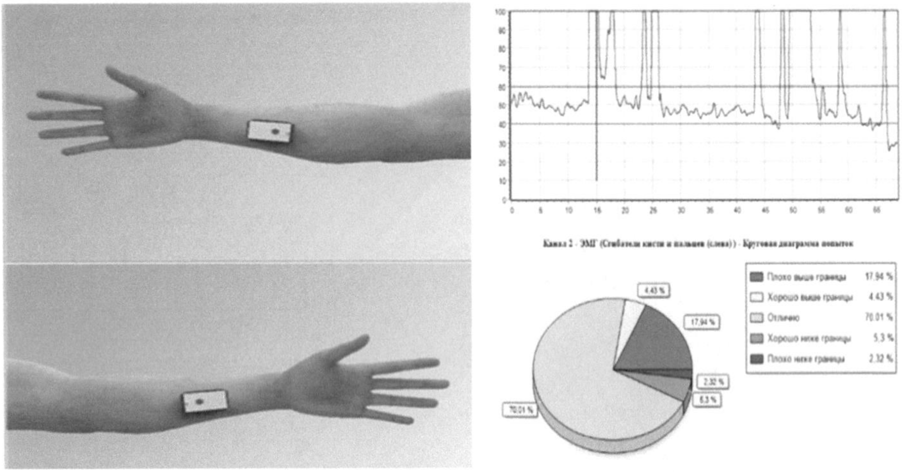

Figure 13.10. EMG monitoring and BFB-training.

On-line transmission of the full amount of diagnostic information is performed, which is recorded during the examination of a patient at the same time using ECG, EMG, EEG and stabilometry methods via Internet channels to the medical subscriber's IP address.

Visualisation, processing and storage of the full amount of diagnostic information recorded from a remote patient on a medical subscriber's PC and the Internet is provided. Comprehensive monitoring is carried out with synchronisation of all channels of registration and remote configuration of hardware and software tools for functional diagnostics. The research results and the preparation of the conclusion are processed on the Web-server.

Specialised software of the Kolibri system registers, displays, processes and stores in computer memory the heterogeneous streams of diagnostic information for a comprehensive assessment of the patient's condition and preparation for BFB training. The high functionality of the software is provided by the following principles of its development:

1. Universality and modularity of implementation.
2. The possibility of a flexible configuration of equipment specifications relevant to the ongoing monitoring studies and biofeedback training.
3. Support of the "hot" update mode of the list of monitoring modules used during the survey session.

4. The possibility of automatic identification of monitoring modules.
5. Equality of techniques implemented by the modules of monitoring and BFB-training.
6. The clarity and transparency of the protocol to identify the specified information.
7. The presence in the protocol of service information.

The IAS implements the following options for the selection of the survey methodology: simple recording of signals over time, Romberg test, BFB-training (games), and definition of individual norms. The selectable biomedical data acquisition channels depend on the survey method chosen. During the BFB-training sessions, the recording of signals taken from the patient also goes into the background.

The developed method of determining the individual norm consists of conducting a special survey designed to form an individual norm in all parameters from all data acquisition channels. This type of examination consists of recording signals from a patient for 60 seconds. The screen at this time for the patient displays a crosshair and a point showing the projection of its pressure centre. For the final formation of an individual standard, at least five surveys are required, preferably on different days. The individual rate is determined for each patient by the first five surveys, each of which has a duration of 1 minute, while the values are averaged and saved across all channels and all states in which the patient was in the process of assessing the norm. After determining the individual norm, the program identifies not only critical states (deviations from the group norm), but also deviations from the individual norm of the examined patient.

Consider the main stages of the information-analytical system in the process of examining students with disabilities.

1. Justification of the quantitative and qualitative composition of the control and studied samples of healthy students and students with disabilities.
2. Surveying a sample of healthy students.
   2.1. Logging into the database of primary data about a healthy student.
   2.2. Defining the individual norm of a healthy student.
   2.3. Passing tests and monitoring parameters of a healthy student.
   2.4. Logging in the database of test results by a healthy student.
3. Surveying a sample of students with disabilities.
   3.1. Logging in the database of primary data about a healthy student with a disability.
   3.2. Determining the individual standard of a student with a disability.
   3.3. Passing tests and monitoring parameters of a student with a disability.
   3.4. Logging in the database of the initial test results of a student with a disability.
   3.5. Individual selection of training for a student with a disability.
   3.6. Conducting training with a student with a disability.
   3.7. Logging in the database of the final test results of a student with a disability.
4. Processing the results of surveys of the control sample of students. Formation of statistical threshold values for normal parameters.
5. Processing the results of surveys of the sample of students with disabilities studied. Detection of deviations from normal values and tracking their dynamics.
6. Analysis of the results and conclusions.
7. Development of recommendations on the individual selection of technical, informational, educational means, as well as rehabilitation and psychological measures aimed at restoring or compensating for impaired body functions of students with disabilities and determining the individual trajectories of their learning.

Currently, a web application for storing and processing unstructured biomedical data and multi-level access to them has been created. This application provides the following features: a unified database for storing data about students and surveys, a convenient interface for working with databases, separation of access rights, ease of adding, editing and deleting data, and quick search through arbitrary data fields, convenient registration, and authorisation of users.

Microsoft SQL DBMS is used to store IAS data due to its high performance, simplicity, reliability, and security. Figure 13.11 shows the structure of the database, designed in the course of work. In the

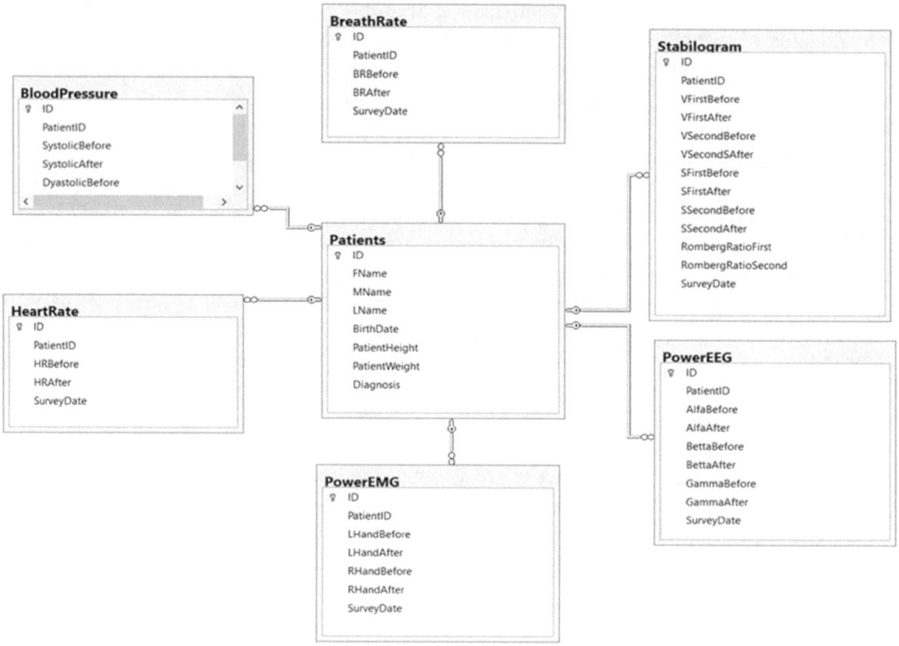

Figure 13.11. DB structure.

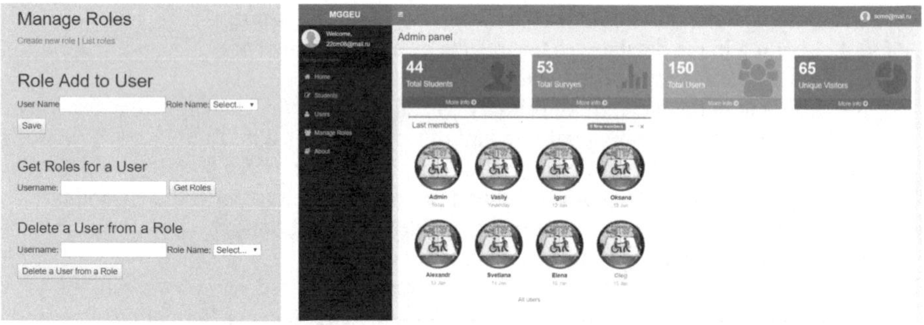

Figure 13.12. Form «User Authorisation».

process of developing a web application, a tool for searching the contents of the form was implemented; forms for editing, adding, deleting and viewing database elements were developed.

To ensure security, the IAS has an authorisation and authentication system that provides access to data only for registered and authorised users; there is a component of access control by roles (Figure 13.12). Currently, the database already contains a large number of records of biomedical data of students of MGGEU. An example of a form administrator is presented in Figure 13.13.

The data obtained in the course of the research serve as the basis for the creation of a statistical base. In the course of further research, it is proposed to make an informed choice of the most effective methods. The selected techniques will be used in the future in the educational process to improve the cognitive abilities of students with disabilities, taking into account their diseases in nosologies, to prevent the development of nervous, musculoskeletal and cardiovascular diseases.

Figure 13.13. Form «Administrator».

13.4 CONCLUSIONS AND RECOMMENDATIONS

The work of the team is aimed at solving the problem of creating an intelligent IAS for processing and storing biomedical data, increasing the efficiency of analysing heterogeneous integrated data using an ontological approach based on the use of cognitive neuro-fuzzy algorithms and allowing for dynamic visualisation of large unstructured data.

As a result of research on the basis of MGGEU, for students with different nosologies methods will be developed and tested for detecting the impact on training and prevention of nervous, musculoskeletal and cardiovascular diseases, as well as the development of cognitive abilities to improve the cognitive functions of students with disabilities, which should positively affect the educational process in general. The application of the proposed approach will allow to create an information-analytical system to support the educational process for people with nosological features.

The system discussed offers the user – a student with a disability – a choice of rehabilitation, technical, informational, educational and psychological measures aimed at restoring or compensating for impaired body functions and disability (Istomina et al. 2019).

Thus, the practical implementation of the present approach to building the information system of support for the educational process will allow building individual learning paths for students, which will affect the improvement of the quality of the educational process and prevent the development risks of nervous, musculoskeletal and cardiovascular diseases.

REFERENCES

Alvarez, J.I., Meyer, F.L., Granoff, D.L. & Lundy, A. 2013. The effect of EEG biofeedback on reducing postcancer cognitive impairment. *Integr Cancer Ther*. 12(6): 475–87.

Aström, K.J. & Hägglund, T. 1995. PID Controllers: Theory, Design and Tuning. 2nd Edition. Research Triangle Park, NC: Instrument Society of America.

Bayramov, E.V. 2018. Razrabotka i primeneniye informatsionnoy intellektualnoy sistemy v edinoy obrazovatelnoy srede universiteta pri obuchenii studentov s invalidnostyu. *Chelovek. Obshchestvo. Inklyuziya* 3(36): 143–146.

Chedvik, Dzh. 2013. Programming ASP.NET MVC 4: Developing Real-World Web Applications with ASP.NET MVC. I.D. Viliams.

Efremov, M.A., Petrunina, E.V., Myasnyankin, M.B. & Miroshnikov, A.V. 2019. Intellektualnyye agenty dlya issledovaniya adaptatsionnogo potentsiala obuchayushchikhsya s nozologicheskimi osobennostyami. *Izvestiya YuZGU. Seriya Upravleniye. vychislitelnaya tekhnika. informatika. Meditsinskoye priborostroyeniye* 9(1): 119–133.

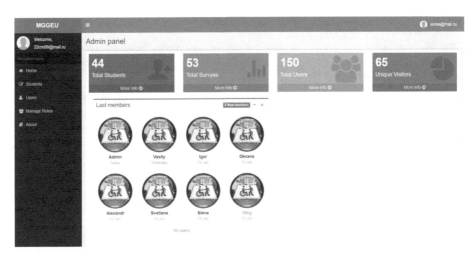

Gaje, P.M. & Weber, B. 2008. *Posturology. Regulation and imbalance of the human body*. S.Pb.: Publishing House MAPO.

Gopalai, A.A., Senanayake, S.M.N.A. & Lim, K.H. 2012. Intelligent vibrotactile biofeedback system for real-time postural correction on perturbed surfaces. *Intelligent Systems Design and Applications (ISDA), Kochi, India, 27–29 November*.

Greenhalgh, J., Dickson, R. & Dundar, Y. 2009. The effects of biofeedback for the treatment of essential hypertension: a systematic review. *Health Technology Assessment* 13(46).

Gusev, E.I., Konovalov, A.N. & Hecht, L.B. 2001. Rehabilitation in neurology. *Kremlin medicine* 5: 29–32.

Hamann, H. 2010. *Spaso-topic Continuous Models of Swarm Robotics Systems. Cognitive Systems Monografs*. Berlin Heidelberg: Springer-Verlag.

Ho, W.K., Hong, Y., Hansson, A., Hjalmarsson, H. & Deng, J.W. 2003. Relay auto-tuning of PID controllers using iterative feedback tuning. *Automatica*. DOI:10.1016/S0005-1098(02)00201-7.

Ho, W.K., Lee, T.H., Han, H.P. & Hong, Y. 2001. Self-tuning IMC-PID control with interval gain and phase margin assignment. *IEEE Transactions on Control Systems Technology*. DOI:10.1109/87.918905.

Holten, V. 2009. Bio- and neurofeedback applications in stress regulation. *Neuroscience & Cognition, track Behavioural Neuroscience*.

Horowitz, S. 2006. *Biofeedback Applications. Alternative and Complementary Therapies* 12(6): 275–281.

Istomin, V.V. 2013. The algorithm behavior of groups of autonomous intelligent agents for biomedical systems based on the theory of swarm intelligence. *Caspian magazine: management and high technology* 3(23): 54–62.

Istomina, T.V., Filatov, I.A., Safronov, A.I., Puchinyan, D.M., Kondrashkin, A.V., Istomin, V.V., et al. 2014. Multi-channel network analyzer biopotentials for remote control of the rehabilitation of patients with postural deficits. *Medical equipment. International Union of public associations Science and Technology Society of Instrument and Metrology* 3: 9–14.

Istomina, T.V., Kireev, A.V., Safronov, A. I., Istomin, V.V. & Karamysheva, T.V. 2011. *Stabilometric Trainer: RF utility model*. Patent No. 122009, application No. 2011137881.

Istomina, T.V., Nikolsky, A.E., Petrunina, E.V., Svetlov, A.V., Chuvykin, B.V., Bayramov, E.V. 2019. Cr internet cyberbiological system for people with disabilities. *International Seminar on Electron Devices Design and Production (SED-2019) Proceedings, Prague, April 23–24*.

Kiselev, A.V., Tomakov, M.V., Petrunina, E.V., Zabanov, D.S. & Zeydan, Z.U. 2019. Slabyye klassifikatory s virtualnymi potokami v intellektualnykh sistemakh prognozirovaniya serdechno-sosudistykh oslozhneniy. *Izvestiya YuZGU. Seriya Upravleniye. Vychislitelnaya tekhnika. Informatika. Meditsinskoye priborostroyeniye* 9(1): 6–20.

Lyons, G.M., Sharma, P., Baker, M., O'Malley, S. & Shanahan, A. 2003. A computer game-based EMG biofeedback system for muscle rehabilitation. *Proceedings of the 25th Annual International Conference of the IEEE Engineering in Medicine and Biology Society*, Piscataway, NJ, USA, 17–21 September.

Meuret, A.E., Wilhelm, F.H. & Roth, W.T. 2001. Respiratory Biofeedback-Assisted Therapy in Panic Disorder. *Behavior modification* 25(4): 584–605.

Nelson, L.A. 2007. The role of biofeedback in stroke rehabilitation: past and future directions. *Top Stroke Rehabil.* 14(4): 59–66.

Nikolskiy, A.E. 2017. Ontologicheskaya model inklyuzii. *Estestvennyye i tekhnicheskiye nauki* 5.

Nikolskiy, A.E. & Petrunina, E.V. 2018. Ontologicheskaya model tekhnologii formirovaniya professionalnykh znaniy i umeniy lits. imeyushchikh nozologicheskiye osobennosti. *Intellektualnyye tekhnologii i sredstva reabilitatsii i abilitatsii lyudey s ogranichennymi vozmozhnostyami (ITSR-2018): trudy III mezhdunarodnoy konferentsii Moskva, Moscow, 29–30 November 2018*.

Rybina, G.V. 2017. Intellektualnaya tekhnologiya postroyeniya obuchayushchikh integrirovannykh ekspertnykh sistem: novyye vozmozhnosti. *Otkrytoye obrazovaniye* 21(4): 44–57.

Sarkisyan, L.A., Latysheva, T., Belozerov, E.K., Gosudarev, N.A., Koryagin, N.A., Olesov, E.E., et al. *Lechebnaya pedagogika*. Moscow.

Torres, V.P. 2013. *Development of Biofeedback Mechanisms in a Procedural Environment Using Biometric Sensors*.

Ziegler, J.G. & Nichols, N.B. 1942. Optimum settings for automatic controllers. *Transactions of the ASME* 64: 759–768.

Author index